WB

KU-202-454

Tools for Practice in Occupational Therapy

H07
Healthcare Library (Room 21.05)
Lymington New Forest Hospital
Wellworthy Road
Lymington
Hampshire
SO41 8QD

To be renewed returned on or before the date marked below

1 1 AUG 2006

2 2 OCT 2007

1 2 FEB 2008

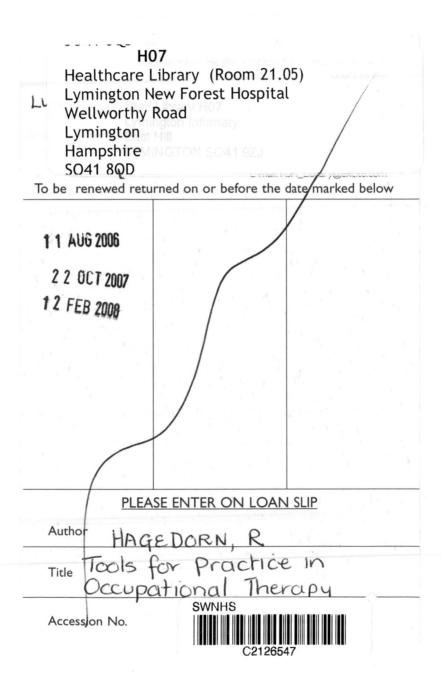

PLEASE ENTER ON LOAN SLIP

Author HAGEDORN, R

Title Tools for Practice in
Occupational Therapy

Accession No.

SWNHS

C2126547

For Churchill Livingstone:

Editorial Director, Health Professions: Mary Law
Project Development Manager: Dinah Thom
Project Manager: Gail Murray
Designer: George Ajayi

Tools for Practice in Occupational Therapy

A Structured Approach to Core Skills and Processes

Rosemary Hagedorn DipCOT DipTCDHEd MSc(AOT) FAOT
Freelance lecturer; former Course Director in Occupational Therapy, Crawley College of Technology, Crawley, UK

030732

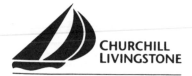
CHURCHILL LIVINGSTONE

EDINBURGH LONDON NEW YORK PHILADELPHIA ST LOUIS SYDNEY TORONTO 2000

CHURCHILL LIVINGSTONE
An imprint of Harcourt Publishers Limited

© Harcourt Publishers Limited 2000

 is a registered trademark of Harcourt Publishers Limited

The right of Rosemary Hagedorn to be identified as author of
this Work has been asserted by her in accordance with the
Copyright, Designs and Patents Act 1988.

All rights reserved. No part of this publication may be
reproduced, stored in a retrieval system, or transmitted in any
form or by any means, electronic, mechanical, photocopying,
recording or otherwise, without either the prior permission of
the publishers (Harcourt Publishers Limited, Harcourt Place,
32 Jamestown Road, London NW1 7BY), or a licence
permitting restricted copying in the United Kingdom issued
by the Copyright Licensing Agency, 90 Tottenham Court
Road, London W1P 0LP.

First published 2000

ISBN 0 443 06159 9

British Library Cataloguing in Publication Data
A catalogue record for this book is available from the British
Library.

Library of Congress Cataloging in Publication Data
A catalog record for this book is available from the Library of
Congress.

Note
Medical knowledge is constantly changing. As new
information becomes available, changes in treatment,
procedures, equipment and the use of drugs become
necessary. The author and the publishers have, as far as it is
possible, taken care to ensure that the information given in
this text is accurate and up to date. However, readers are
strongly advised to confirm that the information, complies
with the latest legislation and standards of practice.

C2126547

The
Publisher's
policy is to use
**paper manufactured
from sustainable forests**

Printed in China

Contents

Preface

Please read this!

Many years ago I was on a management course which began with a timed 'test'. Two sides of A4 paper were covered with a series of complex tasks. The first instruction was 'read everything before doing anything'. Those who followed this found that the final instruction read 'ignore all previous instructions and write your name on the top of the paper'. Those who plunged straight into the tasks had a deeply frustrating time of it. Readers often ignore a preface and dive straight into the book. If you have got this far you are obviously not one of those, and I hope that you will find the comments helpful in understanding the purpose of the book.

For the past 10 years student occupational therapists and practitioners have been grappling with theory, a process which has successively bewildered, challenged and enlightened those involved.

We do, of course, need a sound theoretical basis for practice, but in all the intellectual excitement generated by new ideas there has been a drift away from the previous emphasis on the skills and processes needed to carry out occupational therapy.

Understanding theory without relating it to practice is as useless in real life as knowing everything about the chemical components and dietary values of food without being able to cook.

This book will not tell you 'how to treat a... stroke/amputation/anxiety state etc'. There are plenty of other texts which do this, and in any case there is a move away from this medical-model 'illness-based' approach to the provision of therapy.

This book will also not tell you 'how to treat a patient using the biomechanical/cognitive–behavioural/client-centred etc. approach'. Use of an approach with an individual client is based on situational factors interpreted by clinical reasoning and the needs and wishes of the client. There are too many variables to make a straightforward presentation of 'do this, don't do that' a practical proposition.

What this book does attempt to do is to convey some of the fundamental skills and arts of practice, whilst making connections between these and the principles and theories that underpin their use.

This is, as I always warn readers of my books, a personal view. I have tried to distil 30 years of personal experience into a summary of 'what to do and how to do it'. I have also been concerned to capture some of the skills that I was taught when I first trained, which seem to me to be in danger of getting lost as new generations of therapists develop fresh concerns and interests.

To begin with I wondered why no one had attempted a book of this kind before. I now know. Describing practice has proved far more difficult and challenging than describing theory.

For an experienced practitioner what is done is embedded and integrated into a series of reactions, actions and interactions which automatically come into operation when needed, and which remain submerged to the point of inaccessibility when not in use. The attempt to unpack practice in order to describe it inevitably carries the risk of diminishing it to over-simplified lists of actions, which, without the context in which they are used, may not carry much relevance or conviction.

The book is aimed at students and therefore does to some extent state the obvious – obvious, that is, to those of us who have been doing it for years. There was a point for us all when small but important skills were not obvious at all.

I can anticipate a number of critical reactions to what I have written. The text is based on personal experience, which is inevitably biased and incomplete. Others may see things differently.

I have used my own model of practice as a structure for the description of four central processes. This personal approach is particularly noticeable in the section on occupational analysis. It can be argued that this model is not widely used, or well researched. I think that the test that the reader should apply is whether or not it does illuminate practice and provide a useful analytical structure. If it does, perhaps its use is justified; if not, much of what I have written remains valid and can be used within other approaches derived from person/environment/occupational performance models.

To those therapists who react by feeling 'I don't do it that way', my response is a challenge: please write about what you *do* do and how you do it. Practice cannot develop without dialogue and critique; the evolution of grounded theory is useful, but the description of grounded practice must not be ignored.

Arundel 2000   Rosemary Hagedorn

Introduction

SECTION CONTENTS

1

Introduction: integrating theory with practice

OCCUPATIONAL THERAPY: VALUING SIMPLICITY

Occupational therapists engage people in doing simple things. It is unfortunate that, in the latter half of the 20th century, simplicity, in the sense of being plain and uncomplicated, is undervalued.

This is scarcely surprising. In the span of a single lifetime, scientists and engineers have transformed the world. Humankind has progressed from mastery of flight to landing on the moon. In consequence, 'high tech' is seen as complex, impressive and exciting. 'Low tech', in contrast, is simple, boring and outdated. Occupational therapy (OT), despite computers and environmental controls, remains on the whole 'low tech'.

We live in a culture in which surface appearance is what matters. This has led those who do not use the service of the profession to misinterpret the apparently simple processes of occupational therapy as 'only common sense' or 'doing things to keep occupied'.

There are two errors in this perception. First, simple things do have value. Therapists enable people to dress, cook, shop, work, play, create, construct, because that is what people want and need to be able to do. Commonsense solutions may be simple and obvious – once they have been proposed – but they work. Even 'doing simple things to keep occupied' may have value in the right context and provided that they are the right things.

Second, the appearance of simplicity is, of course, deceptive. To borrow a phrase from computer jargon, occupational therapy has always been presented as 'user-friendly'. Engagement in the process of therapy is what matters, not the professional knowledge and analysis which underpins this.

The metaphor of an iceberg – where only the tip shows above the surface – is often used to convey the idea that occupational therapy has 'hidden' aspects. But an iceberg is a clumsy, inanimate object. Perhaps a computer might offer a better metaphor. Computers are designed to be easy to use but the user knows that underlying the surface simplicity of 'what you see is what you get' is a lot of incomprehensible, impressive, complex, state of the art technology. The problem for occupational therapists is that it is a great deal harder for a lay person to understand that there might be anything complex behind making a cup of tea or planting a geranium.

Yet an apparently simple task is by no means simple when subjected to detailed analysis. Intricate occupations have layers of meanings and symbolism of which even the participant may be unaware.

Occupational therapists may do simple things, but they often do them for complex reasons. Attempts to explain this briefly usually result in oversimplification which confirms the listener's belief that 'there is nothing to it'.

THE PROBLEM OF EXPLAINING OCCUPATIONAL THERAPY

This difficulty in getting others to value the simple task and to understand at the same time that in the context of occupational therapy it may not be simple at all has bedevilled the profession for decades. It has also resulted in defensiveness on the part of therapists.

In the past, in reaction to the hated 'baskets and bunnies' image, therapists have sought to become more 'scientific' and 'high-tech' since these attributes seem to attract esteem. While it would be Luddite to deny that technology has some very valid applications in occupational therapy, the high-tech paradigm has not, on the

whole, proved a comfortable fit. It is interesting to note that, as we enter the 21st century, the wheel is turning back in favour of a more holistic view of human occupation.

The need to explain what we do has also become one of the spurs to the development of a sophisticated rationale for practice. The work of many theorists in the past two decades has greatly enriched the therapist's understanding of the theoretical foundations of occupational therapy, but it has drawn attention away from the core processes and skills which are the essential tools of the therapist. The link between theory and practice has sometimes become obscured in a fog of complex conceptualization.

It may be questioned whether, from the perspective of the client or the uninitiated observer, occupational therapy models and concepts of human occupation have made the connection between the doing of simple things and the reasons why these are done any more comprehensible.

It seems desirable, therefore, to re-establish overt links between 'knowing and doing' and between the simplicity of the therapist's actions and the complexity of the clinical reasoning, principles of therapeutic application and core processes which underlie these actions. It is the intention of this book to re-establish these links.

CONNECTING 'KNOWING' AND 'DOING'

Occupational therapy is a practice-based profession which is based on both art and science. Professional education must be a blend of theory and practical competencies.

The competent therapist is expected to connect 'knowing what to do and why' and 'knowing how to do things' in a relevant manner in order to provide effective interventions. There are a number of organizing structures which assist in making these connections.

These include the problem-based process through which intervention is provided and theoretical structures such as occupational therapy models and applied frames of reference. These structures, together with some of the fundamental principles of occupational therapy, combine to provide a framework for practice which has now been described in many texts.

The core processes and competencies used by the therapist to 'do' have, in contrast, been summarized in somewhat general terms. There is an indication of *what* therapists do, but *how* they do this is not always so clear.

This may be because one often fails to describe the obvious. It may also be due to the fact that 'knowing how and knowing why' is often tacit. Knowing is expressed by the process of doing; explaining exactly what is done and why can be difficult, and the difficulty increases as expertise smooths out and obscures the cognitive links in the chain of decision-making.

What is done must also be grounded in the assumptions on which occupational therapy is based. These assumptions have evolved over time. To begin with, therefore, in order to set the discussion of core processes in context, the development of a rationale for practice will be summarized in relation to developments within the profession and external to it.

THE SEARCH FOR A RATIONALE FOR PRACTICE

A rationale is 'a reasoned exposition, statement of reasons, fundamental reason, logical basis' (Concise Oxford Dictionary). A rationale should link what is done to the reasons why and provide evidence to support these statements.

It is possible to trace a developmental sequence in the search for a rationale for practice which extends over the past 80 years from the adoption of the term 'occupational therapy' in 1917 to the present (2000).

AN EVOLUTIONARY PROCESS

At the start, there was assimilation of 'borrowed knowledge' as the young profession drew on sources as disparate as anatomy, medicine, psychiatry, nursing, sociology, technology and design. During this evolutionary period the focus was on the development of practice, on 'what is done' rather than 'the reasons why'.

The profession then moved on to a period where this knowledge was synthesized, adapted and integrated to form a distinctive and unified body of practice.

At the same time, diversification occurred with the development of occupational therapy specialisms which broadened still further the scope of knowledge and practice. To avoid overload, some parts of occupational therapy were 'hived off' to become monotherapies such as art therapy and drama therapy.

Finally, existing knowledge was reviewed and challenged in an attempt to separate out and define the profession's unique rationale and body of knowledge and practice.

ASSIMILATION, DEVELOPMENT AND REJECTION OF THEORY

From the start, therapists worked under medical direction and therefore assimilated much of the traditional 'biomedical' approach, especially in physical rehabilitation. Various frames of reference used by doctors, psychiatrists and psychologists were utilized to provide approaches to practice. Application of these approaches resulted in adaptation to make them more relevant to occupational therapy; the 'OT version' was gradually created.

In the five decades since the end of the Second World War, the treatment of illness and trauma developed rapidly. Many problems requiring long-term care disappeared from the scene. At the same time, improvements in treatment meant that people lived longer and more disabled people were discharged into community care.

The traditional, somewhat authoritarian model of rehabilitation began to be seen as inappropriate to the needs of people with disabilities living in their own homes. New approaches evolved under the influence of humanistic psychology, sociology and social and political philosophy.

Biomedical rehabilitation continued to be the main approach in acute physical rehabilitation but, in the community and in other care settings, approaches such as client-centred rehabilitation, community-based rehabilitation and independent living (McColl 1997) offered alternative options for service delivery.

These approaches have had a profound effect on the content and process of therapy and the style of relationship with the client. They have produced fundamental changes in values and attitudes, and have been influential in prompting therapists to re-examine the rationale for practice.

Although the four approaches to rehabilitation differ from each other, they may be viewed as a continuum which extends from the acute care setting into the community, and also from directive to client-centred approaches to care.

While the profession has been affected by external developments and theories, it has also been changed from within. The development of degree-level professional education gave impetus to an academic re-evaluation of the profession.

In the 1980s and 1990s, critical enquiry by occupational therapy academics resulted in dissatisfaction with the fact that occupational therapy appeared to be based so much on 'borrowed knowledge'. The search began for a rationale which reflected the unique features of occupational therapy, combining both a desire to 'return to our roots' in occupation and a need to take account of recent thinking.

This critical appraisal led to the development of occupational therapy models and the quest for a unifying paradigm for practice against which the relevance of both practice and theory could be tested and challenged.

It is no wonder that the attempt to unify all this broadly-based material from different sources and periods of professional development causes problems when it comes to making a clear statement of occupational therapy assumptions and practice.

CHANGING VIEWS ABOUT 'OCCUPATION'

Alongside this evolution of theory and practice, and closely connected with it, views about occupation and its value as therapy have also changed.

The founders of occupational therapy were ahead of their time in their holistic view of the individual for whom 'occupation is as necessary as food and drink' (William Rush Dunton's 'credo for occupational therapists' 1917: Miller & Walker 1993). To begin with, occupational therapy was firmly rooted in the use of prescribed, purposeful, productive activities as a means of restoring health, function and quality of life, or retraining productive occupational habits.

In those, less-pressurized, days there was one commodity which is notably lacking in current health care: time. A patient might be available for treatment for weeks, months or even years. It was possible to design programmes of carefully graded activity, to build relationships and to foster achievement. In the absence of television, or even radio, people still relied on making their own amusements through handicrafts, games or hobbies.

During the 1920s and 1930s, technology – films, cars, planes, radio, gadgets for the home, faster, larger machines at work – began to infiltrate everyday life. While some people remained suspicious of anything 'newfangled', to many these innovations must have seemed welcome and excitingly modern. Even so, from the end of the First World War up to the outbreak of the Second World War, neither therapist nor patient had truly been confronted by the 20th century in any very challenging or threatening manner.

After the Second World War, it was a different matter. The pace of change accelerated. Occupational therapists were faced with rapid technological development. At the same time, there was pressure to conform to the positivist paradigm by which scientific validity was judged. Obliged to keep pace with these changes, the profession began to move away from its roots in occupation. The ethos of craftwork and parlour games seemed out of step with contemporary Western culture.

During the late 1960s and early 1970s, the reductionist influence of biomechanical and behavioural frames of reference began to change therapeutic media.

In an attempt to show the link between pre-scribed occupation and therapeutic goal and out-come, assembly work, constructive tasks or games were reduced to their components. In the extreme, this process ended in producing 'thera-peutic exercises' divorced from context, meaning and product.

As the techniques of rehabilitation became increasingly sophisticated and recovery far more rapid, the time for graded treatment pro-grammes became greatly curtailed. The focus of therapy became independent living which nor-mally meant being able to cope with the survival tasks of self-care and basic communication with others.

This led to increasing recognition that adapta-tion of the environment to facilitate occupational performance was as important as the rehabilita-tion of the patient.

At this point, around 1980, the reaction set in, influenced by the growth of the social sciences and the phenomenological paradigm. The move from the professional-centred, medical model to a client-centred, social model of disability in turn influenced perceptions of the rationale for prac-tice; prescriptive 'occupational exercise' was not compatible with autonomy, choice and self-actu-alization.

Engagement in meaningful, productive occu-pations in the areas of work, leisure and self-care again became, at least in theory, the focus of occupational therapy. The influences of the envi-ronment, and the outcome of actions within it, were also recognized.

Theorists began to discuss therapeutic oc-cupation in terms of individual meanings, sym-bolism, context and purpose. The work of anthropologists and ecologists led to a general re-evaluation of so-called 'primitive' cultures which has also influenced views of human occu-pation. Hunter-gatherers are no longer 'ignorant' Stone-Age people who scrape a subsistence living because they know no better, but well-adapted, highly knowledgeable groups who fit perfectly into their often harsh and demanding environments. Their 'simple activities' have meaning and value beyond that which is superfi-cially observable. Perhaps our patronizing and dismissive 'civilised' view of simplicity is about to undergo revision.

It is as if the profession has, over the last 80 years, traced a parabolic arc away from its roots and back again. Perhaps it is necessary to take that journey. T. S. Eliot wrote:

We shall not cease from exploration
And the end of all our exploring
Will be to arrive where we started
And know the place for the first time.
Four Quartets, Little Gidding V

WHERE NEXT?

So where, at the present stage in this continuing journey, have we arrived, and where do we go next? In the past decade (1985–1995 approxi-mately), all these strands of past knowledge and practice have been drawn together.

A new 'family' of theoretical models has been produced which describes occupational therapy as concerned with the individual's capacity to perform occupations within the environment. The nature of human occupation and occupa-tional performance has become the focus for aca-demic enquiry via the new discipline of occupa-tional science. Recent foundation texts (e.g. Christiansen & Baum 1997, Neistadt & Crepeau 1998) have made far more explicit connections between knowing and doing.

Does this mean that we have finally achieved that elusive rationale for practice, and if so, what is it? This question will be further explored in Chapter 2.

2

Competent occupational performance in the environment (COPE)

PERSON/ENVIRONMENT/ OCCUPATIONAL PERFORMANCE MODELS

As described in Chapter 1, a flurry of model-building and theory development occurred in occupational therapy during the late 1980s and early 1990s. Out of this creative and, at times, confusing period, some consensus about the core concerns of occupational therapy seems to be emerging.

A number of similar models has been developed by different theorists. These are like variations on a musical theme which each 'composer' has interpreted in slightly different ways. A selection of the theorists who have published models belonging to this 'family' between 1990 and 1997 is given in Box 2.1.

The central theme which unites these models is the perception that occupational therapy is concerned with people competently and adaptively performing their occupations within the physical and social environment.

For this reason, I have adopted the initials of Christiansen & Baum's (1997) model – Person/Environment/Occupational/Performance (PEOP) – as a collective title to include all models in this group.

There has clearly been an interchange of ideas between these theorists, yet in several cases the originators of models have developed their theories independently in the course of parallel processes of academic analysis and enquiry at about the same time. Each theorist describes the individual, the environment and occupation in subtly different ways, but the similarities of conceptualization are striking.

This is encouraging since such triangulation (obtaining supporting evidence from a number of independent sources) strengthens the validity of the concepts.

THEORETICAL BASIS FOR THIS BOOK

The aim of this book, as previously stated, is to make a very clear link between theory and practice. To do this, I will use a personal version of the PEOP model which I have called COPE (Competent Occupational Performance in the Environment). This model has many similar features to the other models, although it was largely evolved independently during a parallel timescale.

Although I have chosen to use COPE as a theoretical framework, the core processes and the general approach to occupational therapy used in this book are compatible with any of the

Box 2.1	Person/environment/occupational performance models		
Date	Country and theorist	Model title	Content
1992	USA Reed & Sanderson	Human occupations model (3rd edn)	*Individual* — Skills: sensorimotor, cognitive, psychosocial *Occupation* — Productivity, leisure, self-maintenance *Environment* — Adaptation to and with environment
1992	CANADA Polatajko	Enablement model	*Individual* — Cognitive, affective and physical domains *Occupation* — Self-care, productivity, leisure *Environmental dimensions* — Physical, social and cultural
1992	UK Stewart	Model for the practice of OT	*Client* — Active participant in change *Activity* — The medium for change *Environment* — The context for change *Therapist* — Facilitates change
1995a	UK Hagedorn	Core components of OT and occupational competence	*Person* / *Occupation* / *Therapist* / *Environment* — Person relates to therapist in the context of an occupation within environment Balance between the personal abilities, task demand and environmental demand required for competent performance
1995	USA Kielhofner	Model of human occupation (2nd edn)	*Human system* / *Environment* / *Task* — Person interacting (input, throughput, output) with environment to produce occupational behaviour
1997	CANADA Law et al	Person/environment/occupation model: A transactive approach to occupational performance	*Person* — Unique being; variety of simultaneous roles, *Environment* — cultural, socio-economic, institutional, physical, social *Occupation* — Groups of self-directed functional tasks and activities
1997	USA Schkade & Schultz	Occupational adaptation model	*Person* / *Interaction* / *Occupational Environment* — Occupations provide the means by which people adapt

Box 2.1 *(Cont'd)*

1997	USA Christiansen & Baum	Person/ environment/ occupational performance	*Person* *Environment* *Occupation*	Performance results from complex interactions between person, occupations and environment
1997	AUSTRALIA Chaparro & Ranka	Occupational performance model (Australia)	Eight interactive constructs: *Occupational performance* *Occupational roles* *Occupational performance areas* *Components of occupational performance (skills)* *Core elements of performance* (mind, body, spirit) *The performance environment* *Time* *Space*	
1997	Canadian Association of Occupational Therapists	Canadian occupational performance model	*Individual* *Occupation* *Environment*	Spiritual, physical, sociocultural, mental Productivity, leisure self-care Social, cultural, physical

models in the PEOP group. The Canadian Occupational Performance Model (as published in 1997) is particularly clear in its presentation and application and can be used in both clinical settings and community practice. This model is unique in being developed by an Association of Occupational Therapists and adopted as a national framework for practice.

INTRODUCTION TO COPE

The COPE model is used as a basis for this book first because it overtly illustrates the link between the therapist's aim of promoting competent occupational performance and the processes of therapy through which this can be achieved, and second because it enables me to explain a number of important assumptions of occupational therapy.

It is not presented as in any way superior to other models, many of which have been subjected to more rigorous development and testing, but as a contribution to theory which has evolved from, and reflects, British practice and ideas.

The model unites a number of concepts which I have presented previously (Hagedorn

1995a, 1997). COPE is a person-centred, process-driven, occupational performance model which includes the concept of a hierarchy of occupational levels.

It is *person-centred* because the individual is a partner in the process of therapy. The individual participates in the process of naming and framing problems and developing solutions.

Active involvement by the client in the processes of therapy is essential. The therapist has many roles, which may include facilitator, resource provider, advisor, teacher, counsellor, rehabilitation expert, problem solver and designer. Intervention is a shared process in which goals, roles and actions are negotiated between the client and the therapist.

It is *process-driven* because the therapist does not pre-select an applied frame of reference or approach. From the basis of personal theoretical understanding of the core concerns of occupational therapy, as expressed by COPE, the therapist uses the processes of therapy to work with the client to identify areas for action and relevant process of change. Needs and goals can then be specified. The therapist can subsequently select an appropriate approach or approaches and implement actions and solutions within this framework.

KEY ASSUMPTIONS

COPE provides an organizing framework for a number of related assumptions:

1. Competent, adaptive occupational performance is essential to human health and well-being.

2. Competent, adaptive occupational performance depends on a fit between the performance demand generated by the task and the environment and ability of the person to respond to this. If the balance is disturbed, performance will fail to match demand.

3. Humans synthesize skills from the domains of action, interaction and reaction to perform occupations, activities and tasks.

4. Occupations can be analysed using a hierarchical structure based on a developmental analysis linked to episodes of performance in real time.

5. The environment may also be analysed in relation to areas indicating proximity to and ease of access by the user.

6. Performance of tasks and activities places a demand on the individual to learn, adapt and respond. The process of performance, and the perceptions of the consequent product, create changes within the individual. As a result of this intrinsic linkage, the therapist can use tasks and activities as therapeutic media.

7. Occupational therapy takes place when the therapist works with the person in the context of a specific portion of an occupation in a particular environment for a defined purpose.

8. The therapist can intervene to restore balance or 'fit' and promote competence by working with the individual to achieve adaptive change, or by altering elements in the environment or in the way a task is structured and performed.

9. In order to provide intervention the therapist must use four core processes in combination:

- therapeutic use of self
- assessment of individual ability potential and needs
- analysis and adaptation of occupations
- analysis and adaptation of environments.

The remainder of the introductory section will deal with these assumptions, and the core processes will be described in detail in the remaining sections. The organising frameworks of the COPE model will first be described.

THE PERSON/OCCUPATION/ ENVIRONMENT/THERAPIST TRIANGLE

Occupational therapy takes place when the therapist works with the person in the context of a specific portion of an occupation in a particular environment for a defined purpose.

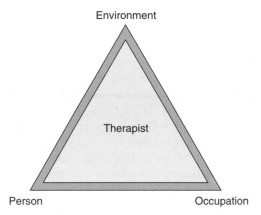

Figure 2.1   The person/occupation/environment/ therapist (POET) triangle.

This simple figure (Fig. 2.1) represents a description of the core components of occupational therapy, the conjunction of the therapist, working with the person, in the context of the person's occupations within the environment in order to restore balance or 'fit'. (This representation can be recalled by the acronym POET.)

THE CONCEPT OF 'FIT'

A theme which runs through the PEOP family of models is the idea that competent or adaptive performance is made possible by an intricate transaction (Law et al 1997), interaction (Christiansen & Baum 1997), or fit (American Association of Occupational Therapists 1994) between the person, his/her occupations and the environment. I prefer to describe this as a dynamic balance between these components, but we are all dealing with similar concepts.

It is tempting to want to give occupational therapists sole credit for the development of the concept that performance depends on the interactions between the person, the task and the environment, but that would be unduly parochial. Ergonomists, who also specialize in the analysis of occupations, long ago reached the same conclusion.

The principles of ergonomics are based on the concept of 'fitting the task to the man' (Grandjean 1988). Like occupational therapists, ergonomists appreciate that competent performance results when the working environment facilitates performance and the worker can meet the task demands.

Singleton (1972) wrote of 'the classic ergonomic procedures of matching men, machines, work spaces and environments.'

I was also excited to discover the chapter by Holm, Rogers and Stone (Neistadt & Crepeau 1998) in which the person/task/environment triangle is presented as a decision-making guide. This material is very similar to the system of problem analysis (SYT analysis, see Ch. 27) which I have used for some years with clients on a pain management programme (Hagedorn 1996, unpublished).

That researchers from different disciplines have come to the same conclusion provides evidence to support the validity of the concept. It should be noted, however, that the P/O/E/ triangle represents the components of *human occupation*. It does not represent *occupational therapy*. For that we must include the therapist in the diagram as shown in Figure 2.1. The therapist acts as the catalyst through whose intervention balance can be restored.

USING THE POET DIAGRAM TO ORGANIZE THE PROCESSES OF THERAPY

The POET triangle prompts the therapist to investigate the three areas which contribute to competent performance: the person, the occupation and the environment. The elements which need to be considered and the ways in which this may be done are described in the later sections of this book.

USING THE POET DIAGRAM TO ASSIST IN THE SELECTION OF AN APPLIED FRAME OF REFERENCE OR APPROACH

The POET diagram also serves as an analytical tool in the selection of an applied frame of reference.

It can be assumed that, if it is to have value, each frame of reference should offer a distinctly different view of the person, the occupation and the environment.

A therapist should be able to analyse these differences and distinguish between these perspectives in order to select a suitable approach.

Table 2.1 gives a simplified version of this analysis for some commonly used applied frames of reference.

A DESCRIPTION OF FOUR PROCESSES OF CHANGE

The therapist can intervene to restore balance or fit by working with the individual to achieve adaptive change.

When a client is referred to, or seeks assistance from, an occupational therapist, it is because there is a problem which affects competent performance of, or balance between, occupations. If adaptive competence and balance are to be restored, something needs to change as a result of intervention.

Change simply indicates an altered state. What once existed has become in some way different. Change is a normal, indeed necessary, process throughout life. Things can, of course,

Table 2.1   Comparison of commonly used frames of reference

Frame of Reference	Person	Aspects important to therapist:	
		Occupation	Environment
Biomechanical			
Graded activities approach	Movement range Strength Dexterity Posture Stamina	Task components which require specified movements, effort, task duration, posture	Height and position of furniture Design of furniture tools and equipment Resistance/assistance leverage; support
Activities of daily living (ADL) approach	Performance skills	Personal and domestic tasks relevant to individual: opportunities for realistic ADL practice	Barriers to performance; adaptations to enhance performance Management of hazards and risks
Neuro-develop-mental	Movement patterns Posture Muscle tone Sensory feedback	Posture and pattern of movement during performance Promotion of sensory input	Height and position of furniture and equipment Promotion of sensory input
Cognitive–perceptual	Ability to perceive and process information	Perceptual and information content of task	Information content: positioning items and people to enhance input
Cognitive–behavioural	Links between thoughts, feelings and behaviour Self-concept Coping strategies	Person's subjective view of task/ activity Indications of positive or negative thoughts and feelings expressed by task performance Potential of successful performance to promote positive cycles of thought and behaviour	Components in used environment which may act as stressors Effect of others on client Situations which reinforce negative thought or behaviour or promote positive reactions
Analytical	Unconscious processes: insight; emotions Past experiences Potential for personal growth	Potential of task to assist in revealing or interpreting unconscious material or resolving conflict	Potential of objects or people to assist in revealing or interpreting unconscious material
Group work	Communication and social skills	Potential of task to teach or provide practice of social and communication skills	Arrangement of furniture, tools, materials, other people to promote social interaction

change for the worse as well as for the better. The therapist is concerned with constructive change, which enhances, enables and empowers.

The occupational therapist cannot 'change the client' (and indeed, if this could be done, it should not be as it would be unethical). All that any therapist can do is to assist the client to change if the client wishes to do so, and in ways that the client decides are acceptable.

The therapist's intervention assists the client to employ one or more of the four major pro-

cesses of beneficial human change – development, education, adaptation and rehabilitation – with their associated approaches and techniques. These processes are shown in Box 2.2. The acronym DARE may be used to recall these processes.

Development means turning potential for performance into usable skill. Development occurs naturally through maturation, but also as an individual is challenged to learn new skills throughout life. Development occurs in a sequence during which more and more complex performance becomes possible. Until the prerequisite developmental level is achieved, the individual cannot perform a task competently.

Education is the process through which a person learns to do new things or acquires new information and understanding.

Adaptation is the process through which a person changes actions, interactions or reactions in some positive manner in response to external demands. Adaptive responses help the individual to cope and survive within a given culture and contribute to feelings of well-being. Maladaptive responses or failure to adapt have negative effects on the individual and/or society.

Development, education and adaptation are the key processes through which individuals normally acquire the ability to perform competently throughout their lives.

When an individual is unable to cope with the demands of daily life, the occupational therapist may work with the individual to identify a problem or deficit in development, education or adaptation which may have led to, or be exacerbating, the problem.

If such a problem or deficit is found the therapist seeks to structure occupations and environments in order to maximize the opportunities for the individual to develop, learn and adapt.

Since, in this context, the therapist is not *treating* the client, this is often referred to as *intervention* rather than therapy.

Rehabilitation differs from the above processes because it is a deliberately structured therapeutic process, normally undertaken by a team of health care professionals. It is aimed at restoring lost skills or function following illness or trauma, and compensating for, or minimizing the effects of, any residual disability. Rehabilitation only applies when the individual previously had an ability, but has lost it, and may involve remedial treatment of the client.

The processes of change are summarized in Box 2.2. (For further description of the four processes of change and associated approaches refer to *Foundations for Practice in Occupational Therapy*, 2nd edition (Hagedorn 1997).)

Box 2.2 Processes of change (DARE)	
Development	The person needs to bring potential abilities into use.
Adaptation	The person, or his/her tasks or his/her environment must change in response to altered circumstances.
Rehabilitation	The person has lost functional abilities or skills which s/he needs to regain.
Education	The person needs to acquire new knowledge, skill or way of viewing his/her situation.

COPE – A MODEL OF THE COMPONENTS OF COMPETENT PERFORMANCE IN THE CONTEXT OF THERAPY

Competent adaptive occupational performance is essential to human health and well-being. Competent performance depends on a balance between the performance demand generated by the task and the environment and the ability of the person to respond to this. If the balance is disturbed, performance will fail to match demand.

The therapist can intervene to restore balance or fit by working with the individual to achieve adaptive change or by altering elements in the environment or in the way a task is structured or performed.

The nature of competence and the importance of competent performance are described in Chapter 7.

The essential feature of the COPE model is the emphasis on the restoration of 'balance' between the abilities of the person, the demands of the tasks and the demands of the environment (Fig. 2.2). The therapist intervenes to restore or create a 'fit' between these elements. Through this intervention competent performance is established, or action taken to minimize dysfunction or disability.

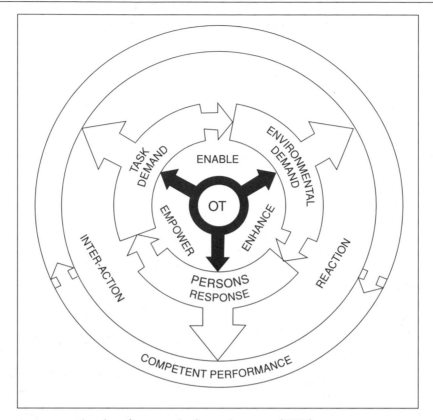

Figure 2.2   Competent occupational performance in the environment (COPE).

PROMOTING FIT – BALANCING PERFORMANCE DEMAND AND INDIVIDUAL RESPONSE

Performance demand

Every time a person attempts a task, three factors come into play: the demands of the task and the demands of the environment, which combine to create *performance demand*, and the abilities of the individual to respond.

Reactions to performance demand are highly individual; people perform at their best when optimally challenged and engaged in what they are doing. But what is optimal challenge? Some people enjoy being 'stretched', having problems to solve, working under pressure, even danger. Others find even minor stressors too much. This presents considerable challenges to the therapist.

Task demand

The task itself places demands on the participant. These demands are intrinsic, that is they are 'built into' the task. Task demand means that the person attempting the task must be physically and cognitively suited to the task. The person must also have the required knowledge, skill and experience to undertake it. Some tasks are very demanding, while others have low demand. The task also places demands on the content of the environment, for the presence of tools, materials or equipment which must be available if the task is to be completed.

Environmental demand

The environment, both the physical content of it and the people within it, provides the context of performance. The context prompts behaviour in response to it – it demands action. The person picks up the cues provided by the environment and the situation and acts accordingly. By taking action the context and situation may be altered in some way, so new responses are called for.

For example, a broken fence panel demands repair. The owner must find new wood to fill the gap. The task of fitting wood demands tools and skills. The fence mender must know how to use these to make an effective repair. Alternatively, the owner must know how to find and employ someone else to do the repair and take steps to do this.

The features in the environment which provide cues for action have been described by Nelson (1996) as *occupational form*. Nelson defines 'occupational form' as 'the composition of objective physical and sociocultural circumstances external to a person that influence his occupational performance.'

The continual dialogue between the person, the person's actions, the results of these and the demand of the environment for new actions is the basis of human behaviour. This is why systems theory has been used by Kielhofner and others to describe human occupational behaviour in terms of input, throughput and output.

While it is useful to analyse the demand from the task and the environment separately in order to understand the dynamics of a situation, in reality these factors combine to elicit performance.

In order for this intricate transaction to take place the individual must be able to act freely within the environment. The individual must be able to interact with others and perceive, understand and react to changes in the situation being faced.

The ability to do this depends on physical and psychological capacities and on past learning and experience. We each bring ourselves into the new situation with all our skills and knowledge, our emotions, memories, interests, values and aspirations. Our reactions are filtered through our individual patterns of perception and cognitive processing.

A person who is unable, for any reason, to perceive the situation, analyse this information and provide an appropriate response is severely disadvantaged.

CORE PROCESSES

In order to provide intervention the therapist must use four core processes in combination:

- therapeutic use of self
- assessment and evaluation of individual potential, abilities and needs
- analysis and adaptation of occupations
- analysis and adaptation of the environment.

The four core processes and associated competencies used by occupational therapists arise directly from this concept of occupational therapy (Fig. 2.3)

The therapist must relate to and communicate with the client to establish the 'therapeutic alliance' or partnership. The therapist forms part of the environment of practice and can use interactions with the client as a therapeutic tool. This requires *therapeutic use of self*.

The therapist attempts to help the individual to understand the individual's current situation and potential for change. The capacity of the individual to respond to the demands of tasks and environments needs to be evaluated. This involves *assessment and evaluation of individual potential, abilities and needs*.

To restore the fit between the person and the person's occupations it may be necessary to adapt the nature of the tasks the person performs, or to use activities and tasks in a therapeutic setting. For this the therapist must be able to employ *analysis and adaptation of occupations*.

Alternatively, it may be necessary to change the demands of the environment to enable or enhance performance. To do this, the therapist must be able to use *analysis and adaptation of the environment*.

LEVELS OF OCCUPATION AND ENVIRONMENT

Human occupations can be analysed using a three-level hierarchy.

Analysis of *occupations, activities and tasks* and the *skill domains* required to perform them, is

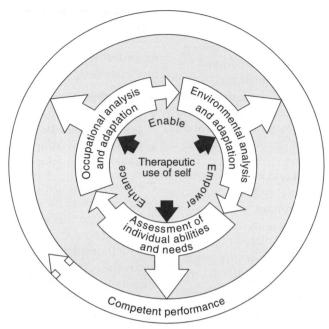

Figure 2.3   Four core processes of occupational therapy.

arguably the most important of the occupational therapist's core competencies.

In order to facilitate analysis, an analytical taxonomy and a hierarchy of occupational levels are proposed. These levels are *organizational*, *effective* and *developmental*, and are based on a combination of developmental theory and an understanding of the way in which different types of performance occur within brief or extended periods of time. This structure assists the therapist with assessment, analysis, teaching and the therapeutic application of activities and tasks. The taxonomy is discussed in Chapter 4 and the levels are described in detail in Chapter 5.

The environment may also be analysed in relation to areas indicating proximity to and ease of access by the user. Levels of the environment are described in Chapter 6.

SUMMARY

The view of occupational therapy adopted by the COPE model can be summarized as follows:

- Occupational therapy is concerned with the acquisition, maintenance or restoration of competent adaptive performance of a balanced and appropriate repertoire of roles, occupations, activities and tasks in order to maintain health and enhance well-being.

- Occupational therapists work in partnership with individuals and groups. The therapist uses specialist processes in order to develop a rapport with the individual and balance the demands of his/her tasks and environments with his/her abilities and skills.

- The therapist may adapt activities or tasks or alter the environment in order to enable the individual to function at his/her maximum level of potential with appropriate assistance or support when necessary.

- Through this intervention, the person is enabled and empowered to gain information and enhance his/her skills in order to achieve competent performance of the things s/he wants or needs to do in the environments s/he uses.

3

Understanding occupation

DEFINITIONS OF OCCUPATION: A CONTINUING DEBATE

As described in Chapter 2, occupational therapy is concerned with the restoration of competent adaptive performance. Competent performance results when the person, the person's occupations and the person's environment are in a balanced relationship.

On the basis of this central assumption, the study of the individual, the individual's environments and, especially, human occupation should form the foundation for occupational therapy. But what do we mean by human occupation, and what words should we, as therapists who specialize in it, use to describe it?

UNDERSTANDING OCCUPATION

Many of the terms and concepts concerning occupation which are in current use have been derived from pioneers in the field of occupational therapy theory.

We owe much to the work of Mary Reilly, a leading American academic. Reilly (1962) coined the term 'occupational behaviour'. She also proposed that occupations could be divided into the categories of play, work, leisure or self-care. During the 1960s and 1970s, Reilly and her associates developed many of the concepts which contribute to current models of occupation and models of occupational performance and the terminology used to describe them.

Reilly's classification of occupations has become widely accepted. It provides a useful 'shorthand' for describing types of occupations.

Recently, however, it has been realized that terms such as work, leisure or self-care are valid as subjective, rather than objective descriptors. The meaning of the occupation to the individual is dependent on the situation and on the participant's personal motivations and experiences. Many occupations do not seem to fit neatly into these general categories.

Human occupations are intricate in structure and organization. They require participants to employ skills ranging from simple to complex. An occupation may be mundane or highly significant. The daily pattern of participation of an individual is woven from many strands and somehow contrives to combine and unite many disparate elements into a continual flow of engagement.

It is inevitable that this rich diversity has generated difficulties for those who attempt to analyse and define occupations. As a result (despite at least 50 years of academic endeavour), there is disagreement about the appropriate words to use when describing different levels of complexity of occupation.

In a position paper on occupation (American Association of Occupational Therapists 1995), the anonymous authors gave a summary of the situation:

Occupational therapy scholars agree that human occupations have emotional, cognitive, spiritual and contextual dimensions, all of which are related to general well-being. However, occupational therapy scholars have not been able to agree on the specific concepts regarding these dimensions or on specific terms to name them.

This paper provides a useful guide to current thinking concerning occupation and other terms such as purposeful activity and function, but definitions of these words are not given.

The position paper is also helpful in indicating the origin of the difficulty over terminology:

One of the problems inhibiting the study of occupations is how to clearly, logically and consistently describe different levels and types of occupation; the term level refers to the complexity of a given occupation.... Even occupational behaviours of complexity, such as dressing or driving are nested within clusters of activity that comprise and are recognized as part of larger sets of organizing behaviour.... This phenomenon of nesting, where simple tasks can be identified as parts of more complex sets of acts is a dimension of occupations which reflects their organization over time and can be viewed as reflecting varying levels of complexity.

The paper goes on to note that various authors (including those cited above) have attempted to solve the problem by proposing that occupations can be described as a hierarchy of different levels.

Occupational science is a recently formed area of academic enquiry which has brought together researchers and theorists from many different disciplines in order to explore and understand the phenomenon of occupation, including the question of whether levels can be identified. This body of knowledge and theory is evolving internationally.

The concept of levels is summarized by Henderson (1996) when describing the systems approach to the study of human occupation. The human system is divided into physical, biological, information-processing, sociocultural, symbolic evaluative and transcendental systems. Henderson puts the position so succinctly that I have quoted her at length:

These systems and the connection among them provide the framework for understanding occupation at different levels... Each level of occupation can be divided into smaller units, and each can be nested in larger units. Occupation is most often defined as work, play, leisure and self-maintenance. Each of these abstract units can be divided into concrete occupations. Concrete units can also be broken down into progressively smaller units... occupation has a long history of this process of activity analysis, consisting of the identification of levels of occupation, of discovering the level at which intervention should occur, of further analysis to determine the need for practice in subroutines or to alter the context of the occupation. However we have not yet agreed a vocabulary to classify all the units of occupation in which we are interested. We do not agree as to the extent to which occupation can be unitized and still be considered occupation. To some of us, the term occupation is used only for larger chunks of activity. To others the term is equated to purposeful activity... progress in understanding the interrelationship between larger and smaller chunks of activity in the physical and spatial world will require that each level be precisely defined and differentiated.

It seems, then, that there is agreement that occupation is a complex, many-layered phenomenon, which may be arranged in levels, but no agreement about how to describe these layers.

My personal view (Hagedorn 1995a) is that there are three levels of occupation: developmental, effective and organizational. These are explained in Chapter 5, together with a descriptive taxonomy to identify different 'chunks' or 'units'.

INSUFFICIENTLY PRECISE DEFINITIONS

It is plain that part of the confusion over the meaning of terms such as occupation, activity and task is due to the fact that usage by therapists is not only inconsistent but it also differs from the dictionary definitions of the words. These definitions are, in turn, somewhat vague and circuitous.

The following definitions are all to be found in the Concise Oxford Dictionary:

- *Action* is variously defined as 'being active; exertion of energy or influence; thing done; mode or style of movement.' It is both a noun and an adjective.
- *Activity* is defined as 'exertion of energy, state or quality of being active; actions; occupations.' Even the lexicographer accepts that activity and occupation are often used as synonyms, and is obliged to define activity as 'the quality of being active'; *active* is, in turn, defined as 'given to action' which takes us on a circular tour of the available words and does not clarify the meaning.
- *Task* is defined with a little more clarity as 'a piece of work imposed: piece of work voluntarily undertaken.' This use of the word task to indicate a defined piece of work implies that it is a more specific entity than an activity. Activity analysis is commonly presented as involving a list of the component tasks. Yet several American taxonomies place 'task' at a higher level than 'activity', which seems to be equated with 'actions performed when being active'.
- *Occupation* is defined as 'means of passing time; employment, business, calling, pursuit.'

None of these standard definitions is of much help to the therapist who wishes to attempt occupational analysis.

DEFINING OCCUPATION

Kielhofner (1995), who studied with Reilly, has defined occupation as:

The dominant activity of human beings that includes serious, productive pursuits and playful, creative and festive behaviours. It is the result of evolutionary processes culminating in biological and social need for both playful and productive activity.

Kielhofner too has to resort to the word 'activity' in this definition.

The definition of occupation used in occupational science is based on one originated by Yerxa and states that occupation is 'Units of activity which are named in the lexicon of the culture' (Zemke & Clark 1996). Other versions add 'occurring within the stream of human behaviour'.

This definition is close to one which I have proposed:

'occupation is a purposeful form of human endeavour having a name and associated role title. It provides a longitudinal organization of time and effort in a person's life. (Hagedorn 1995a, revised)

It seems, therefore, that a consensus view of occupation may be emerging, but it is a gradual process.

Box 3.1 Generally agreed characteristics of an occupation

- Essential to human health and well-being
- Named entity
- Complex structure
- Meaningful and purposeful
- Productive
- Consists of interlocking chunks or units
- Has an organizing function within time
- May be classified situationally as work, leisure or self-care (and other subdivisions).

OCCUPATION VERSUS ACTIVITY

We are *occupational* therapists not *activity* therapists. This simple fact has led to much semantic debate about whether we should describe the media we use as activities or occupations.

Some theorists have expressed strong views that we should avoid the use of the word activity altogether. Darnell & Heater (1994) reject activity as 'much too broad to adequately describe the work we do'. Nelson (1988) also considers that we should avoid the word.

One of the problems, as pointed out by Golledge (1998a), and illustrated by the definitions given earlier, is that 'whilst attempting to define one term "occupation" it is difficult to avoid using other terms, such as activity, in the explanation.'

As we have seen, even the occupational science definition resorts to the word 'activity'. I have attempted in my own definition to avoid the problem by choosing the word 'endeavour' (which the dictionary defines as 'try to do, attempt').

Despite criticism, the word activity continues to be widely used. The third edition of the American Uniform Terminology for Occupational Therapy (American Association of Occupational Therapists 1994) categorizes specific activities under one of three performance areas – activities of daily living; productive activities; play and leisure. A number of textbooks also continue to use the term activity. The most recent edition of *Willard & Spackman's Occupational Therapy* (Neistadt & Crepeau 1998) describes activities of daily living and activity analysis.

Cynkin & Robinson (1990) go against the prevailing trend by describing 'activities health'. They use the words 'creative activity' in preference to occupation. They define creative activity as 'that activity which evolves from one's thoughts or imagination and/or that causes things to happen and/or is constructive and is either originative or productive.' These authors provide a detailed analysis of assumptions concerning activity, the phenomena associated with it, and its role in the maintenance of health and well-being.

COMPETING TAXONOMIES

The debate over the use of 'activity' and 'occupation' is entangled in the debate over whether there are different types or levels of performance, and if there are, which words should be used to describe differing forms of performance.

Ilott (1995) refers to the hierarchy developed by Levine & Brayley (1991) in which they view activity ('any specific action or pursuit') as the 'foundation of the doing process'. Tasks are the next level in the hierarchy. Roles are the highest level, defining and governing tasks and activities. All aspects are influenced by the human and non-human environments.

Kielhofner's model of human occupation (1995) puts roles, routines and habits in the habituation subsystem providing the organizing framework for behaviour. Task performance depends on skills from motor, process, communication/interaction and social interaction domains.

In Christiansen & Baum's (1997) Person/Environment/Occupational Performance model, they propose a hierarchical taxonomy consisting of roles, occupations, tasks, actions and abilities. However, the same authors have also presented a hierarchy in which self-identity is followed by roles, tasks and actions (neurobehavioural and physical).

My own set of terms (Hagedorn 1995a) is broadly similar in structure but uses different words: roles, occupations, activities, tasks and performance units. This is described in detail in Chapter 4.

Johnson (1996) deals with activity analysis, and, although not presenting these words as a hierarchy, describes activities as being composed of tasks. Reed & Sanderson (1992) also describe the process of activity analysis as involving analysis of the tasks the activity can provide, as does Crepeau (1998).

The term activity analysis is commonly used to describe the analysis of a 'chunk of doing'. The term 'therapeutic activity' is also commonly used to denote the 'thing to be done' during the applied use of a portion of an occupation as therapy.

Two Swedish therapists – Haglund & Henriksson (1995) – have explored the available terminology for activity analysis and conclude that it is inadequate. They propose a set of descriptors based on different forms of *action* (intentional, goal-directed movement) which combine to form an *activity* (cluster of actions with an overriding conscious goal).

They note that:

performance of an activity can be analysed at different levels. An activity such as 'having guests for dinner' can be further divided into a number of more limited activities at a lower level such as 'peeling the potatoes', 'laying the table'.

Haglund & Henriksson are also interested in the ways in which activities can be performed simultaneously. This is an advanced form of performance. When a task is being learnt, it requires total concentration but once mastered can be done with half the mind on something else. They note how, in many forms of disability, the ability to do several things at once is lost, with resulting slowing down of performance and loss of independence.

They also propose an adaptation of Nelson's occupational form concept (Nelson 1988), using the terms *occupational norm* (how a certain type of activity is generally executed in a given culture) and *occupational circumstances* (the physical environment and context in which an activity is actually carried out).

Golledge (1998a) distinguishes between occupations (which she equates with the daily living tasks that are part of an individual's lifestyle),

purposeful activities and actions. Her distinction is based on the degree to which these terms indicate the presence or absence of personal meaning and social context: purposeful activities have context and meaning, actions do not.

These competing taxonomies are summarized in Box 3.2.

It will be apparent from the comparisons in Box 3.2 that the underlying concepts concerning the arrangement of these terms is broadly similar. There is a gradation in both complexity of structure and degree of meaning. The components of performance are placed at the bottom, the organizing structures at the top. What differs, very confusingly, is the use of words. In particular, 'activity', 'purposeful activity' and 'task' seem to be used as synonyms. 'Action' is given various meanings.

There is an exact comparison between this use of terminology and the use of words such as 'model', 'frame of reference' or 'approach' to describe models of practice. In both cases, when one gets behind the language, similar ideas are being expressed. The problem is that different authors continue to use different language.

While this situation is understandable, in that it stems from the complexity of human occupation, it is highly unsatisfactory. In particular, it impedes the development of systems of occupational analysis which are essential tools for therapy.

Box 3.2 Hierarchical taxonomies of human occupation

Levine & Brayley	Christiansen & Baum	Hagedorn	Johnson	Kielhofner	Haglund & Henriksson	Golledge
	Self-identity				—	—
Roles	Roles	Roles	Roles	Occupations	Occupations	
	Occupations	Occupations		Roles Routines Habits	Activities	Occupations
Tasks	Tasks	Activities	Activities	Tasks	Action sequence	Purposeful activity
Activities	Actions	Tasks	Tasks	—	Actions	
	Abilities	Performance units	Skills	Skills		Action

A PERSONAL VIEW

Having considered the evidence, I have reached a number of conclusions which are summarized below. Since the topic is still subject to debate, the reader may legitimately arrive at different ones.

Conclusions concerning occupation and activity

1. Occupation can be used as a generic term to cover all forms of purposeful human participation. Thus, we can call ourselves occupational therapists.

2. Occupations are complex entities which occur at different levels. These levels, and the differing types of performance, require specific designations, otherwise accurate analysis is impeded. The word 'activity', provided that it is carefully defined in the context of occupational analysis, can legitimately form part of a taxonomy.

3. The use of the word activity as part of an analytical taxonomy is not inconsistent with our designation as occupational therapists.

In Chapter 4 a system and taxonomy for occupational analysis is proposed.

4

A taxonomy of human occupation

THE NEED FOR A PRECISE TAXONOMY

As indicated in Chapter 3, it is not helpful, in the context of analysis, if we continue to describe performance using the same words to cover many different levels, or if we use words confusingly as synonyms.

The language of analysis must be precise, but it should also be based on normal usage, not seeking unnecessarily to invent new words or to use existing ones with meanings which differ greatly from standard definitions.

It is common for a profession to generate its own scientific or analytical language. It therefore seems legitimate to define the words as used within occupational therapy, and to give each word a specific meaning.

A PROPOSED TAXONOMY FOR OCCUPATIONAL ANALYSIS

The taxonomy which I have proposed is specifically designed to aid occupational analysis (Box 4.1). It has been developed through the experience of conducting activity analysis during which it rapidly becomes apparent that accepted terms run out long before the analysis is completed.

It is recognized that occupational analysis is an artificial process; in reality, performance is experienced as an integrated whole, but it still requires clear description. As previously described, levels of occupation designate different forms of occupational behaviour. The taxonomy relates directly to these levels, so that specifying a level also implies specification of a particular type of occupational performance.

The taxonomy has 11 distinct terms. Social role is an organizational structure which, like occupation, can extend across a long period during a person's life. At the other end of the list, skill components provide the means by which performance can be carried out. The remaining seven terms identify different types of performance at different occupational levels during different episodes of time. These terms are selected to reflect common usage within UK practice, as well as attempting to steer a course through

the minefield of conflicting definitions given in the literature. The definitions and function of the terms used in the taxonomy are shown in Table 4.1.

Box 4.1 Analytical taxonomy of occupation

- Social role
- Occupation
- Routine
- Activity
- Task
- Task stage
- Performance unit
- Actions, interactions, reactions
- Skill components.

Table 4.1 Levels of occupation

Level of occupation	Organizing structure	Definition and function
Organizational	Social roles	Designation of relationships, responsibilities or status within a culture or group which directs the individual's engagement in certain occupations, activities or tasks related to the role over extended periods of time
	Occupations	Named units of daily activity which provide longitudinal organization of time and effort in a person's life and provide that person with an occupational role
Effective	Routines	Habitual and fixed sequences of activities
	Activities	Extended chunks of related performance which take place during a finite period for a particular purpose. The outcome or product of an activity is a change in the previous state of objective reality or subjective experience
Developmental		
Constructive	Tasks	Each task is a self-contained part of an activity. A task is composed of a sequence of stages, often in a predetermined order,
	Task stages	each of which contributes to task completion
Acquisitional	Performance unit	A performance unit is the smallest piece of performance which can be separately identified within a task stage
Proto-occupational	Actions Interactions Reactions	A repertoire of movements and emotional and cognitive responses
	Skill components	Potentials for performance in the areas of action, interaction and reaction. Skill components are divisible into areas or domains: sensori-motor; cognitive; psychosocial

DEFINITIONS USED IN THE ANALYTICAL TAXONOMY

SOCIAL ROLES

A role is 'the behaviour expected of a person occupying a given status or social position... Roles are governed by certain norms or expectations, but are also, to some extent, interpreted by the individuals playing them' (O'Donnell 1992).

The term 'social role' may describe family relationships or general cultural or social concepts (such as 'worker', 'pensioner', 'patient' or 'student'), as distinct from role titles which define occupations, as described below.

Social roles are placed at the head of the hierarchy because they play a large part in directing what the individual does or is expected to do (or not do).

Roles affect perceptions of personal identity, and personal identity and values also direct participation in roles.

Occupational therapists are, arguably, more concerned with what the individual needs to do in order to fulfil role demands, than with the role itself, but the hierarchy would be incomplete without this category.

AN OCCUPATION

An occupation is an organized form of human endeavour which has a name and associated role title. We speak of cooking, accountancy, management, bricklaying, gardening, painting and surfing. We call the participants in these occupations chef/cook, accountant, manager, bricklayer, gardener, artist and surfer.

The participant engages in an occupation over an extended timescale. Usually this means that the occupation is performed on a regular basis over a period of years, possibly for a major portion of the person's life.

In order to sustain this performance over time the individual must retain a mental image of the self participating in the occupational role in the past, present and future. This requires mental planning functions to occur over extended timeframes. For example, if you decide in January to plan and book a late summer holiday, you have to carry with you the image of the holiday and the actions required to get you there. You must plan to get your passport or your injections, to buy suitable clothes and to find someone to care for the cat. These functions occur at the organizational level, and are different in nature from the short-term sequencing or problem-solving which is needed to complete an activity at the effective level.

Because occupation has become accepted as the general 'umbrella' term for all the forms of doing with which occupational therapists are concerned, it is also used as a generic term to indicate occupational performance.

Many occupations may be performed in the context of work, or leisure or self-care, but a few are restricted to one of the classifications. (For a more detailed presentation of my views on the nature of occupation refer to Hagedorn (1995a.)

AN ACTIVITY (CHAINED TASKS)

An activity is a sequence of linked episodes of task performance which takes place on a specific occasion during a finite period for a particular reason. The result of participation in an activity is that some aspect of objective reality or subjective experience is changed; the nature of the change has meaning for the participant.

A completed activity results in a change of some kind. Either something has been added to or subtracted from the environment, or altered within it, or something has changed in the subjective experience of the participant.

The expression 'purposeful activity' is often used. I find this cumbersome, and, given the definition of activity which I have provided, it is difficult to conceive of a 'purposeless' activity (although actions such as random pacing, rocking or plucking may be purposeless). If, however, the reader prefers to insert the word 'productive', that is fine, provided that the nature of 'productivity' is broadly defined.

The product does not have to be tangible. If you 'go to an art gallery to look at the pictures', nothing external changes. The pictures are still on the wall. Yet the activity will have given you visual, cognitive or emotional experiences. Something has changed 'inside you' in your perceptions or memories.

This subjective element is important just because it is so individual. If you go to the gallery with a friend, you may enjoy the pictures but your friend may find them boring. Your own enjoyment may be less if your friend is making disparaging remarks and obviously wishes to be elsewhere.

You can even perform an activity entirely 'in your mind'. Creating the plot of a novel, planning a holiday, composing music, inventing something, all of these things happen in real time within the imagination. At the point at which mental work is taking place, an activity is being performed. The product, however, may remain an abstraction within the mind until at some point the novel is written, the holiday booked, or the invention is committed to paper.

When you decide to engage in an activity you choose when it will happen. There is a time to start and the activity takes a finite period to complete. This definable timeframe is what distinguishes an activity from an occupation.

Any occupation is made up of many activities. These activities may be associated in fixed chains which form *processes* or habitual associations which form *routines*. At any one time, performance of an occupation is expressed in performance of one of the activities of which it is comprised.

When you cook (occupation) you do so at intervals, in the course of a day or a week or a year. The occupation of cooking encompasses a continual series of separate occasions on which you cook. But when you decide to cook a vegetable curry for Tuesday supper, you have specified an activity.

An activity can be identified by a short description of the type of doing and the object – the thing being worked on or the reason for doing it.

'Going for a walk in the woods' indicates action, purpose and product and provides the general context. The context is particularly important. Different intentions and contexts alter the nature of the performance, even when the product is similar.

'Making small cakes to sell in my tea-shop' implies a different set of standards and expectations from 'making cakes for the children'. For the children's tea, the cakes are probably made in a domestic kitchen and standards can be varied somewhat. The cook might be in the role of parent, party-giver or volunteer. Making cakes for sale suggests that the baking is done in a commercial kitchen and that the cook is at her place of work. Standards concerning quantity, productivity, size, weight, ingredients and hygiene must be very strictly met in a work-setting.

An activity is not always linked to an occupational role. Sometimes it is linked to a social role, such as parent or student. At other times there is no associated role title. When we talk about activities of daily living, for example, we describe 'getting dressed' or 'eating a meal', but we do not describe ourselves as 'dressers' or 'eaters'.

Activities of daily living are often linked to form routines. For example, in the morning you may: get clean and comfortable (wash, clean teeth, use lavatory); dress (decide what to wear, get your clothes together and put them on); prepare and eat breakfast; clear up; and get ready for work.

This type of routine is partly determined by practical considerations (one has to wash before one gets dressed) but it has other elements which may vary between individuals. Automated routines (habits) help to streamline the efficient sequencing of frequently needed activities and enable the participant to reserve energy and thinking capacity for other things.

Activities can also be linked in a flexible manner across longer timespans (Cynkin & Robinson 1990). For example, the activity 'going shopping' may be linked to antecedent activities such as 'planning menus for next week', 'planning dinner party for Saturday', 'turning out the fridge and store cupboard to see what is needed'.

Associated tasks may be included in the sequence, such as 'write shopping list' and 'check contents of purse'. In order to shop, one must 'walk/drive to the shops'. After shopping is done, there are consequent activities such as 'unpack shopping and put things away'; 'check household budget expenditure', and, perhaps a day later, 'prepare food for dinner party'.

The ability to organize such chains and sequences efficiently is very important. People who are ineffective organizers are disadvantaged. Loss of cognitive abilities such as short-term memory, planning, sequencing, or problem-solving are very disabling because performance may be reduced to a series of unconnected tasks.

Activities do not, however, have to be undertaken in a neat, single-minded, linear sequence. As pointed out by Bateson (1996), activities (especially for women) are often performed in an overlapping 'enfolded' manner. Tasks from different activities or reactive responses may be interspersed throughout a performance episode. Men, however, are said to be better at performance which occurs in a focused 'chunk' during which one objective is achieved.

A TASK

A task is a 'piece of doing', a self-contained stage in an activity. This is usually described by a simple description of the things to be done. For example, the activity of 'getting dressed' is arranged around a sequence of tasks related to putting on a set of garments.

Activity
Getting dressed to go to work

Dressing tasks
Put on:
    underpants
    vest
    socks
    shirt
    trousers
    tie
    jacket.

A man might choose to vary the sequence somewhat and might omit some items, but there will be a shared understanding with others of what it means 'to get dressed'. A person from a different culture is likely to have a different task list.

A task has meaning in relation to the activity of which it is part but taken in isolation it usually has low meaning apart from that gained by satisfaction when it is completed.

'Putting on a jacket' does not mean very much, except, perhaps, the desire to be warm. But 'trying on a smart new jacket in a shop'; 'putting on a thick jacket to go tobogganing in the snow'; 'putting on a dinner jacket to go to the opera' or 'putting on an old jacket to dig the garden' all have very different contexts and therefore different meanings.

A TASK STAGE

It is a fundamental principle of task analysis that tasks can be divided into stages. Each stage is an act which is complete in itself and also contributes to completion of the whole task.

Task
Put on a shirt

Task stages
    Pick up shirt
    Put one arm through sleeve
    Pull shirt round back
    Put second arm through sleeve
    Do up front buttons
    Do up cuff buttons
    Ensure garment is straight.

In some tasks the sequence of stages is relatively rigid and must be adhered to if the task is to be completed effectively. Other tasks are more flexible. Some tasks have small cyclical patterns where several linked stages are repeated before the next stages can be attempted.

A PERFORMANCE UNIT

A performance unit is the smallest piece of performance which can be separately observed or described (previously, in Hagedorn (1995a), I have used the term task segment).

For example, if one is teaching a small child to do up buttons, the child must learn each unit as a separate skill and then put the units together to complete the task stage.

Task stage

Do up buttons

Performance units
- Grasp button between finger and thumb
- Grasp material of buttonhole between other finger and thumb
- Bring button and buttonhole together with button underneath hole
- Push button through buttonhole from beneath
- Catch button as it passes through to top of hole
- Pull button completely through hole
- Settle button firmly across hole to ensure closure.

You will note that much longer descriptions become necessary in order to define each performance unit with precision. Even simple tasks have an extraordinary complexity at this level. The individual cannot undertake such sequences of actions, perceptions and judgements until the necessary level of neurological and motor development has been reached.

ACTIONS, INTERACTIONS AND REACTIONS

When we examine small units of performance lasting for only a few minutes, we find that individuals continually *act, interact and react*.

ACTIONS

Actions are intentional and goal-directed. The individual decides to 'do' something; performance follows in a seamless flow. Actions are the 'building blocks' of performance which can be re-assembled in infinitely variable patterns and sequences.

Humans recognize the importance of actions by giving them names – verbs. With these 'doing words', we describe what we do to ourselves and others. We acknowledge the subtle variations in the way we act by qualifying the verb with a descriptor – an adverb. So we run, hold, twist, push; we can do these things quickly, gently, firmly, strongly.

The skill to perform an action has, at some point, to be developed. Each action needs co-

ordinated use of *skill components*, sensori-motor, cognitive and perceptual.

REACTIONS

We not only do things because we want to, we also do things in response to what happens around us; we react to people, situations and events and to the organic and inorganic content of our surroundings. Some of our reactions are innate, while others need to be learnt.

Some reactions are automatic, based on protective physiological responses. Other reactions take the form of physical actions. We also react emotionally or cognitively. Once again, we name these responses: we speak of being hurt, angered, surprised, shocked, pleased, happy or disappointed.

INTERACTIONS

Humans communicate with each other, verbally, and through expression and gesture. Interactions are a mixture of action and reaction; we both intend to communicate and react to the communications of others. We may also interact with animals.

A FLOW OF BEHAVIOURS

The way in which actions, interactions and reactions combine in a flow of behaviour woven into and around occupational performance is best illustrated by an example:

A woman is making a cup of coffee in the kitchen. She lifts the kettle, takes it to the sink and fills it. She notices a dirty mark on the sink and washes it off, and then takes the kettle back to plug it in. As she does so, she looks out of the window, and smiles to see the sun brighten the flowers in the garden. She can take her coffee outside and have it in the sun. She switches on the kettle, goes to the refrigerator to get some milk. In the fridge she sees a bowl of left-over, wilted salad which she removes and puts in the bin. Meanwhile the kettle is starting to sing; she finds a mug, puts a spoonful of coffee into it, and mentally notes that the jar is almost empty and she needs to buy another. She is about to make coffee when the cat comes in from the garden. The cat winds round her legs and she bends to make a fuss of him: she greets him by name and asks 'Are you hungry?' The cat miaows and rubs harder. She goes to the cupboard, gets a tin of cat food, opens it, fills the cat's bowl and places it on the floor. As she does so, she talks to the cat about what a good cat he is and what a nice dinner she has for him. Once the cat is happily settled and after watching him enjoy his meal for a moment, she finally pours hot water onto her coffee, fills it up with milk, and goes out into the garden.

The way in which, in real life, we act, interact and react in this spontaneous and fluid manner, even when engaged in task performance, is important. It is an aspect which is often ignored in formal task analysis, and which it is hard to recreate in a synthetic occupational therapy environment. As noted by Haglund & Henriksson (1995), the inability to do more than one thing at a time can be disabling.

Equally, it is disabling to let attention wander too freely between competing actions and re-actions so that the task is uncompleted.

SKILLS AND SKILL COMPONENTS

The terms which I have just explained relate to the *analysis of an occupation*. It is also necessary to be able to analyse the abilities of the individual when engaged in skilled performance.

Skill is another loosely used word which can mean anything from a specific domain of performance to something nearer to the dictionary definition 'expertness, practised ability, facility in an action or in doing something; dexterity' (Concise Oxford Dictionary).

In general, therapists understand 'a skill' to mean 'a piece of practised and competent performance'. Skill describes *how* a thing is done, not '*the thing being done*'. One may also analyse skill in relation to the occupational taxonomy.

To give an example: driving is a skill. One may drive well or badly. The occupational role is 'driver', an activity may be 'drive to work'. There will be many tasks associated with this, each of which is divisible into stages which can be subdivided into performance units.

There are levels of skill. A basic skill (used to complete a performance unit) would be one that is the foundation for others. Expertise is highly developed complex skill which much exceeds competence.

As one learns to be a driver, at each level skills must be mastered and integrated to achieve competence at the overall skill of driving. One must then practise and hone the skills of driving over time in order to become an expert.

All these uses of the word relate to the *integrated use* of skill. It is important to distinguish this from the *components of skill*.

Skill components are sometimes referred to as *domains* of skill. They are the basic physical and cognitive building blocks of performance. To perform even the simplest performance unit, the individual must access, integrate and employ many different skill components.

Many authors have produced extensive lists of skill components (see Ch. 28). These are usually classified under headings. Those given in Box 4.2 are the ones commonly used, but the skill components listed under each heading vary from one text to another. The reader is advised to refer to these lists in order to gain an understanding of the scope and complexity of human skill components.

A more extensive list of these components is given on pages 223–226.

If we analyse the performance unit 'grasp button between fingers', we can identify many skill components.

Performance unit — Grasp button	
Skill components	
Sensori-motor	e.g. pinch grip; fine touch, pressure
Cognitive–perceptual	e.g. object recognition; figure and ground discrimination; concept formation; memory; process sequencing
Psychosocial	e.g. recognizes/enjoys social approval of task completion.

The ease with which humans normally acquire and master such a complex synthesis of behaviours and judgements and then chain

Box 4.2 Skill components	
Sensori-motor components	Those required for the execution of movement and the reception of input from the environment.
Cognitive–perceptual components	Those involved in learning and the application of knowledge or processing of information from the environment.
Psychosocial components	Those required for communication with and response to others. Awareness of self and of self in relation to others.

them into task performance is remarkable in the light of this level of analysis. The outstanding feature of skilled human performance is the ability to combine these skill components adaptively into an infinitely variable series of behaviours.

While many animals exhibit intricate behaviours such as nest-building, hunting or mating, these tend to be relatively fixed and unadaptable. Only the behaviour of the higher primates, such as the simple tool-making and learned food-gathering techniques of some of the great apes, comes close to the behaviour of humans. Even these primitive skills are, in evolutionary terms, several millions years behind our own.

Levels of occupation

A HIERARCHICAL APPROACH

Human occupations can be analysed using a hierarchical structure related to three occupational levels.

A 'level of occupation' is an artificial construct. Occupations entwine, nest and enfold. Occupational behaviour has ebbs and flows and patterns. These normally unite performance into a more or less seamless flow as the performer moves from one area of activity to another interspersed with periods of repose.

A division into levels is simply a tool to facilitate occupational analysis. It helps to illustrate the developmental and temporal features of occupation. It serves to give a language to describe the position of one action within a series.

Analysis of levels of occupation may also help the therapist when teaching skills or tasks and during the assessment of occupational performance. It can aid the provision of therapy. It may help to indicate appropriate approaches.

The structure which I will use in this book is a development of the three-tier hierarchy which I described in 1995. This hierarchy reflects the normal sequence in the acquisition of occupational behaviour, and also the different timespans within which performance can take place. It does not imply incremental levels of complexity, for occupational analysis demonstrates that complexity – albeit of different kinds – exists at all levels within the hierarchy.

	Box 5.1 Performance complexity related to timeframe (examples are based on estimated timings)
Time	**Type of performance**
0 – 10 seconds	Simple actions leading to completion of part of task, e.g. pick up pen; do up button, hit several keys on keyboard, eat one mouthful, catch ball; add short sequence of numbers
10 – 60 seconds	Completion of simple task or task stage, e.g. fill kettle and plug in; open car door, sit, fit key in ignition; switch on TV and select channel; put on jacket; comb hair
1 – 10 minutes	Completion of chained sequence of tasks or several short unconnected tasks, e.g. make a sandwich; walk to local shop; draw quick sketch; play short game with child
10 – 60 minutes	Undertake one long sequence of tasks in relation to an extended activity, or several extended, but unrelated tasks, e.g. drop children at school, drive to petrol station, return home, have coffee; mow the lawn and complete other gardening tasks; go out with friends, have drinks and snack
1 day	Undertake many different tasks and activities related to personal care, leisure, work role or social role as influenced by age of participant, environment, temporal and seasonal conditions. Use the results of these performances to enhance personal health and well-being, or to contribute to that of others or to change aspects of personal environment
1 year	Engage in a repertoire of performances connected with social roles and personal occupations. Discard some roles and occupations and acquire others

BASIS FOR THE DESIGNATION OF OCCUPATIONAL LEVELS

The concept of different occupational levels is based on two important perceptions about the nature of occupational performance:

1. it follows a developmental sequence
2. it occurs within real time.

A DEVELOPMENTAL SEQUENCE

We learn our occupations over time according to an observable, developmental process which is followed from birth to maturity. During this process, we extend our occupational repertoire from simple actions through the use of basic skills for simple task performance into complex co-ordinated and integrated sequences of occupational behaviour.

This learning sequence is repeated whenever the individual needs to adapt to changing personal or environmental circumstances by acquiring a new behaviour. This developmental process is sometimes referred to as the ontogenesis (development over time) of occupations.

TEMPORAL INFLUENCES

The temporal dimension of occupation has been described by numerous occupational therapy theorists, who draw attention to the way in which people use time, and the temporal patterns, long and short, which affect and organize performance throughout life.

The nature and complexity of performance and outcome depend on the timeframe. If we 'freeze-frame' an episode of time, we can study the performance which takes place within it. Simple examples are given in Box 5.1.

This analysis suggests that occupational behaviour moves and changes along complex temporal pathways. If one isolates a single short episode of performance, it appears quite different from when one views it in the context of a long organizational sequence. As in all hierarchical systems, changes at one level resonate up and down throughout all levels.

One of the indicators of dysfunction is that performance takes much longer than it should. A simple action such as doing up a button may take a minute or more; a simple task sequence needed for meal preparation may take two or three times as long as normal; the variety of occupations and activities which can be fitted into the day becomes much reduced, performance becomes more linear, with one thing being done at a time, instead of nesting and enfolding several different tasks.

The hierarchy which evolved from this analysis has three levels:

Three	Organizational	Roles and occupations which organize and unify performance over 1 or more years
Two	Effective	Routines and habits which organize performance over weeks or days Activities which last for an extended period during a day or link one time period with another
One	Developmental (proto-occupational, acquisitional and constructive)	Tasks and task stages which last 3 to 10 minutes Performance units which last from a few seconds to a few minutes

LEVEL THREE: ORGANIZATIONAL

At this level, different roles and occupations are woven together to make the pattern of a person's life. The pattern will change as the person moves from childhood to adulthood and into old age or as the individual is challenged by new opportunities or goals.

For most of the time, the flow seems relatively uninterrupted. Occasionally, however, change is marked and even abrupt. Such noticeable changes occur when circumstances in the life of the individual alter, or when one of the culturally significant points in life is reached, such as coming of age, starting work, marriage or retirement.

These points at which new roles are adopted and occupations change in consequence are marked in many cultures by rituals and ceremonies to indicate their importance.

Roles and occupations provide the structures by means of which the different strands of a person's life can be organized over time.

Occupations and roles help the individual to develop a concept of self as an actor in the physical and social environment. The experience of 'doing things' within time provides a perspective on the past, a structure for the present, and a means of planning and influencing the future.

At the organizational level, process skills predominate; the individual must plan, problem-solve, organize and sequence. The individual may also imagine, create, and construct mental images of the past present and future. Individuals must arrive at an understanding of the world and their relationship with it.

LEVEL TWO: EFFECTIVE

At any one time, individuals are concerned with a portion of living – extending for an hour or two – in which they do things which will make a difference to their lives. This immediate sense of 'doing things today' is linked to the remembered past and the foreseeable future.

This form of 'present doing' is productive. It has an *effect* – a result or consequence. 'To effect' means to bring about, accomplish, cause to exist or occur (Concise Oxford Dictionary). Thus the name 'effective' has been chosen to describe this level.

As a result of action, something is changed. The thing which changes may be something tangible in the person's surroundings, the quality of a relationship, or something abstract within the inner experience of the individual or another person.

The activity being performed may contribute to some long-term goal but that may not be at the front of the person's mind when the person is engaged in performance. What matters at the time is the current experience of being involved in action, the immediate purpose of acting, and the achievement of the desired result.

Nevertheless the relationship of this piece of performance to others and the consequences of the actions taken will be consciously evaluated at some point. The person may act because of factors unrelated to present performance, for example when undertaking a disliked activity which will, however, lead to a desired future outcome.

It is at this level that subjective, situationally influenced meanings are experienced in connection with personal activities.

LEVEL ONE: DEVELOPMENTAL

The developmental level is where the building blocks of performance are learnt and assembled. Taken in isolation, performance at this level is relatively ineffective.

A single task or task stage achieves little unless it is related to a set of other tasks sequenced to form an activity, which in turn relates to other activities, occupations or roles.

This level has three subdivisions which indicate the type of performance at each level:

- proto-occupational
- acquisitional
- constructive.

PROTO-OCCUPATIONAL LEVEL

The prefix 'proto' means first or original. At this level, nothing productive is achieved, for the skills required for performance have not yet been mastered.

The individual must convert potential abilities into usable skill components which are the precursors to and foundations for skilled performance.

The timeframe at this level is only 'now' as concepts of past and present in relation to actions have not yet been developed.

When we are born we can do nothing. We experiment with our limbs and senses, define the limits between ourselves and the outside world. We explore objects and develop the first concepts of things and the primitive awareness of cause and effect, and likes and dislikes.

This is also the level to which a person may return if seriously damaged in body or mind, and the level past which an individual may be unable to progress if born with severe learning difficulties.

ACQUISITIONAL LEVEL

An acquisition is something useful which one has gained. At this level, skills are developed.

This is done by acquiring small units of 'doing', actions, interactions and reactions, and building them into blocks of performance which will contribute to completion of task stages and simple tasks.

Each small piece of performance at this level takes only a few seconds or minutes.

This is the first rung on the ladder which leads to the development of the person into a fully rounded, 'occupational being'.

In normal development, acquisition is rapid and new skills are continually integrated into the repertoire causing incremental development of complex skills and consequent gains in competence in an increasing repertoire of tasks.

CONSTRUCTIVE LEVEL

To construct means to fit together, frame or build. At this level, the person performs simple task stages and chains these together into short sequences to complete a task. Tasks can be chained into more complex sequences. Each task contributes something to the chain and together they combine to achieve a purpose or product.

The timeframe for task performance is still relatively short – the 'here and now' – with just the immediate past and near future kept in view.

Meanings are derived from the context of task performance rather than the nature of the task. If appreciation of context is limited, meaning is restricted and gratification resulting from the task may become the most important motivator.

Skills are more complex at this level and may take longer to master. A period of practice is needed during which 'bumps and joins' in the sequence of skilled performances are smoothed out.

It is possible to function adequately at the constructive level, since things 'get done', but a person who cannot perform above this level needs guidance in order to relate current tasks to a wider picture.

Such individuals need prompting to consider an extended timeframe and may have difficulty in foreseeing the consequences of their actions. They may also be unable to cope with more than one task at a time.

This is a phase which children naturally go through, but in an adult such performance would probably be dysfunctional. The person would be likely to function below the higher levels of competence, rather as described in Allen's cognitive level 5. (Allen 1985).

HOW THE HIERARCHY RELATES TO DYSFUNCTION

Deficits of function can occur at any level. Deficits at each level can be related to other analytical structures or hierarchies as shown in Table 5.1.

The occupational level specifies the level at which dysfunction first becomes apparent. The National Centre for Medical Rehabilitation and Research (NCMRR) definitions (Christiansen & Baum 1997) indicate the nature of the dysfunc-

tion (societal limitation is excluded as it originates within the environment). Maslow's hierarchy of needs (Maslow 1970) indicates the type of need likely to be unmet if dysfunction occurs at that occupational level. Allen's six cognitive levels (Allen 1985) describe performance deficits caused by damage to cognition.

It will be apparent from Table 5.1 that the 'match' between these hierarchies is not perfect, for they are dealing with different descriptions of dysfunction. Despite this, putting these different views together helps to present a picture of the effects on competent performance of deficits or damage at each level.

The significance of this composite picture is more obvious when the effects of damage at each level are identified as shown in Table 5.2.

For a person to function at organizational level, societal limitation or disability must not

Table 5.1 A comparison of three hierarchical models of human needs and function/dysfunction in relation to levels of occupation

Occupational levels – normal ability at each level	NCMRR levels – description of dysfunction	Maslow's hierarchy – description of personal need which may not be met	Allen's cognitive levels – description of performance deficit associated with cognitive level
Organizational Able to cope with social roles and occupations	*Disability*	*Self-actualization* *Cognitive and aesthetic needs*	*Level 6* Planned actions
Effective Able to cope with daily activities	*Disability*	*Need for esteem* *Need for love and belonging*	*Level 6* *(Level 5)*
Developmental *Constructive* Able to perform tasks and task stages	*Functional limitation*	*Safety needs*	*Level 5* Exploratory actions *Level 4* Goal-directed actions
Acquisitional Performance units	*Impairment*	*Safety needs*	*Level 3* Repetitive manual actions
Proto-occupational Able to develop skill components	*Patho-physiology*	*Physiological needs*	*Level 2* Postural actions *Level 1* Reflexive, automated actions

Table 5.2 Effects of damage/dysfunction at each level of occupation

Expected development		Nature of damage/dysfunction		
Occupational level	Expected achievement	Nature of damage	Area of need affected	Dysfunctional performance
Developmental				
Proto-occupational	Skill components developed Skill domains established	Damage to cells and tissues; interruption of or interference with normal physiological and developmental processes Damage to organs and systems	Not able to meet physiological needs	Only able to make simple automated responses: awareness of environment much diminished
Acquisitional	Able to complete task segments and build simple skilled performance	Restriction or lack of ability to perform an action or task within normal range	Not able to meet safety needs	Only able to complete simple, repetitive actions with cues and demonstration
Constructive	Able to complete task stages and tasks Able to chain tasks	Dependent with PADL and DADL		Only able to complete single task stage at a time with prompts and cues Can complete one simple repetitive task
Effective	Can chain tasks to form activities Can organise activities in relation to past/future	Inability or limitation in performing PADL, DADL Limited productivity, leisure etc.	Partly able to meet safety and higher needs	Can initiate action and perform tasks Poor planning judgement, organisation, problem-solving
Organisational	Can manage varied and appropriate repertoire of activities, occupations and roles	Societal limitation and disability affect performance in some areas	Most needs met	Complex activities and chains of activities can be completed; shows creativity, reasoning, symbolic thought and problem-solving but has some areas of limitation

DADL, domestic activities of daily living; PADL, personal activities of daily living

affect ability to cope with roles and occupations. All needs should be met (in so far as is reasonable within normal human life) and the person should be able to demonstrate competent performance in a range of occupations and activities.

SUMMARY

Conceptualizing occupational behaviour as occurring at different levels is artificial, but it does provide a useful analytical tool.

Accurate occupational analysis is a fundamental prerequisite for intervention. Analysis leads to the naming and framing of problem areas and the selection of appropriate approaches which are relevant to the developmental level being addressed.

There is a need for further research to validate this structure, but pending international agreement on a taxonomy for the description of human occupation, use of these levels may illuminate and facilitate occupational analysis and adaptation.

6

Environmental levels

WHY DO WE NEED TO CONCEPTUALIZE THE ENVIRONMENT IN LEVELS?

The concept that occupations are divisible into levels has been presented as an artificial construct which assists analysis. In the same way, an understanding of the environment in terms of levels or layers also aids analysis of its content and impact on the user by focusing the attention of the therapist on what is relevant at any given time.

Analysis of the environment is usually presented in terms of its constituents, physical, organic, human, social and cultural, and the effect of this content on human actions and reactions. Like occupational analysis, a full environmental analysis can be daunting. Where does one start or stop?

At present, few theorists have paid much attention to forming a structure for environmental analysis. Bronfenbrenner (1979) (cited in Christiansen & Baum 1997) has proposed a three-level, systemic structure for analysis. He suggests that *macrosystemic analysis* considers society as a whole; *mesosystemic analysis* deals with the community and *microsystemic analysis* with the environment used and inhabited by the individual.

A similar idea has been explored by Spencer (1998) who uses the terms *immediate scale, proximal scale, community scale* and *societal scale* to designate levels radiating outwards from the user. Spencer provides examples of analysis of the physical, social and cultural components at each level.

My personal system of environmental analysis has some similarities. I propose that three environmental levels can be described in terms of *proximity* to and *accessibility* by the user, and the *significance* of the content to the user.

The structure is hierarchical because the environment closest to the user depends on the content and organization of the next layer out, which in turn depends on the layer beyond that, and so on out into the universe.

PROXIMITY, ACCESSIBILITY AND SIGNIFICANCE

For the purposes of occupational therapy, the environment needs to be considered in relation to the user who is the focal point from whom 'layers' can be imagined to radiate outwards. The proximal layer is centred on the user. Environmental content changes as users move from one part of their environment to another or changes the focus of their awareness. The more remote areas remain in a more stable relationship which may change slowly over time. Environmental levels are shown in Figure 6.1.

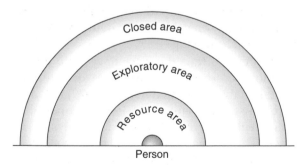

Figure 6.1 Environment levels.

The environment surrounds the individual, expanding in size and scale from the immediate, easily accessible surroundings, to the known and accessible area inhabited and used by the individual, and beyond into the wider world where varying degrees of accessibility are encountered. Ultimately it extends to the as yet unknown and inaccessible universe.

Analysis of the environment in terms of its proximity to the user is based on the assumption that individuals engaged in occupational performance normally pay attention to, and utilize elements of, their environment in proportion to its proximity, as modified by the requirements of the task and the significance of the content.

Human perception is geared to organize what is perceived into meaningful patterns and recognizable objects. The relationships of objects to each other in space and to the position of the user are also evaluated as the individual seeks information about resources, risks, barriers and access.

Through experience, the individual constructs awareness of the external environment, and combines this with awareness of the personal 'internal landscape' in which the individual's knowledge of the external world is mirrored, to form a 'world in the mind'.

Although the therapist can only analyse the observable aspects of the external environment, the 'internal landscape' is important. A brief description of the internal environment is therefore included on page 44.

I will use the terms shown in Figure 6.1 to designate the three levels in the external environment:

- resource area
- exploratory area
- closed area.

RESOURCE AREA

This area consists of all the places, objects and people frequently used by and familiar to an individual. The individual can move easily through this environment at will, interacting with it, adapting and changing it through actions, obtaining from it the things the individual needs.

This is the area with which the therapist is principally concerned, and which may require detailed analysis.

The resource area can be divided into three levels (Fig. 6.2), indicating proximity to the individual at any given moment:

1. immediate environment
2. near environment
3. used environment.

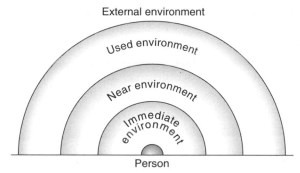

External environment

Used environment

Near environment

Immediate environment

Person

Figure 6.2 Levels within the external resource area.

IMMEDIATE ENVIRONMENT

This is the area of easiest access which can be reached by the user by stretching out arms, hands or body without moving away from the starting position. (For the adult, this means approximately a 1 to 1.50 metre circle pivoted on the central axis of the body.)

This is the environment where performance units and task stages are carried out.

The most important features of the immediate environment are objects, people, and physical conditions (heat, light etc.). The general content of the environment is perceived by the senses. Tangible content can be explored and manipulated by the hands.

The immediate *physical* environment affords the practical requirements for the task which is being done now, and cues to tasks which may be required in future. It may include information about threats and risks to be avoided.

The immediate *social* environment includes contact with and communication with others, cues to social interactions and behaviours and again, potential risks or threats from others.

This is the first part of the external environment to be discovered and explored during infancy, when objects are highly significant.

Cognitive impairment can cause the individual to return to (or never leave) this primitive level of awareness and exploration (Allen 1985).

NEAR ENVIRONMENT

This is the area which a person can explore within a few steps, for example a room or a defined outside area. The near environment can be conceptualized as a cube about 2 metres high by 4 metres wide and deep, which shifts with the person as the person moves from place to place.

The nature of the near environment may be static for a time, or may change rapidly as the person moves through different areas. The person is focused on the content of this near space, but may remain peripherally aware of events and objects in the resource area beyond.

For example, a housework task may take the participant from the kitchen to store cupboard in the hall, out to the back garden and back into the kitchen again. Awareness of the kitchen is maintained while in the hall or garden. Use of the environment is organized in relation to task sequences.

The near environment is made up of physical and sociocultural components and provides the user with much of the information which is responsible for environmental demand. Symbolic material, cues for roles and occupational behaviour, subjective reactions or perceptions based on memory become important at this level. Behaviour of others is an important component.

The near environment usually contains resources which may be needed to support or complete the tasks in a series. The presence of or lack of such resources and ease of access to them are important.

USED ENVIRONMENT

This includes all the external areas with which an individual is familiar and which the individual routinely uses and moves within.

During infancy and early childhood, this area is limited to home and a few nearby places. As the adult develops patterns of occupation, the used environment expands to include adjacent areas, places where shopping is done, places of recreation and entertainment, the place of work, and homes of friends and relatives.

These are the areas which have been found useful in the past and can be predicted to be useful in the future. Some of these areas will be used according to a definite temporal pattern, while others will have only intermittent use. Areas which remain unused for a long period begin to fade in importance until they finally get omitted from the resource area.

The individual normally sees these areas as predominantly safe, familiar and comfortable to use. There are few surprises here. Risks if they exist, are usually well-known so that they can be readily anticipated and action taken to avoid them. Unexpected risks may provoke considerable anxiety because they violate the established pattern.

The used environment also contains the local cultural and social influences which will affect the individual.

The richness or poverty of the used environment is believed by some theorists to have very significant impact on the self-concept, attitudes and abilities of the individual. Lack of opportunity because of environmental deprivation is held by some social scientists to be a primary cause of social marginalization and dysfunctional or antisocial behaviour.

EXPLORATORY AREA

This area contains, in theory, the whole of the rest of the accessible world, although in practice access is limited by many factors. The area contains new information, challenges, the stimulation and excitement of the unknown. It also contains threats and dangers, some known and some unknown.

Exploration has been proposed as a strong motivator for human action (Kielhofner 1995). From the moment a child is born, it begins to explore and humans continually seek to push outwards the boundaries of the exploratory area. As soon as an area is thoroughly explored, how-ever, it is likely to become part of the individual's resource area, and the sense of discovery is lost.

Attitudes to exploration vary widely. Some people are very cautious and timid 'explorers' who are satisfied with a well-known territory. Others seek to push the boundaries (and themselves) to the extreme in their attempts to penetrate the unknown.

As the person ages or becomes incapacitated, the exploratory area may shrink again because the desire or ability to access it is reduced. Ultimately, aged people may return to a state where the immediate and near environment is all that matters.

The exploratory area can be divided in several ways: for example, in terms of distance, in terms of feasibility of access, or by geographical or political area.

The exploratory area affects the individual directly only when the individual visits it, but its contents constantly affect the individual indirectly. Culture, government, politics, economics, production of food, artifacts or fuels, natural disasters, wars or famines in areas far from those we use in daily life can have far-reaching effects on people's lives.

CLOSED AREA

This is the part of our world which we either do not know about or which is closed to us. It includes a (rapidly shrinking) part of our planet – the deepest ocean; the most inaccessible jungle; the highest mountains. It also includes all that we see or believe to exist in the universe.

A notable feature of 20th century life is the ability of people to construct mental models of the 'unknown' world based on vicarious experience and learned information. We may never have been to Africa or Australia, but we know a good deal about these places. We have some expectations of what we might find if we were to go there. We can contact people and places we have never seen through communication media or via the Internet.

We are the first generation of humans for whom this is true for many rather than few, and it is likely to have a profound influence on our perceptions of the world.

It was very difficult for people who lived before the age of easy travel and global communication to conceptualize places which they had not personally visited. Their world view was bounded by blank spaces on the map and imagined terrors – 'Here be dragons!'

Now this unknown and inaccessible level has been pushed into outer space, and aliens have replaced dragons in our imagination. Even here, the exploratory area is being extended both by actual space exploration and by the work of cosmologists bent on revealing the nature of the universe.

The closed areas, real or imagined, physical or metaphysical, seem to present the ultimate challenge to human imagination and understanding.

SUBJECTIVE VIEWS OF THE ENVIRONMENT

INFORMATION-PROCESSING BY THE BRAIN

People act, interact and react in response to the environment. The environment *provides information* which enables the user to judge the nature of the situation, the roles of those within it, and the actions which are required in order to respond.

We know that most human behaviour is learnt. The effect that behaviour has on the environment will contribute to it being repeated or discontinued. However, human beings behave as they do for complex reasons which take account of more than a simple feedback loop between behaviour and effects on environment.

In order to 'know what to do', the brain continually *samples* both the environment and its own store of experiences, makes a 'best guess' about what is going on and whether it is significant and should be attended to, and directs action in response to this judgement. It then samples the results in order to gain feedback and judge what to do next.

The user of an environment may focus attention on one area to the exclusion of others when engaged in an absorbing task. More frequently, attention moves focus from the near to the peripheral to the distant, continually cue-gathering and processing in a manner which moves across levels in a seamless flow.

The individual may not be aware consciously of this scanning action, and one of the functions of the brain is to filter out unwanted, irrelevant or distracting information so that attention can be directed to the matter in hand.

If the individual is unable for any reason to gain and interpret cues or 'filter out' unwanted information, this can be very disabling. For example, a person with cognitive dysfunction may be unable to perform a simple task because of overload of information from the peripheral levels of the environment.

The therapist needs to appreciate the impact which the information in an environment is likely to have on an individual, in order to judge whether modifications are needed to enhance performance or promote a specific physical, cognitive or social response.

ROLES, RULES AND MEANINGS

People are 'social animals'. From birth, each individual begins to learn to interpret social signals from others. The small child rapidly learns a repertoire of roles and rules. Experience builds in the mind the ability to recognize a pattern of physical, social or symbolic information in the environment as having special and consistent meaning. A repertoire of appropriate responses and scripts is stored which will be brought into use when triggered by the right cues.

This purely information-processing model of meaning is, however, incomplete, because meaning also has an emotional content. It is bound up with feelings, beliefs, attitudes and values. It becomes significant.

Some situations have very clear significance; the roles and rules within them are widely accepted by a culture, and the majority of people produce similar and predictable responses to them. Such situations may have formal labels which help rapid recognition of what is going on.

For example, you understand what is likely to happen at a wedding, or a funeral, at a party or a picnic or an interview for a job. If you encounter a black hearse with a coffin, or a group of people eating a meal sitting on the ground in the countryside, you, as an adult, have no difficulty in knowing what is going on. A child will, however, at some point, have to learn what is meant by 'funeral' or 'picnic', and how to behave appropriately in these different settings. Meaning is added through experience; grandad's funeral or a birthday party picnic modify the individual's view of each type of event.

We also designate areas of our used environment with functional titles and design these to contain a set of tools and artifacts to support this designated use. We have bedrooms, bathrooms and living rooms. We have shops, cinemas, theatres, churches, mosques and temples. We have farms and factories.

These titles tell us what the environment is *for*, what we are supposed to *do* in it, and how to *interact* with and respond to others in that area. We define purpose and process, roles and relationships in a single nominal cue-word.

Other situations, however, are more ambiguous and open to a wide range of personal interpretations. These in turn depend on previous experience. Two individuals meeting within such a situation have to undertake a rapid summary of what is going on and reach a mutual, but undiscussed, acceptance of how to deal with it. It is a tribute to the rapidity of our ability to process such information that we usually come to a very rapid and similar agreement about 'what is going on'.

If we get it wrong we are mutually embarrassed. If the cues are really ambiguous, we fall back on very safe, acceptable, social responses which can 'keep us out of trouble' until we have 'sussed' what is happening and how to respond. This mutual 'mind reading' is a useful social response, but in closer relationships it can lead the individuals to act on a set of incorrect assumptions.

The therapist does need to consider how well the environment is providing information about roles, rules and meanings, and whether changes in the environment will promote more accurate cue acquisition.

THE 'WORLD IN THE MIND'

Understanding the ways in which we perceive and process information about our surroundings leads to appreciation of the ways in which we shape the 'inner landscape' of the mind.

It is important to recognize that for each one of us 'the environment' exists as a construct within our own brain. Even though we live on the same planet, come in contact with the same tangible objects, and find that elements of our experience coincide, your view of the world will differ from mine.

I have proposed (Hagedorn 1995a) a model of the environment which shows that we construct an inner environment, a personal world mirroring the levels of environmental reality (resource area, exploratory area, closed area) in 'inner space' (Fig. 6.3).

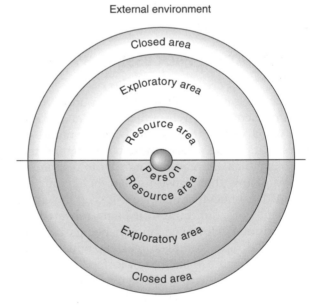

Figure 6.3 Environmental levels: internal and external environments.

This inner environment can never be entered or fully understood by any other person (or, arguably, even by the self who inhabits it). This inner world may also contain landscapes of the imagination, places which never existed and never could. We can create visions of heaven, or hell, or another world. Sometimes these mental images become very real, even to the extent of blurring the boundaries between reality and imagination.

Perhaps we need this mental, 'world-building' capacity as a means of creating and testing out images of future changes to the real world. To build a house, one must first imagine how it will look.

If one can imagine a house which has not yet been built, but could be, one can also imagine a magic castle on a cloud mountain. If one can imagine a house built of stone, one may also imagine a house built of glass. A thousand years ago, one would not have been able to build this; a hundred years ago, it became possible to work out how it could be constructed. Today, we may imagine what it would be like to live on another planet; in a hundred years time, we may do so.

A person builds a mental image of the world at any one moment which starts with the concept of the self as conscious of its own being in a specific location, at a particular point in time: 'I am here; it is now.'

The task of the moment is performed within a defined space close to the performer, which is the focus of the performer's attention. At the same time, there is peripheral awareness of the near environment, which is within sight or touch. There is also awareness of the 'world outside'.

As I write this paragraph, my attention is focused on my word processor screen and keyboard. I am aware at the edges of my vision that there are books and papers and box files on shelves and on the floor.

I can glimpse the blue walls and the rug on the floor. I know this is my study, upstairs in my house. This is a room where I expect to work. I know that if I turn my head I can see the door and a picture on the wall. If I look out of the window, I see the trees in the front garden and get a distant view of fields across the neighbouring rooftops. If I stop to think about it, I know I am in Arundel, West Sussex, England, United Kingdom, Planet Earth, The Universe.

The last two locations may rarely be considered but they are quite important to me in surviving as an organism. I need the oxygen in the atmosphere and the light of the sun. But the content of the universe is not helping me directly with my task, nor is my awareness of the world.

If I drift into an imagined replay of my last visit to Venice, or my plans for my next holiday, or consider my anxieties about the loss of the rainforest and the problem of global warming, or think about a forthcoming visit from a friend who lives at a distance, that is not helping me to write a book. I must dismiss these parts of my internal landscape for the time being.

The fact that I am in England is important to me as a social and cultural being; it affects what I write. It means that I am writing in English and not in French. It is important for me to know that my publisher has an office in Edinburgh; without this resource, my book would not be printed or distributed. There are professional colleagues or friends scattered across England and Scotland to whom I can turn for advice.

Arundel, and some nearby places in West Sussex, contain the resources for my daily life: the shops I use; the garage where I get my car repaired, my doctor, my dentist, the local hospital, my place of work, my friends, the places I go to relax. These places are coloured by the meanings they have for me.

My house and my garden have special meaning because they belong to me. They are places where I can feel safe. I have the things around me which I need and things which I do not need, but which please me. I possess things which have memories hooked onto them which give them added significance. I do not have to be in the same room as these things to know they are there.

I can explore this whole landscape of familiar existence 'inside my head'. I can try to describe part of it to you, but ultimately it is a private world which you can never enter.

If, as a therapist, I want to help clients to make more sense of their personal world, or in some way change their perceptions of it or the meanings they attribute to it, I can only do so indirectly.

THE 'OCCUPATIONAL INTERFACE'

This model of the external and internal environments reminds us of the intensely subjective nature of our experiences and perceptions, but it also illuminates something of even more fundamental importance to the therapist.

The individual needs to connect a personal inner world with external reality. The world 'inside the head' is the place where wants, desires, dreams, physical and psychological needs originate. 'Out there' is the world of action and interaction where the individual can do things which change both the world and the individual's perceptions of it.

The things we do – our occupations – form the bridge between the inner and outer worlds. We act, and by acting we set up the dynamic interplay of reaction and interaction by which we create ourselves as occupational beings.

The therapist cannot enter or directly change the 'inner environment' but, by altering the nature of occupational performance, and the effect which performance has on the environment, the performer may be enabled to find new meanings and gain new personal understanding. By adding to the stock of the inner resource area (knowledge, skills, positive attitudes), the individual can become more competent in achieving goals. By managing external reality more competently, the individual may find it easier to understand and manage the inner world.

ENVIRONMENTAL ANALYSIS

Many complex interactions take place between systems at each level. The therapist can study these interactions and systems as a means of enriching understanding of person–environment interactions. In daily practice, however, the therapist is primarily concerned with the analysis of the resource area, of environments familiar to and used by an individual. The skills needed to undertake this kind of environmental analysis are described in Section 5. A summary is shown in Table 6.1.

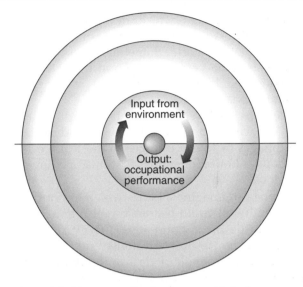

Figure 6.4 The occupation/environment interface.

Just as any system of occupational analysis is an artificial construct imposed as an aid to description, so any system of analysis of environment is simply a convenient set of labels.

Forms of environmental analysis include:

Content analysis	Objective observation and recording of who and what is there: geographical features, organisms, objects and artifacts. It may include an evaluation of resources, risks barriers/ access, proximity, position and quantity or nature of information provided.
Demand analysis	Appraisal of the effects of the content on people and their perceptions and behaviours. This may include social and cultural influences, roles, rules and situational meanings.
Adaptive analysis	Identification of elements which need to be altered and the means by which this may be done.

These forms of analysis can be related to Bronfenbrenner's *microanalysis* category. They are used to analyse the immediate environment and the used environment.

Mesoanalysis could be used to describe the exploratory area in so far as this impacts on a particulalr individual.

Table 6.1 Summary of environmental analysis

Environmental level resource area	Type of analysis	Level of occupation
Immediate environment	Microanalysis	Actions Interactions Reactions Performance units Task stages Tasks
Near environment	Content analysis Demand analysis Applied analysis	Tasks Activities Routines
Used environment	Mesoanalysis	Activities Routines Occupations Roles
Exploratory area	Macroanalysis	

Macroanalysis, exploring the wider implications of the known environment on human behaviour – political, economic, sociocultural, geophysical – is undertaken by researchers from a number of disciplines and is beyond the scope of this book.

The closed area is incapable of analysis because it is unknown.

Competence

Competent, adaptive performance is essential to human health and well-being.

Since promoting competent performance is a central aim of occupational therapy, it is clearly necessary to understand what is meant by competence and some of the issues and debates which surround it.

In this chapter, four related aspects of importance to the therapist will be considered:

- the nature of competence
- competent adaptive performance as the aim of therapy
- professional competence
- problems in measuring competence.

WHAT IS COMPETENCE?

A starting point is a simple explanation. The state of 'being competent' is defined as being 'adequately qualified to perform a task' (Concise Oxford Dictionary).

This appears straightforward, but unfortunately competence is yet another term with debatable meanings. Competence is a word much used in education, but teachers appear to have the same problem defining it as therapists do with occupation, and for much the same reasons.

Ashworth & Saxton (1990):

consider the meaning of competence as an aspect of the *description of human activity* has not yet been coherently specified. In particular, it is not clear whether a competence is a personal attribute, an act, or an outcome of action; moreover the idea of competence as currently used is open to complaints that it is atomistic (reductionist), individualistic, and unable to cover all types of relevant behaviour or mental activity.

These authors provocatively describe how the concept of competence, as well as being confused, ill-defined, and hard to assess, can place constraints and limitations on teaching.

Their analysis provides a useful warning to avoid overly reductionist interpretations of competence. Competence is complex, many layered and situational. They go on to cite the definitions produced by the Training Agency (1988) in their guidance on National Vocational Qualifications.

Competence is a wide concept which embodies the ability to transfer skills and knowledge to new situations within the occupational area. It encompasses organization and planning of work, innovation and coping with non-routine activities. It includes those qualities of personal effectiveness that are required in the workplace to deal with co-workers, managers and customers.

This places competence within the organizational and effective levels and draws attention to the need for adaptive responses.

The Training Agency then goes on to specifiy how competence can be divided into elements or competencies. A competency is:

an element of competence which describes what can be done; an action, behavioural outcome which a person should be able to demonstrate. Or an element of competence may describe such things as the knowledge or understanding which is essential if performance is to be sustained, or extended to new situations within the occupation. Each element of competence has associated performance criteria which define the expected level of performance.

This seems to bring the idea of competence to lower levels of performance, perhaps the acquisitional and constructive levels, where particular tasks or performance components can be specified and evaluated. It also illustrates how competence can be a matter both of 'knowing how' and also 'knowing about'.

Part of the problem of defining and measuring competence stems from the fact that the nature of competence changes from one occupational level to another. At the constructive level, for example, it is relatively easy to specify

what is to be done and to judge how well it has been achieved. The components of performance are mainly overt and observable. At the organizational level, however, competence involves much more cognitive processing that is not only hidden from an observer, but intrinsically far harder to evaluate.

Barnett (1994) provides a comprehensive discussion of the limits of competence and the problems of defining what it is. He contrasts two concepts of competence, 'an internal or *academic* form, built around a sense of the student's mastery within a discipline; the other is an *operational* conception of competence, essentially reproducing wider societal interest in performance.'

Academic competence deals with 'knowing that', where theories and concepts are aimed at developing a discipline and achieving better cognitive understanding. Operational competence is to do with 'knowing how'. It is defined pragmatically and situationally. It is connected with issues of economics and organization, measured by outcomes indicating better practical effectiveness.

Barnett concludes that both of these accepted forms of competence, while valid within higher education, are inadequate. He proposes that education needs to extend beyond notions of competence into an area which he designates as *'life-world becoming'*. This is based on *reflective knowing*, and a critical, dialectic, ethical approach to achieving the common good, and attaining better practical understanding.

Occupational therapists are as much educationalists as they are therapists, and familiarity with the literature on competence is an essential part of an informed understanding of the ways in which occupational therapy seeks to enable and enhance competent occupational performance.

COMPETENT ADAPTIVE PERFORMANCE AS AN AIM IN OCCUPATIONAL THERAPY

The aim of occupational therapy can be summarized as:

To enable the individual to achieve competent adaptive performance in whatever occupations, activities or tasks are important, meaningful or necessary to him or her, in the environment he/she uses, in a manner that the individual considers satisfactory, meeting any essential performance standards within accepted cultural boundaries.

Hagedorn 1995a, rev 1998

The educational use of the term has spilled over into areas of practice concerned with teaching and learning. Thus, in the context of learning disabilities, Fleming et al (1997), state:

The occupational therapist assists the individual by teaching specific competencies, leading to an overall level of competence which is effective and has relevance to his or her specific environment.

Kielhofner (1995) expands on his previous work, defining a continuum of levels of occupational function, stretching from exploration (a phase of learning and development) to competence (consistent adequate performance) and achievement (high level or expert performance). He states that:

Persons operate at a competence level of function when they strive to be adequate to the demand of a situation by improving themselves or adjusting to environmental demands and expectations. Individuals at a competence level of functioning focus on attaining, improving and organizing skills into habits that allow consistent, adequate performance.

Matheson & Bohr (Christiansen & Baum 1997) define competence as 'the ability to interact effectively with the environment while maintaining individuality and growth.' They describe a model of occupational competence which fits with the PEOP paradigm. This model:

describes how individuals adapt to changing capacities and assimilate new roles across the lifespan and how that development influences behaviour… it emphasises the ecological nature of occupational performance which inextricably links the person and the environment, specifically through the role challenges that the environment provides.

These authors view occupational competence as based on five related concepts: capacity, effectance, affordance, competence and self-efficacy. These are quite complex concepts and the reader is advised to return to the original texts to gain a full understanding of them. Competence

has already been defined. Only the basic definitions of the other four terms are provided here.

Capacity	'the immediate potential of the individual to perform tasks.'
Effectance	'the sub set of the individual's abilities pertinent to the task challenges posed by role demands.'
Affordance	'anything which the environment can offer the individual which is pertinent to the role challenge and can facilitate role competence.'
Self-efficacy	'the feelings people have about their ability to be successful in using a particular coping strategy or problem-solving approach.'

Matheson & Bohr take a developmental view of occupational competence throughout the lifespan, which they analyse as variations in the interactions between the person, the person's roles and the environment. They conclude that:

occupational competence is role directed. It develops because humans, as social beings, feel the need to look for and accept challenges that are part of their social roles.

Despite some differences in terminology, these different authors do seem to agree on the general importance of competence and its characteristics.

Competent performance is:
- Linked to social or occupational role
- Adequate, consistent and effective
- Adaptively meets environmental or task demand
- Meets specified standards or criteria.

It includes:
- Organization and process skills
- Skilled task performance
- Ability to transfer skills to new situations
- Specified knowledge and understanding.

It is important to understand that competence is not perfection, simply consistent and adequate performance which 'gets the job done'. It meets the demands of roles, occupations or tasks and the demands of the environment in an adaptive manner. It utilizes personal response in an optimum way.

COMPETENCE AND INDEPENDENCE

In occupational therapy, independence is generally understood to mean 'functional independence' – the ability to perform a selected task without help, prompting or supervision.

Christiansen & Baum (1997) note that 'Rogers (1982) declared that functional independence is not only the core concept of occupational therapy but also the goal of the occupational therapy process.' It is true that much of the therapist's time is devoted to promoting functional independence, as defined in the previous paragraph.

The relationship between competence and independence is not direct. One cannot say for certain that an incompetent person is also dependent although when lack of competence extends across a large proportion of the individual's performances, independence is bound to be compromised. Equally one cannot be sure that an independent person is fully competent.

Independence (like freedom) is as much a matter of attitude of mind as it is of behaviour. The dictionary defines being independent as 'not depending on authority or control'. If a person has severe physical restrictions, yet maintains a sense of self-efficacy and autonomy despite the need to rely on others, that person may feel independent.

It is also possible to imagine a situation in which a person is living independently (in the sense of wanting no help) but performing many tasks 'incompetently', at a level which is not adequate or consistent.

The person may deliberately have chosen to accept lower standards of performance in some areas because the person values independence (in the sense of being autonomous) more highly than competent task performance, or because the person wishes to reserve available energies for tasks which the person values more highly.

We are social animals and in that sense none of us is totally independent; 'interdependence' might be a better description. Much of what we do depends on our ability to co-operate with, and use the resources of, others. Furthermore, the meaning of independence is affected by culture, gender and status. This entangles the link between independence and competence. It becomes easier to see how the two concepts are related if we examine what happens at each occupational level. Consider the following example.

A man is involved in a serious accident and becomes tetraplegic. Minimal facial movement and a flicker in one finger are all that is possible; breathing requires assistance. Cognition and perception are, however, intact. This man is able to harness several sources of assistance. All necessary personal care is provided. The home environment is adapted so that he has some control over it through automated equipment.

The man retains a loving relationship with his wife and children and keeps in touch with a network of friends. A previous interest in information technology enables him to develop a new business. Despite being confined to a special bed or wheelchair, he manages to run a successful company.

Does this man perform competently and independently? The answer varies depending on how one defines competence and independence, which level of occupation is being considered, and which skills are assessed.

At the developmental level, physical task performance is neither competent nor independent. He is totally reliant on others. However, cognitive task performance is competent and independent; choices and decisions can be made. He is orientated and in control.

At the effective level, the picture is less easy to describe. Although delegating the actual performance of tasks and activities to others, productive performance does take place. He is able to procure what he needs. Things get done; items which are wanted are obtained, and business is conducted. Life has meaning beyond the immediate necessities of survival.

At the organizational level, looking at the whole pattern of his life, despite the enormous challenges he has faced, this man is undoubtedly both competent and independent. He has maintained a varied repertoire of occupational and social roles. Although disabled, one could not in any way describe him as dysfunctional: his reactions to his disability have been very positive and highly adaptive.

This example shows that, as discussed by Ashworth & Saxton (1990), to view competent performance simply in terms of independently 'doing or not doing' to a specified standard is too narrow.

COMPETENCE AND ADAPTATION

Many theorists, particularly those who belong to the 'person/environment/occupational behaviour' schools of model builders, stress the importance of adaptation.

Adaptation is used by occupational therapists in two senses: to convey the process whereby a therapist changes a task or an environment to enhance performance, and to describe changes which take place within an individual in response to challenging external circumstances and situations. It is the latter sense with which we are concerned here.

Schkade & Schultz (1997) (who have based their own model around this concept) state:

a close look at occupational therapy literature confirms that adaptation is a concept so fundamental to the field that it is recognised as a universally accepted treatment goal… and also as a measure of therapeutic effectiveness… however, the profession's understanding of adaptation is varied and perhaps elusive.

After a closely argued review of what adaptation means, its theoretical assumptions and importance, Schkade & Schultz list ten beliefs concerning adaptation and conclude by proposing that 'adaptation is of such significance that it functions as a paradigm within occupational therapy'.

One of the ten beliefs states that 'demand for adaptation appears when the fit is inadequate'. As long as the person is competently able to respond to performance demand, the need for adaptive response is low. Everything is working fine. However, when the demand from the task or the environment overloads the person's ability to respond, something must change to restore competent performance.

The change must first occur within the individual who must decide whether to change the task, the environment, or some aspect of the individual's own actions, interaction or reactions.

People who are highly adaptive cope competently with a wide range of circumstances; they seldom require the assistance of a therapist unless faced by exceptional challenges which have temporarily overwhelmed their ability to adapt.

Individuals who have low adaptive abilities find it very hard to cope with anything outside the routine. Personal change is difficult or threatening. Setting personal goals is an overwhelming task. Because individuals cannot adapt they are less likely to act, react or interact in a way which will resolve their problem situation or reduce the challenge they are facing.

Experienced therapists are well aware that the degree to which a person has previously acquired adaptive skills predicts the duration and success of intervention.

In the example of the tetraplegic businessman, we saw that it was difficult to assess his level of independence and competence. It was, however, very clear that he was highly adaptive.

Ashworth & Saxton (1990) offer an interesting example of a similar kind: suppose that good communication is specified as a desirable competency for a manager. Manager A has good personal communication skills and communicates directly. Manager B does not have such good personal skills, but recognizes this and delegates communication to another individual who has good skills. Both managers achieve the goal of good communication. Which is competent?

As the authors point out:

if competence only refers to an individual mental capacity or a personal skill, then only the first manager has communicative competence. If the focus in crediting a person with competence is the overall success of their performance, then both managers would be deemed competent.

An occupational therapist might prefer to describe manager B as adaptive; manager B has recognized that the situation demands a response manager B is unable to provide and has procured the required action from someone else.

This kind of problem frequently occurs during functional assessment; a simple assessment of whether or not the person *can* perform a task does not give the whole picture.

One recently developed instrumental activities of daily living (IADL) measures the Assessment of Living Skills And Resources (ALSAR: see p. 155) and has recognized this problem; it takes account of both the resources available to support performance and the ability of the client to *procure* services. For example, the client may be unable to cook, but arranges for meals to be brought in. The client is not a competent cook, but adaptively meets the need for regular meals.

The higher up the occupational and environmental levels one goes, the greater becomes the need for adaptive responses. When performing simple tasks in the immediate or near environment, the need for adaptive reponses is relatively low.

When fitting together whole patterns of interlocking activities and routines in the course of a day, and coping with unexpected events or problems, the need for adaptive responses becomes much greater.

At the organizational level, where imaging, reasoning, planning, prioritizing and problem - solving are needed, the individual must change to meet the challenges of the wider physical and social environment, with regard to the individual's whole repertoire of roles and occupations. Here effective use of high-level, adaptive responses is essential.

COMPETENT ADAPTIVE PERFORMANCE

It is apparent, therefore, that at higher occupational levels competent performance is intrinsically adaptive. It therefore seems redundant to use both words to describe the aim of occupational therapy. However, the traditional educational concept of competence as expressed by behavioural or learning objectives, is, as we have seen, reductive and restricted.

Competence of this basic kind, while essential developmentally, is insufficient to describe the nature of the adaptive performance required at higher occupational levels. The word adaptive is added in order to emphasize this more holistic view of competence.

This has to be interpreted each time with regard to specific individuals, their occupations and their environment and the situation in which performance takes place.

PROFESSIONAL COMPETENCE

The term 'competent' is often applied to professionals: the aim of occupational therapy education is to produce a therapist who is 'competent to practise'.

As soon as one specifies that someone should be competent, one is obliged to define competence and then to identify specific competencies and to find a way of assessing or measuring the degree to which competence has been achieved.

As we have already begun to recognize, this presents many problems. The more complex the task and the more it requires the use of specialized cognitive processes such as reasoning, decision-making or problem-solving, as well as observable skills, the harder it becomes to define and measure performance.

This is partly a problem of defining the level of performance; different levels require different types of description.

Professional competence is a particular kind of 'high level' competence.

The College of Occupational Therapists' Code of Ethics and Professional Conduct (1995) has a section on professional competence and standards.

Therapists must ensure personal competence to practise by being state-registered. They should only provide services, or use techniques, for which they are qualified by education or experience, which are based as far as possible on research or evidence. They must comply with any relevant standards, policies and procedures, seek appropriate supervision, and ensure through continuing personal development that they keep up to date.

This makes it plain that competence is essential, and describes some of the mechanisms by which it may be achieved – approved qualification; standards of education and practice; personal monitoring of level of skill and knowledge; a lifelong commitment to learning – but it does not state what competence consists of.

It is easy to recognize the extremes: we know when to describe a therapist as 'highly competent' (exhibiting consistent, high standards of practice and/or expertise). We also know when to rate a person as 'incompetent' (unable to perform adequately, or potentialy causing damage or risk).

In occupational therapy texts, the words competence and competency have been defined in relation to the practice of occupational therapy. For example:

Competency   'having the cognitive and psychological abilities to make the right decisions that are judged to be rational by other members of one's society. Can also include having the physical abilities to act on those decisions.'
(Hansen 1993)

'A single knowledge, skill or professional value.'
(Fleming et al 1997: 409)

Competence   'The repertoire of competencies'
(Fleming et al 1997: 409)

CORE COMPETENCIES AND CORE SKILLS: TERMINOLOGY

In an attempt to define the nature of occupational therapy practice and to set standards for professional education, the terms 'core competency' and 'core skill' have been widely used.

The concept of a 'core skill' or 'core competency' is found in both education and industry.

The idea of a 'core' or central skill is straightforward. Any trade or profession must have certain specified skills which either separately or in combination are unique to that trade or profession and essential to it in carrying out its business.

One definition from a business management textbook states that:

the core competencies of the organisation are the unique bundle of skills it possesses which permit it to offer a sustainable competitive advantage.
Doyle (1994)

The words *skill* and *competence* tend to be used as synonyms, but they are not truly interchangeable.

As just described, there has been considerable interest in educational circles in *competence-based training*. Generally, this means that students are taught to master a set of *skills* which combine to make them proficient in some situation or task.

The degree to which students are proficient is their level of *competence*. The shortcomings of this approach have already been noted, none the less there is no satisfactory alternative method of describing what a profession should know and do.

A simple way of separating competence from skill is to consider that a *competency* is a cluster of skills performed in a situation, whereas a *skill* is a piece of performance which may be used in many different settings and rearranged to perform different competencies. *Competence* is the degree to which performance meets set standards and requirements in a range of situations.

The occupational therapy literature has tended, (probably because therapists often think about their clients' performance in terms of skills) to speak mainly of the *core skills of the occupational therapist*. However, occupational therapy educationists commonly use the term *competency* because this better describes the integrated level of performance.

I prefer to see the descriptive terms as a hierarchy:

Core process	A set of related practices and procedures structured to contribute to a distinct set of purposes or products within an area of occupational therapy practice.
Core competency	A set of related skilled performances, knowledge, and values which produce a defined result to a specified standard in a particular context or setting, or several settings.
Core skill	A piece of performance completed to a specified standard. A skill involves the ability to integrate, organize and sequence skill components within the domains of action, interaction and reaction to achieve smooth and effective performance of a task with few or no errors. Core skills can be adaptively combined and used in different settings.

Therefore, assessment is a *process*; one of the *competencies* needed for assessment is interviewing; the *skills* required to conduct an interview include asking relevant questions, recording information and putting the person at ease. These skills are not, however, restricted to use in the competency of 'interviewing'.

This makes it clear that occupational therapy has a number of processes, numerous competencies and very many skills. The skills can be assembled flexibly as required to form a competency. A particular skill will be used in connection with many competencies, but the skills required for a particular competency remain as a related cluster.

Therefore, a therapist will use the skill of recording information in many different contexts while performing different competencies. However, if recording information was left out of the competency of 'interviewing', or if performance of that skill was poor, the interview is unlikely to be conducted to the required standard.

Within this text, the word 'competency' will be used as a generic term in preference to 'skill' which will be restricted to the narrower sense defined above.

Other words used in occupational therapy include technique, and modality and definitions of these terms can be found in the glossary.

MEASURING COMPETENCE

As described in the above section, the need to measure or assess performance is implicit in the concept of competence. There are a number of inter-related issues in discussing assessment of competence, and these are fundamentally the same, whether one is assessing a patient or a student therapist.

First, what is to be measured, process or product, or both? Second, how does one set standards or criteria against which these items are to be assessed? Third, is it possible to measure these items reliably, consistently and in a valid manner?

PROCESS OR PRODUCT?

Competence relates both to process – *how* things are done (how efficiently, how fast, best method or sequence etc.) – and to product – the *result or effect* of what is done.

One therefore needs to specify both how the task is to be done and the expected result or standard; one may choose to assess either, or both. The specification has to be done with clarity and precision.

WHO SETS THE STANDARDS?

Standards may be set by the assessor, the participant, or with reference to generally accepted norms of performance.

Standards set by an assessor

In education, or in the workplace, assessment of competence is still mainly undertaken by an assessor who must strive to be objective and impartial.

The assessor measures both process and product against some pre-determined criteria or standard. Has the task been completed? Is the product satisfactory? Could the standard of performance be improved? Were risks taken? How many errors were made?

The assessor needs to select the right level of performance for the situation, and then find a means of checking performance against that level. This does not necessarily mean that performance is errorless. Occasional minor errors may occur, but these are recognized and corrected.

In the same way, the criteria by which the product is judged must be clearly set out so that the result can be objectively measured.

This need to set clear criteria has led to the use of statements of competence as used in National Vocational Qualifications.

A statement of competence should incorporate assessment of:
skills to specified standards
relevant knowledge and understanding
the ability to use skills and to
apply knowledge and understanding to the performance of relevant tasks.

This kind of statement, cited by Ashworth & Saxton (1990), is often phrased as a behavioural objective; for example 'the student will demonstrate, using an anatomical model, the muscles used to extend the elbow.'

The Training Agency (1988) also introduces the idea of setting standards as an aid to assessing competence:

Standards will form the prime focus of training and the basis of vocational qualifications. Standards development should be based on the notion of competence which is defined as the ability to perform the activities within an occupation.

While it is possible (but not easy) to specify competence in this way at the acquistional and constructive levels where performance can be observed, the higher up the occupational levels one progresses, the more difficult it becomes.

It is also very difficult to apply external assessment to the internal, unobservable aspects of process. The product may be completed, but the quality of processes such as problem-solving, creating, information-processing can only be inferred; even the participant may find it hard to articulate all the stages of the process as they actually happened.

Standards set by the participant

In student-centred models of learning, or in client-centred therapy, it may be the participant who sets the standards. The participant has a subjective viewpoint. Personal standards and attitudes towards competent performance are highly variable. This means that the degree to which process or product, or both, are valued also varies.

The product of the task may be rated as important and the participant may only be satisfied with 'perfection'. On the other hand, the task may be part of a hobby in which the experience of participating is more important than the end product; being a 'bad artist' can be as satisfying as being a 'good one'.

The author recalls hearing a famous pianist give a radio interview in which she said that to perform 'badly' in public was agony, but to perform in a less than perfect manner when she

played for her own pleasure at home did not disturb her; she only wanted to be totally immersed in the joyful process of music making.

Self-perceptions concerning performance are, by their nature, subjective and biased. People with low self-esteem and low self-efficacy ratings typically undervalue their performance and may rate it as incompetent even when it is not. Over-achievers may set themselves unrealistically high standards and are dissatisfied with anything less. Faulty feedback can be as disabling as an actual functional limitation.

It is clear that previous experiences are of fundamental importance in influencing perceptions of performance as competent.

The therapist has to take account of the person's own view of what is competent, but may need to help the person to modify that view if it seems inappropriate.

One might assume that the participant would at least be in a good position to evaluate the intellectual components of performance, but this is not simple. Since one has no access to others' patterns of thinking, one has no criteria against which to compare one's own.

In addition, as one becomes more expert, the brain 'smooths out' the links in the reasoning chain until, in some cases, the conscious basis for action has disappeared. This type of tacit knowledge, which is expressed in doing, is very hard to access without prolonged reflection and analysis.

Standards set by society

Society provides the cultural context for performance. There are cultural 'norms' and standards which influence both therapist and participant. Such norms can vary widely between subcultures. Occasionally, the assumptions which society makes about competence need to be challenged, but they cannot be ignored.

THE SITUATIONAL CONTEXT

Ashworth & Saxton (1990) point out that one of the drawbacks to the traditional model of competence is that it is based entirely on the performance of the individual. It is difficult to take account of elements in the environment, or contributions from other people which may adversely (or beneficially) affect performance.

For example, a performer may cope well in a simulated environment if nothing unexpected happens, but badly in a realistic environment where there are distractions, interference from other people, or pressures to complete to an imposed timescale.

Competence should be transferable from one situation to another, yet inevitably the assessment of a competency takes place on one occasion in one context. The degree to which competence is transferable or generalizable can be hard to assess.

RELIABILITY OF ASSESSMENT METHODS

From the above discussion, it should now be clear that the assessment of competence is fraught with difficulties.

It is probable that a totally accurate and reliable method of assessment has yet to be developed. All forms of assessment are partial, limited and subject to a degree of error. The very act of having one's performance observed changes the nature of the performance and the meaning of the situation.

The problems of assessment and available methods will be discussed in more detail in Section 3.

8

Core processes in occupational therapy

VIEWS OF THE CORE SKILLS AND COMPETENCIES USED IN OCCUPATIONAL THERAPY

The debate over core competencies – what are
they and are they different from those of related
professions? – has occupied occupational therapy theorists for a long time.

The first extensive presentation of occupational therapy core concerns and competencies
was produced by Mosey (1986) in her comprehensive description of the psychosocial
components of occupational therapy. Based on
her previous work, she lists the 'domains of
concern' of the profession as: performance
components; occupational performances; the life
cycle; environment. Mosey then describes the
'legitimate tools' of occupational therapy as
follows:

'The permissible means by which the practitioners of
a profession fulfil their responsibilities to society.
Although legitimate tools may change… at any given
time members of the profession are expected to
use only those tools that are currently defined as
legitimate for the profession. The legitimate tools
for occupational therapy are the non-human
environment; conscious use of self; the teaching–
learning process; purposeful activities, activity
groups and activity analysis and synthesis.'

The American Association of Occupational
Therapists has done much work on the definition of occupational therapy processes and
service competencies. An Appendix to *Willard &
Spackman* (Hopkins & Smith 1993), the standard
text, defines the processes of service provision

and lists the competencies expected of an entry level practitioner.

An entry-level competency is defined as 'minimal competence acceptable upon completion of a technical or professional education program'. These are classified under the headings: assessment; program planning; intervention; documentation; service management; research; professional competence; promotion of the profession; ethics.

In the 9th edition (Neistadt & Crepeau 1998), this subdivision was altered to a list of entry level skills, intermediate skills and high proficiency skills. At entry level, the focus of role performance is summarized as: 'the development of skills; socialization in the expectations related to organization, peers and the profession; acceptance of responsibility and accountablitiy in role relevant activities.'

In 1994, the College of Occupational Therapists published a position statement on 'core skills and a conceptual framework for practice'. The anonymous authors defined core skills as 'the expert knowledge at the heart of the professional'. The unique core skills of occupational therapy are listed as:

Use of purposeful activity and meaningful occupation as therapeutic tools in the promotion of health and wellbeing.

Ability to enable people to explore, achieve and maintain balance in their daily living tasks and roles of personal and domestic care, leisure and productivity.

Ability to assess the effect of, and then to manipulate, physical and psychosocial environments to maximize function and social integration.

Ability to analyse, select and apply occupations to use as specific therapeutic media to treat people who are experiencing dysfunction in daily living tasks, interactions and occupational roles.

(A number of subsidiary skills are also listed.)

It seems that, just as ideas concerning the core concerns of occupational therapy are beginning to cohere, so a similar process of consensus building is happening in relation to core skills in the areas of personal relationships, assessment, occupation and environment.

In Chapter 2, I described the POET 'triangle': the interactions of the person, and the person's occupations within the environment, which, with the introduction of the occupational therapist into the situation, provide the components of occupational therapy.

The COPE diagram attempts to convey the nature of the 'balancing act' which is at the heart of occupational therapy in which the demands of the tasks and the environment and the ability of the person to respond are harmonized to enable competent performance.

This requires the therapist to use four core processes (Box 8.1).

Box 8.1   Core processes of occupational therapy

- Therapeutic use of self
- Assessment of individual potential, ability and needs
- Analysis and adaptation of occupation
- Analysis and adaptation of environment.

The art of practice is the appropriate selection and synthesis of elements of these processes for each individual. In combination, these processes define the unique contribution of occupational therapy within health care.

In addition, there are generic processes. These are used by many health care professionals. I have described these (Hagedorn 1995a) as 'meta-processes' because they are used to organize and integrate the core processes. These processes are: case management; implementation of therapy or intervention; service management. To these may be added 'the three Rs' of occupational therapy (Hagedorn 1995b) – reasoning, reflection and research.

These processes and their associated competencies and skills are described in many occupational therapy texts and in management textbooks, and they will not be considered in this book.

There is a further set of generic competencies and skills which would be used by anyone who deals with people, whether they work in health care or a service industry. These include:

- ensuring the comfort of the client
- being welcoming and polite according to cultural norms
- showing respect to the client

- listening to what the client wants
- providing reassurance and explanation
- ensuring that the client understands the nature of the service to be provided and the expected results
- providing information and promoting choice.

In addition, there is a set of competencies which are needed by anyone who works with people who are frail, elderly or unwell. These include:

- assisting with personal care
- providing for basic needs
- ensuring safety
- assisting the patient to move
- monitoring signs of stress or discomfort
- ensuring autonomy and personal dignity.

These skills are generally acquired by student occupational therapists during fieldwork placement and it is important that the student should be provided with opportunities for practice and feedback on performance.

INTRODUCTION TO THE CORE PROCESSES DESCRIBED IN THIS BOOK

The next four sections of this book are aimed at providing detailed guidance on the essential core processes of the occupational therapist.

THERAPEUTIC USE OF SELF

A key factor in any therapeutic intervention is the therapist's ability to communicate with the client and to develop an appropriate therapeutic relationship or 'therapeutic alliance'.

Mosey (1986) described 'conscious use of self' as one of the legitimate tools of practice. She defined this as:

the use of oneself in such a way that one becomes an effective tool in the evaluation and intervention process. Conscious use of self includes but is greater than rapport and the art of practice... (it) involves a planned interaction with another person in order to alleviate fear or anxiety, provide reassurance, obtain necessary information, provide information,

give advice, and assist the other individual to gain more appreciation of, more expression of, and more functional use of his or her latent resources.

The term 'therapeutic use of self' is preferred only because 'conscious use' implies that therapists are continually aware of what they are doing. While this may at times be the case, when interactive reasoning is consciously directing the quality and content of the dialogue with the client, there are also many times when interactions appear, and feel, spontaneous.

This does not mean that therapeutic processing is absent from the mind of the therapist, simply that this is submerged in the flow of events, although it may be recovered later.

There are many levels and styles of relationship, from the traditional and relatively formal professional approach to more complex and prolonged client-centred models of interaction.

In order to use the self in the context of therapy, therapists must possess emotional maturity and good insight into their own needs and styles of relationship. They must learn – like an actor or a politician – to exploit personal characteristics which are of benefit in a therapeutic relationship. They must also be able to cope with the personal stresses and reactions which may be the consequences of some relationships and situations.

This is an art which is probably 'caught' rather than 'taught'. It depends to a large extent on the intelligence, personality, attitudes and communication style of the therapist. One can improve one's style of communication by learning the necessary skills, but one cannot change one's intelligence or personality. Empathy and the ability respectfully and uninvasively to care about another person are special attributes which cannot easily be taught.

Therapeutic use of self is sometimes said to involve making intuitive judgements about people and situations. 'Intuition' is an over-used word. It is based on complex, very rapid cognitive processing, involving cue acquisition, interpretation and response, but it does convey the delicate nature of the judgements and interactions required in a therapeutic alliance.

Many of the interactive skills which form the basis of therapeutic use of self are learnt during childhood. By the time a person decides to train, patterns of cognitive processing are well-fixed, and it may prove very difficult to unlearn patterns of interpretation and response.

Therapists need to recognize their own needs, and yet must be able to submerge them in order to create appropriate boundaries to the intervention. They must be aware of all the psychological 'traps' such as over-identification, transference or projection which can interfere with a prolonged therapeutic relationship.

ASSESSMENT OF INDIVIDUAL POTENTIAL, ABILITY AND NEEDS

The foundation for therapeutic intervention is a clear and accurate evaluation of the potential and abilities of the individual in relation to the individual's needs and goals. This is essential for the provision of relevant interventions which can be justified and seen to be effective.

Assessment may be conducted by the therapist, or by the client, or as a partnership between them. There is a bewildering array of tests, checklists and other assessment tools, and the therapist must understand the basic theory of assessment, and know how to discriminate between tools on the basis of validity and reliability.

Assessment is influenced by the use of objective or subjective approaches.

In an objective approach, assessment may require detailed observation, measurement and repeated testing. The functional effects of impairment may need to be identified in relation to the multitude of daily activities in which an individual engages.

With a subjective approach, assessment may be a more holistic, descriptive process. The therapist needs to see the individual as a person with thoughts and feelings, motivations, interests and aptitudes. That person has a history which makes the person unique. The person is capable of choice concerning the person's own future. The person needs to be appreciated in the context of the person's own culture and environment, doing the things the person wants and needs to do. The person is a partner in the process of assessment.

The occupational therapist is concerned with the whole spectrum of human skills, through all ages. Add to this the complexity of occupational behaviour at all levels, and the tangled psychological and social interactions of a human being and the potential range of assessments and investigations is very large.

Assessment may sometimes be an end in itself, for example when a report providing a 'snapshot in time' is required by someone who needs to understand the situation of the client 'right now'. More usually, it is needed as part of the occupational therapy process, to guide and measure intervention.

Assessment also has some predictive value, but this must be treated with caution unless using an instrument which has been shown by research to have reliable predictive value.

Possibilities and probabilities need careful evaluation which requires experience and high-level, clinical reasoning. It is seldom safe to say with complete certainty 'I know what will happen in this case', but it may be acceptable to say 'These are things which may happen'.

ANALYSIS AND ADAPTATION OF OCCUPATION

The unique feature of occupational therapy is the use of normal tasks and activities as media for therapy. A fundamental assumption of occupational therapy is that engagement in occupations promotes health and well-being, provides opportunity for personal development and skill acquisition and assists recovery from illness or trauma.

Occupational analysis takes place at each of the three levels of occupation.

At the developmental level, analysis breaks down the task into the smallest units of which performance is composed. The individual skill components can be identified, and the therapist can map how these build into competence.

Task demand is an important component in the person/occupation/environment transaction. To analyse demand, it is necessary to tease out the constituents of which demand is comprised in a specific situation.

To do this, the therapist must observe, record and analyse elements of performance. There are many approaches to this, from comprehensive analysis to all possible features and parameters of a task to highly focused analysis of the need for particular skills or movements.

At the effective level, the therapist becomes interested in integrated performance or work, leisure and self-care activities and a more broadly based, analytical approach is needed.

At the organizational level, the therapist seeks to understand the rich complexity or occupational behaviour across a person's life, and the interaction between occupational roles and social roles and relationships.

Adaptation of occupations may be required to achieve therapeutic aims or to facilitate performance so as to improve the match between the task and the ability of the participant. Adaptation may concern the sequence, timing or structure of the task, the tools and materials, or the standard of performance.

To apply a task or activity as therapy, a further set of analytical procedures is required matching the needs, abilities and interests of the individual to the performance demand of the selected therapeutic occupation, in order to achieve a specified goal. If any of the core competencies can be said to be unique to occupational therapy, it is this one.

ANALYSIS AND ADAPTATION OF ENVIRONMENT

Analysis of an environment takes account of the physical setting – the buildings, objects or natural features – but it also considers the less obvious features which contribute to environmental demand such as people, cultural expectations and rules of behaviour.

Therapists in a community setting may spend much of their time making specific adaptations to a disabled or elderly person's home to enhance well-being, remove barriers to performance and promote safety and facilitate daily living. Such adaptation extends from the provision of simple tools or items of equipment through to major alternations to buildings.

Therapists recognize that the environment has subtle effects on behaviour. Using environmental cues and settings, it may be possible to facilitate interaction, reduce stress or promote engagement. Even small changes in the positioning of chairs and tables within a room may impede or facilitate engagement in a task.

In rehabilitative settings, adaptations may need to be provided in the early stages and then progressively withdrawn as improvement in function occurs.

THE ART OF PRACTICE

In combination, these core processes, guided by clinical reasoning and practical experience, form the unique art of practice of occupational therapy.

Why is engagement in occupation therapeutic?

Performance of tasks and activities places a demand on the individual to learn, adapt and respond. The process of performance and the perceptions of the consequent product create changes in the individual in the domains of action, interaction and reaction. Because of this intrinsic linkage, the therapist can use tasks and activities as therapeutic media.

The belief that engagement in occupation is therapeutic is the historic core of professional practice, and yet it is paradoxically difficult to explain how or why engagement in occupation is effective and few texts attempt to do so.

Much of the explanation is implicit in the discussions of the nature of human occupation. It seems to be assumed that engagement in occupation produces beneficial change and that, as therapists who understand occupation, we should all know why. But as we have seen, our understanding of human occupation is still imperfect, and in consequence, our understanding of the dynamics of therapeutic occupation continues to evolve.

One of the problems is, of course, that the 'how and why' of occupational therapy is a very complex question with many different answers. The brief statement above can only provide an indication of some of the most significant mechanisms.

At its best, occupational therapy is individualized, a unique process for each patient. Also, it must be admitted that, while every therapist is convinced that occupational therapy *does* work, the objective evidence to support this is still insufficient.

This is partly because the quantitative, reductionist research paradigm is inapplicable in much of occupational therapy practice, and partly because therapists' time is taken up by treating patients, and research time is not allocated as an expected part of the job as it is in some other professions.

None of these problems should be used as an excuse to prevent us from stating the basic assumptions on which the therapeutic use of occupation is based.

EXPLANATIONS BY THEORISTS

Theorists who have attempted to answer the question 'how does it work?' tend to do so in terms of their preferred model of practice, or as part of a philosophical exploration of human occupation.

Many theorists (for example, Reilly, Mosey, Reed, Kielhofner, and Wilcock) have presented explanations of the fundamental importance of human occupation, descriptions of what participation in occupation achieves, or summaries of underlying assumptions.

There is a general agreement that participation in appropriate, selected activities and tasks:

- promotes learning (knowledge, attitudes and skills) and enables a person to perform competently
- provides or supports personal role and identity in the context of a particular culture or society
- involves skilled use of the hands through which a person can productively explore and use the environment to promote survival, health and well-being
- challenges and changes the internal organization of the organism in ways which promote adaptive responses
- provides a means of structuring and integrating the totality of a person's performances
- assists in the acquisition of a balanced repertoire of necessary or meaningful occupations
- diverts attention from unpleasant physical or psychological symptoms
- promotes recovery from illness and trauma.

These statements, however, tend to focus on *what* occupational therapy achieves, rather than explaining *how* it does this. An explanation of some of the mechanisms involved will now be attempted.

ENGAGEMENT IN OCCUPATION PROMOTES LEARNING

Much of what happens during occupational therapy can be explained by reference to theories about how people learn.

Behavioural theories explain the acquisition of behaviour in terms of externally generated rewards and sanctions.

Developmental theories describe the sequence in which humans acquire skills and a range of behaviours, practical, social and cultural. Most developmental theories explain how the intrinsic potential of the organism is challenged by interaction with the environment to produce behaviour. The degree to which environmental opportunity and intrinsic (genetically determined) ability dominate in this interaction is still the subject of debate.

Cognitive learning theories describe the ways in which the human brain learns to perceive, process, store and recall information. Situations trigger responses, scripts are developed and behaviours acquire meanings and symbolisms. Cycles of adaptive and maladaptive behaviours are set up on the basis of the ways in which we think and feel about our actions and their consequences. Positive experiences promote adaptive learning.

Social learning theories deal with the ways in which humans relate to others as individuals and especially in groups. Social customs and roles also have to be learnt.

Humanistic theories describe the importance of motivation and individual styles of learning, and the need to learn in one's own way at one's own pace, in an environment which facilitates learning.

All these theories give partial explanations which have to be combined to give a full understanding of how people learn. What they all agree upon is that *the natural way for people to learn is through 'doing things'*.

Lower organisms are pre-programmed. A worm does not need to learn 'how to be a worm'; it is born to be a worm and to do the things worms do. It may, through the nature of its reactions to the contents of its environment, become a worm with a better capacity for survival, but that is probably the extent of its ability to learn.

The higher up the chain of evolution one moves, the longer it takes for an infant to become a fully functioning adult. Young chimpanzees or elephant calves take years to develop all the skills they need to survive socially and physically.

How do they do this? It is plain that, while they are born with the capacity to do many things, they rely to a large extent on watching adults engaged in the tasks of being elephants or chimpanzees, and trying to copy them.

They also play, investigate, experiment and explore with other infants and adults. As they do so, they develop adult bodies and adult skills. In fact, the only way to become a competent chimpanzee or elephant is to spend a long time practising 'doing and being' a chimpanzee or elephant.

For humans, also, the long period of play, experiment and learning through experience is essential for the development of a repertoire of skills. Repeated performance of tasks develops and integrates skills and finally produces competent performance (Schwammle 1996).

This is no new concept. Cynkin & Robinson (1990) note that Aristotle wrote 'what we have to do, we learn through doing'.

Kielhofner (1995) states that:

We are not born carpenters, teachers, therapists, guitarists, fishers... but we may become them by behaving as such. Our forms follow our functions. By taking up new occupations we reconstitute ourselves.

So, we learn through doing. Learning produces long-lasting changes in our skills, our thoughts, and the way we understand and feel about the world. In a real sense we 'are what we do', and by doing, we become what we are.

Learning does not happen in unrelated episodes; it is a product of the totality of experience which the individual integrates and organizes. There are no short cuts.

Competence has to be gained by experience. Appreciation of the results of performance on the environment and the rewards or sanctions this provides for the performer shapes future performance. Success promotes success. Success fosters satisfaction. Failure may promote avoidance or frustration.

Learning depends on opportunity. To become a piano player, one must play the piano (and acquire specific skills by playing scales or sight-reading music). It is of no use simply to have the genetically determined aptitude to play the piano; one must also have the piano and a piano teacher. If no piano is available, one will not become a pianist. One must be born into a culture where piano-playing is an accepted skill. If one has never heard or seen a piano being played, piano-playing will have no meaning.

What the occupational therapist does is (literally or metaphorically) to 'provide the piano' – to provide the opportunity for positive learning in the form of tasks to perform, instruction, practice, information, analysis of problems, challenges to meet and meanings to interpret.

The therapist/teacher helps to 'engineer' positive outcomes and to provide feedback to ensure these are appreciated by the individual. Occupational therapists believe that all individuals (provided that they are conscious) have the capacity to learn.

ENGAGEMENT IN OCCUPATION PROVIDES A ROLE IDENTITY

In animal groups there are social roles, usually expressed by degrees of dominance or submission. It is much more debatable whether there are any occupational roles. Sometimes, it seems as if these do exist but this may be due to the human tendency to anthropomorphic interpretation of instinctive behaviour as indicating 'worker', 'playmate', 'nanny', 'watchman' or 'pathfinder'.

Human social roles bring with them the need to perform tasks appropriate to that role. We need to learn to do what children, parents, lovers, students or grandparents are expected to do in our culture.

For a human, an occupation also becomes a means of expressing identity. We tell others (and ourselves) who we are by giving ourselves occupational titles. We participate in jobs, hobbies, interests and sports. We become journalists, factory workers, model builders or footballers. When we retire, we continue to develop roles as volunteers, students or artists. If we lose our occupational roles, we may lose our sense of identity as well.

The therapists seeks to maintain and expand the repertoire of occupations in relation to the roles of an individual.

USE OF THE HANDS

The ability to use the hands to perform an amazingly adaptive and skilled range of activities is a defining characteristic of humans. Loss of hand function not only affects the ability to survive and thrive, it also affects wider perceptions of the self as a competent and effective performer in the world.

A number of occupational therapy theorists, including Reilly, Cynkin and Wilcock, have stressed the importance to the human being of the use of the hands in constructive and creative activity. These theorists have argued that the act of using the hands in a skilled manner is in itself therapeutic. This has a neurophysiological basis.

It takes time to acquire and integrate performance skills because these require the development of complex patterns of connections between nerve cells. The 'wiring' of the brain has to change to establish and connect skills.

The large amount of motor and sensory cortex occupied by control of the hand suggests that numerous interconnections must be developed between hand function and other areas of the brain. It is not clear whether these neural linkages change because of the totality of experience, or because of repetitive use of specific neural pathways and interconnections.

Perhaps this widely integrative network is part of the therapeutic mechanism? At this stage in our knowledge we can only speculate.

At this period in Western culture much of the skilled work of the hands has been taken over by machines. It has even been suggested that people will ultimately evolve into some kind of synthesis of human/machine in which physical capacity to act becomes irrelevant.

Others argue that technology is proceeding at a faster pace than our stage of evolution is capable of matching; perhaps we need to reserve space in our lives for skilled use of our hands as an anchor in this world of automated virtual reality.

Improving or restoring skilled use of the hands, or compensating for loss of hand function, is an important aspect of occupational therapy.

CHANGES IN THE HUMAN BRAIN THROUGH OCCUPATIONAL PERFORMANCE

Evidence is growing to support one of the fundamental assumptions of occupational therapy, that participation in particular occupations produces changes in the individual and the way in which the human brain operates.

The television documentary series 'Why men don't iron' (UK Channel 4 1998) demonstrated that recent studies of how the brain responds to different tasks show differences in cortical function between men and women. During dichotic listening tests, women, for example, used both hemispheres to process language whereas men used one.

Men, on the other hand, have better developed spatial perceptual discrimination. A persuasive argument (controversial from the prespective of those who believe such differences to be learned) was put forward to support the view that these fundamental differences are intrinsic, a matter of genes and hormones.

From the perspective of occupational therapy, however, the significant finding was that men who do jobs which are usually stereotyped as 'female' (such as nursing) develop female patterns of brain use when undertaking dichotic listening tests, whereas women who do 'male' jobs (such as engineering) show masculine patterns when doing spatial tests.

The obvious question is whether these are people who selected their jobs because they already have brains which function in the 'transsexual' manner for biochemical reasons, or whether participation in the occupation actually changes the way the brain operates. If the latter were proved to be true, it would have enormous implications for therapists.

ENGAGEMENT IN OCCUPATION PROMOTES SURVIVAL AND WELL-BEING

We each need to do things in order to be able to stay fit and healthy and to obtain the necessities of life.

We also do things because they 'make us feel good' about ourselves or the world around us. Humans are the only animals to make things or do things which have no use other than a symbolic or aesthetic one.

Loss of the ability to do what we want and need to do independently and effectively not only puts us at risk but also damages our perceptions of ourselves and adversely affects our roles and relationships. Occupational therapists seek to maximize the individual's functional abilities and to enhance independence in all areas of performance.

ENGAGEMENT IN OCCUPATION PROMOTES ADAPTATION

When a person performs a task within an environment, the person must meet a specific performance demand which is generated by a combination of the nature of the task, the situation and the environment. If problems are encountered, the individual is challenged to find ways of surmounting them; the individual must adapt in some way.

It is accepted that people need a certain level of stimulation before they are prompted to act. If stimulation is low, motivation tends to be low and either nothing is done, or what is done is not done well. On the other hand, if stimulation is too high, the individual feels stressed and performance may again be adversely affected.

Each person's perceptions of and reactions to stimulation from the task and the environment is intensely individual. One person's pleasant thrill may be another's terror. What seems mundane and boring to one may be experienced as a reassuring routine by someone else. The reactions of the body and mind to stress are now well-understood and are affected by many factors.

In order to perform at the optimum level, challenges must be just right. There must be fit between the person, the task and the environment. The nature of the task must motivate the person to respond. The environment must facilitate performance by providing the material necessities for it, the right prompts and cues to elicit it, the right amount of stress, and a situation in which the behaviour produces results which are experienced as satisfying.

When all these factors coincide, optimum performance results. This does not mean that the task is always perceived as easy. Adaptive responses are best provoked by situations which challenge the individual's ability to respond. The individual not only reacts to the situation but also acts within it and contributes to changing it.

The successful results of participation build confidence and self-image, engender positive feelings of being in control and make future successful participation more likely. Working at a level of optimum challenge and maximum engagement has been described by Csikzentmihali (1993) as *flow*.

The challenge for the therapist is to judge how best to provide a situation in which adaptive responses will be stimulated and practised.

OCCUPATIONS STRUCTURE AND INTEGRATE TOTAL PERFORMANCE

Occupations provide structure to human life by organizing the way in which the individual uses time and sequences tasks. Occupational performance makes the varied facets of personal experience cohere and relate to each other.

A BALANCED LIFE

Occupational therapists believe that well-being is promoted when an individual engages in a varied repertoire of occupations and activities, including work, leisure and self-care, and those with spiritual or transcendental aspects, interspersed with appropriate periods of rest and relaxation.

There is no 'ideal balance' or formula; the individual needs to work out what best suits personal needs. The therapist's role is to introduce the idea of balance and facilitate new experiences and ways of organizing time and energy.

A feature of dysfunction is that the repertoire of activities becomes impoverished and restricted. This impoverishment may take several forms.

At one extreme, there is the chronic 'couch potato' slumped in front of a television (or, these days, 'mouse potato' in front of a computer screen) who is inactive and uninvolved with wider aspects of daily life. At the other end of the spectrum is the over-achieving 'workaholic' whose single-minded engagement in work leaves no room at all for any other form of relationship, role or occupation.

More common is the individual who, because of illness, pain or disability, finds even simple tasks an effort. All the waking hours are devoted to the struggles to accomplish the 'musts and oughts', the chores of basic survival. Almost all endeavour is at the level of task performance. This pattern removes from life most of the things which occur at the effective level and 'make life worth living'; friendship, adventure, creativity, leisure and, most important, simple enjoyment.

Through therapeutic intervention it may be possible to adjust patterns of activity in order to reinstate some variety and improve the quality of living. The experience of varied activities and roles feeds back into the perceptions of the self as gaining some pleasure and satisfaction from life. This in turn improves motivation and coping strategies.

OCCUPATIONS PROVIDE MEANING WITHIN AN INDIVIDUAL LIFE

The concept of 'meaning' in relation to activities or occupations is much discussed, but what do we mean by 'meaning?' It is one of those words which we understand intuitively but have trouble defining.

Christiansen & Baum (1997) offered the following description:

Meanings reflect our overall interpretations of life events. Most of our intentions and actions are filled with meaning. This meaning comes from the nature of a situation and how we interpret its significance based on our current goals, values and past experiences. There are individual meanings and collective or shared meanings.

The most important features of meaning are that it is highly individual and also predominantly contextual. Meanings are conveyed by objects, by signs and symbols, and by events and actions.

I have proposed (Hagedorn 1995a) that simple tasks taken out of context have low meaning, while chained tasks and activities occurring within varied contexts and in relation to the continuing stream of individual human experience can be rich in meanings and symbols.

It is a problem for the therapist to retain meaning in therapeutic occupation. Therapy often takes place in simulated, protected environments in circumstances which are in some respects artificial.

The meanings of a task done 'as therapy' cannot be the same as the meanings of that task when performed in another setting. The most that can be achieved is the creation of a convincing replica of a 'normal' situation which draws on the meanings which the individual had previously generated when doing that task.

The meaning of an activity can be positive or negative. In therapy, one normally seeks to provide positive experience for an individual, because adaptive responses are more likely to occur during positive engagement.

However, because familiar activities can become connected with negative meanings from the past, this 'luggage' may burden the new performance of the activity. This may be used to provide opportunities for exploration of negative meanings and ways of dealing with them. Sometimes, however, the 'luggage' gets in the way.

There are benefits to be gained, therefore, from engaging the individual in unfamiliar activities because the individual then has a chance to develop new meanings, relatively uncontaminated by the preconceptions of previous experiences and expectations.

ENGAGEMENT IN OCCUPATION CAN REDUCE AWARENESS OF PHYSICAL OR PSYCHOLOGICAL SYMPTOMS

One of the mechanisms which may contribute to the therapeutic effects of engagement in occupation is that the capacity of the brain to pay focused attention to several things at once is limited.

If the brain is totally engaged in coping with a challenging flow of engagement, the scope for it consciously to register distractions such as unpleasant physical sensations, memories, emotions or thoughts unconnected with the task in hand is reduced. The passage of time is not monitored. Awareness resides in the processes and products of performance. This engrossed engagement or flow is experienced as pleasant and rewarding.

It is plain, however, that in order to 'lose oneself' in an occupation one must experience it as an integrated whole. As soon as the focus becomes 'this movement' or 'that perception', flow is lost. In order to monitor parts of performance, the brain must pay attention to physical movements or sensations thereby opening sensory channels which may bring awareness of discomfort or tension.

This leads to a paradox which has troubled therapists for several decades: in order to be specific as therapy, an activity must be structured to produce particular, relevant movements or responses. However, the further one travels down the route of highly specific adaptation, the more one risks losing the benefits of focused engagement in a task as a whole.

PRESCRIBED OCCUPATION PROMOTES RECOVERY FROM ILLNESS OR TRAUMA

Occupational therapists are concerned with occupations in two distinct, but overlapping ways.

The therapist can *intervene* to solve performance problems. In this approach, action is directed towards adapting factors *external to* the client, such as features of the environment or aspects of the task.

So, for example, when the individual cannot bend to reach the feet, the therapist may provide a suitable dressing aid, or may modify clothing or footwear or show the client how to change the position in which dressing takes place.

Alternatively, the therapist may *treat* the individual by means of *prescribed occupation*.

Therapists believe that it is possible to turn task performance into therapy by creating a situation in which a task must be performed in such a way that a desired response is achieved. The performer must move, react, reason and engage with others in a particular way.

In the above example, the therapist might aim to improve the range of movement and strength in the client's lower limbs, or to increase confidence in balancing and reaching, through performance of tasks which *demand* these components.

The assumption is that, as the performer participates in the prescribed task, the performer is enabled to develop skills, learn new information, recover lost function, adapt the mode of behaving, thinking or reacting, solve practical problems or experience something of value and relevance to the performer's situation.

If performance demand is to be used in this precisely structured manner, it is plainly necessary for the therapist to have control over at least some elements of the situation in which the task is to be performed. The demand must be, like Goldilock's chair, 'not too large, not too small, but just right'.

To recover physical function, therefore, one must do physical tasks which require movement, strength and exertion, at an appropriate level. To improve attention span, one needs a task which requires an amount of attention and concentration. To become more able socially, one needs to encounter others in a variety of social situations.

Applied occupational therapy is based on these principles. Tasks are adapted or *synthesised* to provide specific demand.

However, the therapist must also consider the individual's interests, experiences, values and motivations. The task must not only be therapeutic, it must also be acceptable and relevant to the client.

Creation of performance demand for therapeutic purposes is therefore a subtle art and not an exact science, which requires many factors to be kept in balance. When used well, it can produce real benefits.

The art depends on the proficient use of the central core skills of occupational analysis and adaptation and environmental analysis and adaptation, through which performance demand can be analysed and adapted.

LEVELS OF OCCUPATION AND THE BENEFITS OF OCCUPATIONAL THERAPY

Another way of untangling the intertwined assumptions about the benefits of engagement in prescribed occupation is to look separately at each occupational level.

DEVELOPMENTAL LEVEL

At the developmental level, the therapist is concerned to promote skill acquisition and the organization of separate skills into integrated complex patterns of performance. Unless the individual can achieve this, it will be impossible for higher level function to be achieved.

At this level (actions, interactions and reactions, performance units, task stages and simple tasks), participation is focused on the present and the immediate past and future.

Therapy using simple tasks:

- develops (or restores) skill components in the domains of action, interaction and reaction
- integrates skills from the three domains into smoothly sequenced performance
- improves skill and promotes competence
- connects effective action and successful outcome
- promotes well-being by improving performance of tasks which are essential to health and survival. (e.g. basic, personal self-care; basic communication)
- enables exploration of the environment
- promotes exploration of and recognition of personal skills.

When working at the developmental level, one is concerned with small episodes of performance. It may well be appropriate at this stage to take a reductive standpoint, utilizing tasks which provide the opportunity to train or regain specific aspects of function.

EFFECTIVE LEVEL

At the effective level, the performer engages in chained tasks and activities. Activities involve the performer across a longer timespan. The performer needs to plan, anticipate, predict and problem-solve. Activities mesh to form patterns across the day and over longer timeframes.

Participation in therapeutic activities:

- contributes meaning to situations
- promotes interaction with others
- requires skilled use of the hands
- provides a means of experiencing creative, imaginative and symbolic aspects of performance
- produces products valued by the participant or by others
- promotes structured and well-balanced use of time
- enables the individual to practise techniques of task analysis, pacing and problem-solving
- builds the individual's ability to engage in performance of increasing duration or difficulty
- provides personal challenges which stimulate effort, motivate adaptive participation and provide rewards
- provides opportunities to experience flow and be diverted from physical or cognitive discomfort
- helps individuals to explore their environment and widen the boundaries of their resource area
- provides experiences other than the mundane
- contributes to identity as a performer of an occupational role
- promotes perception of the self as an effective actor within the social and physical environment.

ORGANIZATIONAL LEVEL

At this level, the therapist can engage the client in a review of past, current, and future social and occupational roles. The balance of differing roles and occupations, (work, leisure, self-care, spiritual and transcendental) and periods of rest or relaxation, can be reviewed, but changes have to be made at the effective level if necessary.

By telling the story of their life (in 'occupational terms'), clients can gain insight into personal perceptions and can identify needs, interests and abilities and check if opportunities to meet these are present in the current situation.

The pattern of a life also has cultural, social and symbolic relevance. It is part of who the person is and how the person is perceived in a particular culture.

These analytical exercises do not need to involve 'doing things' but are a means of context setting and of evaluating and understanding occupational aspects of the life of an individual.

THE NEED FOR RESEARCH

It is not sufficient for the profession to depend on a set of assumptions and theories about the benefits of occupational therapy.

There is an urgent need for research to support these assumptions.

Somehow therapists must find ways of evaluating practice which avoid inappropriate reductionism and yet stand up to academic scrutiny. A starting point may be to use rigorous qualitative techniques to develop a body of grounded theory and documentation of cases which demonstrates effects. This is a huge challenge for practitioners in the 21st century.

10

Synthesis: the art of practice

THE THERAPIST AS ARTIST/CRAFTSPERSON

Occupational therapy has, from the beginning, required a synthesis of science, philosophy, craft, technology and design. The comparison of the therapist with the artist or craftsperson seems apt. Artists also need science as well as technique, imagination and innovation along with a set of rules and procedures.

Each time an artist attempts a picture, whether the artist is traditional or at the cutting edge of some modern movement, the basic components of materials, tools and techniques must be assembled in a fresh configuration. Each time a potter throws a pot upon a wheel, the potter must re-assemble a personal armoury of techniques and skills to engage with the clay to produce a new form. Throwing techniques may be taught, but only the creativity of the potter can achieve the transmutation which turns the 'pot in the mind' into 'the pot on the wheel'.

Similarly, occupational therapy has defeated attempts to render it down into a series of standardized techniques and methods. Where these exist they can, like the painting of drapery or background landscape in an old master, be delegated to a competent technician.

Occupational therapy remains holistic, innovative, a process which is re-invented and re-interpreted each time a therapist and client collaborate within the therapeutic alliance.

The art of practice lies in the therapist's ability to make a fresh combination of the core processes in the context of an individual life, in order to enable, empower or enhance competent performance.

The ability to do this can only come through the experience of actually doing it. No-one can ultimately teach an artist to paint a new picture; it must be born from a personal and internal process of focused engagement with materials and subject.

There is also one highly significant difference between the therapist and the artist. Few artists collaborate in producing their work. Clay and paint are passive media. In occupational therapy, there are two 'artists' – the therapist and the client who seeks to arrive at a new impression or image of his or her life.

To describe the process of therapy in terms of art may appear to overemphasize the creative and spontaneous aspects of it. But art, even modern art, is primarily a conscious, intentional and structured process. Things are included and excluded. Even accidental effects are deliberately sought. Tools are used; materials are selected.

Therapy, therefore, does need both tools and structure to assist therapist and client in working through the processes and making decisions.

SYNTHESIS

Synthesis is a 'building up of separate elements (concepts, propositions, facts), into a connected whole' (Concise Oxford Dictionary).

The synthesis which is created by an occupational therapist when working with an individual is daunting in its underlying complexity, and yet must appear simple and natural.

The therapist must first contribute an understanding of people, occupations and environments.

The therapist must fully understand the scope and limitations of occupational therapy, its theoretical basis, specialist techniques and applications. The therapist must know how doing, being and becoming interact and combine, and how, through clinical reasoning, to use this dynamic process as therapy.

The therapist needs to bring to bear a repertoire of personal practical abilities, and artistic, creative and technical skills, for in order to enable competent performance one must first be able to perform competently oneself.

The therapist has to use these skills, insights and understandings to inform the creation of a new therapeutic alliance, with a unique and valued individual, in a particular local environment, in a way which will direct future actions and decisions.

That individual, the pivot point of the whole endeavour, is an expert in the situation being faced, contributing knowledge, experience and potential, and a desire, however dimly perceived, to make something happen.

Somehow, together, therapist and client need to find a way to understand their situation and to embark on the risky journey towards change.

TOOLS AND STRUCTURES WHICH PROMOTE SYNTHESIS

The organizing frameworks for knowledge in occupational therapy are the theoretical models and approaches. These assist and direct the synthesis of the art of practice.

The organizing structure which directs practice in real time is the occupational therapy process, which sequences and formalizes the processes of problem naming, framing and solution, and the delivery and evaluation of intervention.

The tools for practice are the core processes through which the therapist and client can build the therapeutic relationship and explore occupations, environments, and personal abilities and needs.

COPE AS A SYSTEM TO PROMOTE SYNTHESIS

The POET, DARE and COPE structures can provide the therapist with an analytical framework (Fig. 10.1). This structure can be used with the core processes of occupational therapy in order to organize information-gathering, and assist the therapist and the client to identify problems, select priorities and goals and take actions in a logical sequence of enquiry and decision-making (Box 10.1).

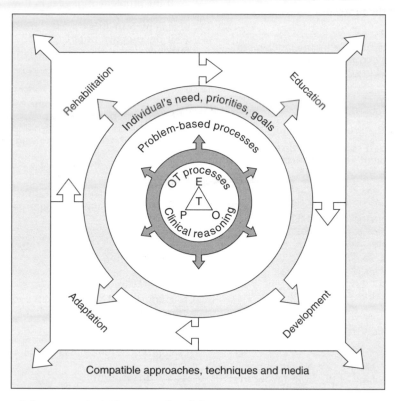

Figure 10.1 Processes of change used within occupational therapy.

Box 10.1 A SYSTEMATIC APPROACH TO OCCUPATIONAL THERAPY – INITIAL STAGES

Stage one: Profiling

Aim

To obtain a profile of the client as a past, present and future performer of roles and occupations in the environments which the client uses, and to form some basic assumptions about the nature of the situation and the relevance of occupational therapy.

Action by client

Describe past and current abilities and skills, present needs and situation, and future wishes and intentions. Describe activities and tasks which the client wants and needs to do which are a current cause of concern or dissatisfaction. Describe relevant features of the environment which the client uses or inhabits.

Action by therapist

Analyse this information with the client and make some preliminary assumptions or hypotheses about the situation and the likely course of the intervention.

Outcome

A written record of relevant facts and impressions.

Baseline data about the situation at the start of the intervention.

Analysis by the therapist of whether or not intervention is required and the probable general areas for further investigation or action.

Acceptance by the client of the need for intervention.

Box 10.1 *(Cont'd)*

Stage two: Naming the problem

Aim

To work with the client to specify the problems in achieving competent occupational performance. To define the nature and origin of these problems in relation to the client's own condition, tasks or environment.

Action by client and therapist

Determine whether the problem is due to:

- some present or past condition or circumstance which limits the client's ability to act, interact or react
- task demand which is in some way inappropriate in relation to the abilities of the client to respond
- environmental demand or societal limitation which fails to enhance, or imposes a barrier to, competent performance.

Outcome

A problem list indicating problems affecting the client, the client's tasks or environment.

Stage three: Diagnosis – framing the problem

Aim

To define the nature of the situation within the rationale and terminology of the COPE model and according to any appropriate frame of reference.

Action by therapist

To evaluate the quality and sufficiency of information available. If it is inadequate, decide what further investigations or assessments will be needed and undertake these.

If the problem has its origin with the client, is this because the client:

- has not developed (or must recapitulate development) in one or more skill domain
- has failed to adapt behaviour or psychological processes in response to changing circumstances
- has physical or psychological pathophysiology, impairment, functional limitation or disability resulting in the loss of previous knowledge or skill
- has not acquired necessary information or skill or has not had necessary experiences in which to apply skill and knowledge?

Decide which sector(s) of the DARE quadrant is(are) applicable, and which approaches may be effective in the light of this analysis.

Decide whether engagement in therapeutic activity may be appropriate for this client or whether functional adaptation is required.

If the problem originates in the environment, how might the environment be adapted to enhance or enable performance?

If the problem originates in the nature of the task, how might the task be adapted to enhance or enable performance?

Action by client

Explore with the therapist some of the likely causes of the current performance problems; begin to frame these problems in a way which improves understanding and facilitates problem-solving or adaptive action.

Outcome

The problem is framed, the results of this analysis are recorded and an applicable approach or approaches are selected.

Stage four: Prioritize

Aim

To identify what should be done in the course of the intervention and to decide what should be done first.

Action by client

Exploration of personal priorities, needs and goals.

Action by therapist

To negotiate with the client about the client's wishes, expectations, and priorities for action. To agree with the client the parameters for intervention.

Outcome

A record of agreed priorities.

Stage five: Action plan

Aim

To work with the client to explore alternative solutions and actions, define objectives and agree an outline action plan.

Client and therapist

Undertake prelimin*ary problem-solving and discuss alternative solutions where available. Discuss goals, objectives and actions and establish the agreed outcome measures so that success of the intervention can be measured.

Outcome

A record of the goals/objectives, outcome measures and action plan.

Flexible use of the structure

These five stages in Box 10.1 are not time-limited: they may take 5 minutes or 5 weeks. Stages 2, 3 and 4 of this structure need not be used as a rigid sequence. The enquiries, analysis, discussion and decison-making may take place in the course of a fluid and dynamic process of interaction between therapist and client. However, at some point in that process, the essential diagnostic reasoning, naming and framing, prioritizing and solution-generating must take place using the POET and DARE structures.

Subsequent stages

Therapy or intervention progresses through the application and synthesis of core processes. At intervals in the process new problems may be identified and new goals can be set. Progress is evaluated jointly by client and therapist so that outcomes can be measured and decisions can be taken about whether to terminate or continue intervention.

SECTION 2

Therapeutic use of self

SECTION CONTENTS

Introduction to therapeutic use of self

WHAT IS THERAPEUTIC USE OF SELF?

The therapeutic use of self is arguably the most important of the core processes of occupational therapy. So much hangs on the way in which the therapist carries out the professional role and develops appropriate and effective therapeutic relationships.

What is meant by the phrase 'therapeutic use of self'? Mosey (1986) began her chapter on 'conscious use of self' with the statement that it is 'the use of oneself in such a way that one becomes an effective tool in the evaluation and intervention process. (This) involves a planned interaction with another person… it includes, but is greater than rapport and the art of practice.'

Mosey goes on to distinguish between spontaneous response which is essentially unplanned, and use of self which is planned for a therapeutic purpose.

The use of aspects of oneself for a therapeutic purpose is certainly an important part of what I mean by therapeutic use of self, but it is only a part of the picture.

Schwarztberg (in Hopkins & Smith 1993) notes that 'the clinician's therapeutic use of self is a necessary requirement to the (therapeutic) relationship. This is similar to the use of purposeful activity in occupational therapy. As single elements of the process the activity and relationship are each insufficient when used alone.'

I have used a variation of the POET diagram to indicate that occupational therapy is based on a *triad* which enables the therapist to form a therapeutic relationship with the individual in the course of performance of an activity. The relationship facilitates performance while the shared experience of the activity enhances the relationship (Fig. 11.1).

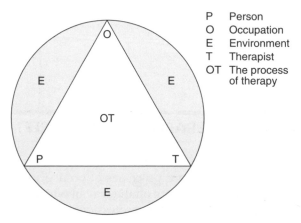

P   Person
O   Occupation
E   Environment
T   Therapist
OT The process of therapy

Figure 11.1 The occupational therapy triad – therapist, person, occupation – interacting within the environment.

THE SELF

We need to begin with an understanding of what is meant by that elusive concept 'the self'.

Each of us has many aspects of self. There is the self which others see but we do not and the social self we show to others, which changes as we adopt different roles in different situations. There is the private self 'inside our heads' which others do not see, and the invisible aspects of self, buried deep, which even we do not know about (Hargie et al 1994). All these different 'selves' impact upon our work as therapists.

In the context of therapeutic use of self, we are mainly concerned with the professional self, the aspects of self which the therapist uses when performing a professional role. The social self and the private self contribute to this professional persona but need to be governed by it.

THE PROFESSIONAL SELF

What does it mean to 'be professional'? When the therapist offers services to a patient or client,

the therapist does so in the context of an implied 'contract' between a professional person and the person who seeks a service.

This contract places obligations on both parties. The therapist is expected to be skilled, efficient and competent in the service of the client. The therapist will 'do good' and 'do no harm'. The therapist will behave honourably, ethically and honestly, and treat everything said by the client with total confidentiality.

The client is similarly expected to treat the professional with respect, to listen to what the therapist says, to negotiate agreed action and to carry this out.

In the past, this social contract made it plain that the power and authority lay with the professional. This professional power was partly the result of social status, and partly 'sapiential authority'; there was a certain mystique; the professional 'knew more' and 'knew best'.

During the past decade, this implicit contract has altered significantly. Influences as diverse as post-modernist deconstruction of authority, political expediency, the disability rights movement and the increased emphasis on client-centered practice have combined to weaken professional authority.

There are both benefits and losses in this situation. In many ways, it is an improvement; a more balanced relationship facilitates communication and should enhance therapy. The professional relationship is viewed more as a partnership between equals, a *therapeutic alliance*, where two people come together to share knowledge and experience.

However, it also means that, while the professional remains tightly bound by a strict set of ethical and legal constraints, the professional is now liable to be challenged and questioned. 'In my professional opinion' is no longer a sufficient justification for actions or assumptions.

The client still expects safe, skilled and competent service, but compliance with and respect for professional authority is no longer automatic. The loss of social status and respect for sapiential authority has made professionals far more vulnerable. They are now open to abuse, assault, and legal action in ways which were unthinkable a few decades ago.

These changes make the dynamics of the therapeutic relationship even more crucial and the skilled therapeutic use of self even more essential.

VALUES AND ETHICS

To use aspects of oneself in a planned manner, one must tread a fine line between being an effective therapist and being a person who uses interactive skills to achieve conscious manipulation, or control, of others.

The key to the therapeutic relationship is that therapists must first understand and value themselves, and second, value and seek to understand their clients. Valuing someone ensures beneficial intent and positive action and counteracts imposition or control.

Because therapists deal with people who may be vulnerable and open to exploitation, it is essential for them to adopt the highest standards of personal probity and ethical behaviour.

The ethics of practice and the core values and attitudes which organize the practice of occupational therapy have been extensively described. Values are important because they influence both interactions and clinical reasoning.

In an earlier book, I have summarized 39 values mentioned in occupational therapy literature (Hagedorn 1995a: 30) in relation to the person, the occupation, the environment and the therapist.

The American Association of Occupational Therapists (Kanny 1993) lists seven core concepts which guide practice. These are presented below in abbrieviated form:

Altruism   Unselfish concern for the welfare of others.

Equality   All individuals must be perceived as having the same fundamental rights and opportunities and must be treated fairly, impartially and with respect.

Freedom   Allows individuals to exercise choice and to demonstrate independence, initiative and self-direction.

Justice   Places value on moral and legal principles such as fairness, equity, truthfulness and objectivity. Laws must be complied with and legal rights must be protected and respected.

Dignity   Emphasizes the importance of valuing the inherent worth and uniqueness of each person.

Truth   Requires that we be faithful to facts and reality.

Prudence   Is the ability to govern and discipline oneself through the use of reason.

The presentation of this list of values concludes with a summary which provides an important reminder that the application of a value system is less easy in practice than in theory:

The emphasis or priority given to each value may change as one's professional career evolves and as the unique characteristics of a situation unfold. Although we have basic values that cannot be violated the degree to which certain values will take priority at a given time is influenced by the specific situation and the environment in which it occurs. In one instance dignity may be a higher priority than truth: in another prudence may be chosen over freedom… The practitioner faces dilemmas because of conflicting values and is required to engage in thoughtful deliberation to determine where the priority lies in a given situation. The challenge for us all is to know our values, be able to make reasoned choices in situations of conflict and be able to clearly articulate and defend our choices.

The Canadian Occupational Performance Model (Canadian Association of Occupational Therapists 1997) lists a set of strongly humanistic values and beliefs under the headings: about occupation; about the person; about the environment; about health; about client-centred practice.

A clear set of values is essential as a unifying bond for any group. It is not, however, sufficient to have values. One must put them into practice, and, as Kanny points out, that is not easy. The therapist is continually challenged by moral and practical dilemmas.

AN ETHICAL CODE OF CONDUCT

The College of Occupational Therapists has issued a Code of Ethics and Professional Conduct (1995) which gives detailed guidance on ethical practice and behaviour. The code deals with:

- client autonomy and welfare

- service to clients
- personal/professional integrity
- professional compliance and standards.

This code of conduct makes it clear that therapists must provide high quality services in an organized and efficient manner. Therapists must pay continual attention to the development and maintenance of their therapeutic skills; they must at all times strive to do their best for their clients within the ethical framework of practice.

These are not small demands. The therapist has to demonstrate the highest standards of personal, moral and ethical behaviour, keep the law, respect human rights, and ensure that no harm befalls the client either by acts of ommission or commission.

The difficulty of putting ethics into practice is described at length by Seedhouse (1988). He states that:

there remains much uncertainty and room for conflicts of values within the ethics of health. But this is simply the nature of ethics. *The* right course of action cannot be prescribed as if it were a pill for a specific ill. There will always be legitimate alternative courses of action that might be chosen.

Seedhouse proposes an 'ethical grid' to guide the practitioner through the maze of ethical decison-taking.

The formation of a therapeutic relationship is therefore constrained and directed by the adoption of the professional role and the values and ethics which accompany this. These impose boundaries which must be overtly recognized.

The professional relationship must be distinguished from friendship or any other form of interaction. Expressions of sexual interest or intent between professional and client are explicitly forbidden.

The therapist may be friendly, but not become a friend; show caring concern, but maintain separation; may need to mask negative reactions, yet must remain authentic; seeks to facilitate change, yet not impose control. This implies considerable insight and maturity on the part of the therapist.

In the past, 'being professional' carried an implication of extreme self-discipline in terms of personal reactions and emotions. The professional person was expected to be unshockable, unmoved by the disasters of others. Professionals were expected, somehow, to construct a barrier between their private and professional selves. Above all, professionals had no need of any kind of help themselves.

This expectation has not wholly disappeared, but it is more readily accepted that 'the professional' is also a person who has feelings and needs which should be recognized.

THE COMPETENCIES OF PROFESSIONAL SELF-MANAGEMENT

The therapist needs to be able to:

- monitor personal behaviour and emotions in order to practise in a disciplined and professional manner
- modify interactions with others through the use of interactive reasoning and interactive skills
- set appropriate boundaries to relationships in professional settings
- reflect on personal performance and development to maintain high standards of service
- seek personal supervision when necessary
- organize work in an efficient and effective manner
- monitor ethical aspects of practice, seeking to work in accordance with the code of conduct and within an ethical framework.

THE SOCIAL SELF

Therapists usually like people and get on well with them. A misanthrope would be unlikely to seek out a career as a therapist, and would certainly not succeed as one.

Good social skills are an essential prerequisite for a therapist. There are many aspects of a therapists's interactions where good manners, politeness, and all the small verbal and non-verbal tricks used by any successful host or hostess to 'oil the social wheels' can be used to good effect.

There is, however, a difference between 'being sociable' and 'being a therapist'. The difference, as Mosey suggested, is to do with planning and intention.

Social skills are essentially reactive and spontaneous responses to situations and other people. They are useful during informal interactions, or during brief, formal, therapeutic interventions where the therapist is not required to develop any continuing relationship with the client, for example, a telephone call, answering a question or providing a short piece of advice.

In any ordinary social situation, an interaction between people who have not met before may lead in many directions. The interaction may be due to pure happenstance and the participants may never meet again. They may meet intermittently in contexts which do not foster the development of a deeper relationship. They may 'click' and decide at once to move further towards a sharing intimacy. One or both may equally decide to avoid all future meetings. Numerous other possibilities exist.

In a therapeutic relationship, most of these possibilities are excluded. The relationship exists for a shorter or longer duration for a particular purpose in a specific context which sets boundaries which are (or should be) understood by both parties.

One may develop a certain affinity, even an intimacy born of propinquity in difficult circumstances, but one is not moving towards a deeper relationship. This does not mean that the therapeutic relationship is artificial or inauthentic. It simply means that it is a special kind of relationship with definite boundaries.

In a therapeutic relationship, the therapist uses, or suppresses, aspects of the 'social self' in a deliberate manner in order to further the relationship or move it in a specific direction.

THE PRIVATE SELF

The therapist is also a person. That person has needs for attachment or safety, desires for connection or separation and unconscious fears which affect every new relationship.

Each of us has mental suitcases full of the unwashed laundry of past relationships, locked rooms inside the mind into which we will not go, and skeletons which stubbornly rattle in their cupboards.

It may take a lifetime to come to terms with the private self, or even to acknowledge its existance. While it would usually be inappropriate for an occupational therapist to be required to undergo years of personal analysis in order to be able to practise (we are not, and should not seek to become, psychotherapists), some degree of insight is essential.

To be human is to be imperfect, but also to have the potential to aim for a kind of perfection. We all have gifts to bring to others.

The therapist may be able to use the private self as a means of gaining insight into a situation, or empathizing with a client, but the therapist must be very wary of using deeply personal experiences in the context of a therapeutic relationship. In no way is it likely to be helpful for the client if the therapist is attempting to work out some personal need or past experience in the course of a therapeutic interaction.

Being honest and truthful in a relationship also means being honest and truthful with oneself. It means not expecting the impossible of oneself or of others. We cannot like all other human beings. Sometimes, we cannot help liking another human being too much. There will be clients (or even colleagues) with whom we cannot (and should not) work.

The therapist needs to be able to recognize when the private self is intruding into the professional self and to ensure that this is not to the disadvantage of the client. If it affects the therapeutic relationship to an unacceptable degree, the therapist must either pass the client on to someone else, or must seek personal help from someone uninvolved with the situation.

Anyone who seeks to meet the needs of others without paying any attention to personal needs is heading for burnout. Being a therapist may be deeply satisfying but it can also be hugely stressful. There are times when the private self has needs which must be recognized and met; that too is part of being professional.

PERSONAL CHARACTERISTICS WHICH PROMOTE THERAPEUTIC USE OF SELF

The therapeutic alliance is a form of 'helping relationship' (Carkhuff 1969). The helping relationship requires the use of a set of facilitating skills derived from humanistic psychology and psychotherapy (Carkhuff & Berensen 1977). The way in which therapists may develop and use these skills has been discussed by Lloyd & Maas (1992). They list the following qualities or dimensions of the helping relationship: empathy, genuineness, facilitative genuineness, respect. In addition, the therapist must possess other personal qualities and the skills to use these to enhance the relationship.

INSIGHT

To use themselves effectively in a therapeutic relationship, therapists must first have a degree of insight: an accurate understanding of their own strengths, needs, attitudes, emotions and 'hang-ups'. This is not won easily, or in a short time.

Insight is gained through a continued process of reflection and self-critical awareness in which therapeutic relationships are monitored and checked to ensure that personal motivations do not intrude at the expense of the client.

The therapist must deal with issues raised by reflection, for personal growth is important. In areas of practice where relationships may become intense or stressful, good supervision is essential.

The therapist must cultivate an ability to submerge aspects of the self which may be unhelpful to a client, while bringing to the fore aspects of self which will be helpful. Some people find this impossible. Such people usually have difficulty with their own relationships and they cannot easily form therapeutic ones.

PATIENCE

Building a therapeutic relationship can take time. If a client has had mainly negative experiences with others, there is no reason for the client to suddenly trust a therapist.

Failures of communication litter human life. Watching clients struggle to find words to explain what they want or how they feel, without leaping in and putting words into their mouth can be as difficult as sitting on one's hands while someone struggles to fasten a button.

Trying to find words to say the same thing yet again in a different way in the hope of communicating something important is equally taxing.

It is worth remembering that the client who has insight, is articulate and keen to adapt and has clearly formulated goals, scarcely needs the therapist.

HUMOUR

The appropriate use of humour with a client is a real gift. Laughter can change lives. The skill is in knowing when to laugh and how to get the client to laugh with you.

Therapists often strive to lighten a situation with humour, but therapy is not 'a laugh a minute' and to attempt to make it so trivializes the process. It is better to remain serious than to make a client feel diminished or patronized by the inappropriate use of humour.

Therapists do need personal reserves of humour to counteract the stresses of practice, even if it is sometimes of the 'graveyard' variety. The bitter humour of the cynic, however, may be a danger sign. Cynics are usually more than halfway towards burnout.

ENERGY

Physical energy is certainly necessary; the therapist needs stamina and the ability to keep going. It is also important to be able to put mental energy into a situation in order to promote change. A static situation cannot easily alter. The client who is confronted by difficult circumstances often lacks the kind of energy necessary to make new things happen – either it has all been used up in the effort of coping, or the circumstances have combined to drain what was available.

Mental energy is not some esoteric, 'psychic' force. It is a combination of personal well-being, motivation, confidence, belief in self-efficacy, determination and enthusiasm which powers action and makes things happen.

The therapist needs to be able to muster sufficient reserves of this kind of energy to 'transfuse' the client, so that by 'borrowing' from the therapist's reserves, action is given a kick start. This does not mean that the therapist should always act with the loud and synthetic enthusiasm of a holiday camp leader (although this may occasionally be required). The transfer of energy needs to happen subtly, by osmosis.

Mental energy is not inexhaustible. It has to be replenished and its use has to be controlled and limited to some extent. A continual, unreserved pouring out of personal energy can eventually lead to burnout. Some clients act as energy-draining 'sponges' which are never filled.

HONESTY

Honesty is concerned with telling the truth and keeping promises. It underpins the ethical approach to professional life. While it may sometimes be necessary to be 'economical with the truth', a therapeutic relationship with a client can only be built on personal integrity and trust.

Honesty may also help both therapist and client to deal with strong emotions. Professionals are traditionally instructed to repress expressions of anger, disgust, sorrow or pity in front of the client. There are many times when this is necessary-although it may be wise to go somewhere later and 'explode' privately or with someone you trust.

There may be occasions, however, when it is honest and right in the circumstances to say 'what you tell me (or what you are doing) makes me feel angry, (or sad, or horrified or whatever)' because failure to acknowledge the reality of the situation would be a failure of common humanity.

VALUING THE INDIVIDUAL

Occupational therapy is founded on a set of humanistic values concerned with respecting other people as individuals who have potential. The humanistic approach of 'unconditional positive regard' is often quoted as essential in the therapeutic relationship.

The therapist does need to accept the client at the starting point in an uncritical and nonjudgemental manner. This does not mean approval of every aspect of the client's life or behaviour. There may be behaviours or attitudes that need to be challenged.

Valuing the individual means regard for the person as a unique being who is entitled to all human rights including the right to choose.

This includes the client's right to choose not to take the therapist's advice, and the right to decide not to act to change the client's own way of living or thinking, however 'desirable' this may seem to be.

Empathy

In her chapter on the therapeutic alliance, Pelonquin (Neistadt & Crepeau 1998) describes empathy as consisting of: 'a turning of the soul; a recognition of likeness; a recognition of uniqueness; an entering into the experience of the other; a connection with feelings; a power to recover from the connection.'

Pelonquin emphasizes the deeply personal nature of empathic contact, but goes further in this direction than I would be prepared to travel.

Empathy does require the ability to see a situation from someone else's point of view. This understanding informs the therapeutic relationship. The therapist is able to 'be with' the person to the extent that the therapist can appreciate feelings or reactions, but crucially, the therapist does not share these feeling. The therapist remains 'at one remove', simultaneously connected and yet disconnected.

Empathy enables the therapist to act as an advocate for the client, putting forward the client's point of view if the client is unable to do this effectively alone.

The wise therapist does not, however, rely uncritically on empathy or 'intuition' as a means of assessing the form a relationship should take. Humans are not thought-readers, although they often behave as if they think they are.

Assumptions about other people may be accurate; human interactions are based on rapid appraisal of others and these judgements are often correct, but equally, they may be mistaken.

Intuitions and empathetic reactions depend at least in part on correct perception and interpretation of behavioural cues and these perceptions can be muddled by prejudice, preconception, and personal beliefs or feelings.

Assumptions about patients need to be treated as hypotheses to be reviewed or challenged.

CARING

This is a minefield of a word for it has many, emotionally loaded meanings. We care for children or pets; we care deeply for loved ones; we care about issues in which we believe. Care is not a neutral word; it may imply protection, commitment, concerned action, even passion.

In the general sense of being concerned for the welfare of other people, and motivated to help them, caring is important to anyone involved in health provision: it is no coincidence that such provision is commonly called 'health care'.

Pelonquin writes that 'without caring in the relationship occupational therapy is a sterile technique'. But in which sense of the word should occupational therapists 'care' when dealing with their clients? We need to distinguish between caring *for* and caring *about*.

To care *for* another person often means 'to do things for the person' or to promote the person's safety and well-being; nurses care for their patients. Occupational therapists may need to provide care at times but the value systems which underlie therapy and this form of caring are fundamentally different. Occupational therapy is not about 'doing things for someone' but about 'getting people to do things for themselves'. The differences are sometimes a cause of conflict and misunderstanding between professionals and between the therapist and another carer.

Caring *for* may be an impersonal and practical matter; one may care for a machine, with a view to just keeping it running. Caring *for* may also become a form of emotional bondage sometimes removing control from the person being cared for to the carer and at other times allowing the dependent person to dominate the carer. None of these aspects of caring is in any sense therapeutic.

Caring *about* the client is another matter. A therapist who 'does not care' in this sense is a useless therapist; one cannot be detached and indifferent to the person one seeks to assist because that would inhibit the therapeutic alliance. We need to care about the client by showing humanistic values of regard and respect, not being '*on the client's side*' but being '*alongside the client*' in whatever situation the client is in.

Caring *about* clients in a therapeutic context facilitates those people in taking control of themselves as fully functioning, valued, unique human beings.

BEING ONESELF

Of course one cannot be other than oneself: even actors admit to using aspects of themselves when playing an apparently dissimilar character to their own. In the same way, therapists must at times become actors and play a part, yet, like actors, remain authentic and essentially themselves in the process.

Being a therapist is 'being oneself' in a special context with particular 'rules'. In this respect, it is no different than 'being oneself' in all the other roles one may have in life – boss, employee, lover, friend, child or parent – but it may require a more conscious and disciplined approach than other aspects of one's life.

The therapeutic relationship

WHAT IS A THERAPEUTIC RELATIONSHIP?

When describing the therapeutic relationship we are primarily concerned with dyadic interaction, the dynamics of communication between two people. Therapeutic relationships in group contexts, while important, are different in several respects. This will be discussed later.

A therapeutic relationship is more than the transient professional contact which one may have with a client or patient when providing straightforward information or services. It is a relationship which develops over time and may last for days, weeks or months.

There are many possible styles of therapeutic relationship. These are influenced by models of practice, by psychoanalytical theories, and by the context and environment in which the relationship is taking place.

In occupational therapy, the relationship is normally a partnership between the therapist and the individual which evolves when that individual seeks the assistance of the therapist to promote joint exploration of, and action on, some problem affecting daily life.

The boundaries of the relationship are set by the need to intervene in the problem situation. Once intervention is completed, the relationship is naturally ended.

This style of relationship is also described as the '*therapeutic alliance*', a phrase which neatly captures the collaborative nature of the process.

HOW DOES THE THERAPEUTIC ALLIANCE INFLUENCE THE OUTCOMES OF THERAPY?

There is general agreement in the literature that the therapeutic alliance is an important factor in the effectiveness of therapy.

Krupnik et al (1996) cite a meta-analysis of therapeutic alliance studies (Horvath & Symonds 1990) in which the authors concluded that 'the therapeutic alliance has been significantly associated with outcome not only across a number of investigations but also across different types of psychotherapy.'

Krupnik et al point out, however, that it is difficult to compare studies because of the differences in style and techniques used by the therapists, and also because a significant factor in whether the outcome is successful is the degree to which the patient is able or prepared to contribute.

In their own study, which compared the relationship between therapeutic alliance and treatment outcome for depressed outpatients who received interpersonal psychotherapy or cognitive–behaviour therapy or a drug or a placebo, therapeutic alliance was found to have a significant effect on outcome for both psychotherapies and active and placebo pharmacotherapy.

An important finding in this study was that, while ratings of patient contribution to the alliance were related to treatment outcome, ratings of therapist contribution to the outcome were not linked.

It is clear, therefore, that a successful therapeutic relationship is at least as important as the treatment on offer. It is not, however, simply a matter of the therapist's skills. It also depends on how far the client participates actively in the process (although one might argue that the degree of participation is influenced by the therapist's skills in promoting this).

It is possible for the elements of an interaction to be measured by a trainer observer. Krupnik et al used a modified version of the Vanderbilt Therapeutic Alliance Scale which measures three subscales: therapist, patient and therapist–patient interaction. This is, of course, only practical in a research setting. In everyday practice, the therapist has the hard task of attempting to monitor, analyse and reflect on the components and outcomes of an interaction both as it occurs and after the event.

While every therapist is aware of clients who, for various reasons, are unable or unwilling to participate, this study also raises interesting questions about the therapist's ability to motivate and enable the client to do so.

It is also (perhaps discouragingly) clear that an effective therapeutic relationship may be the most important part of therapy. It may matter less *what* is done than *who* is doing it and *how* the relationship develops.

To some extent occupational therapists have always understood this. They have sought to build bridges across the relationship void by involving the client in an activity through which the relationship can naturally evolve and be expressed and facilitated.

COMPONENTS OF A SUCCESSFUL RELATIONSHIP

So what are the components of a successful interpersonal relationship? In a review of interpersonal relationships and individual outcome, Lewis (1998) lists ten basic relationship concepts. These relate to dynamics within the relationship, and to aspects of balance and include:

Attachment	The need for a relationship which provides security, satisfaction and meaning.
Connection and separation	A greater or lesser individual proclivity for both closeness and intimacy and independence and autonomy.
Negotiation	In the early stages of a relationship, there is a complex negotiation to balance connection and separateness.
Unconscious fears	These play an important part in negotiation as each person attempts to achieve a balance that provides maximum satisfaction and freedom from fear.

Power	Each person attempts to influence the other to accept a balance congruent with his/her proclivities and fears.
Values	Shared beliefs and cultural factors influence the relationship and become established within it.

These components are discussed by Lewis in the context of marital relationships, but they underpin any prolonged relationship to a greater or lesser degree, and require consideration.

Lewis describes maintenance of balance and changes in balance and then deals with health-facilitating balances and the optimal balance as follows:

Health-facilitating balances	Although any balance of connection and separateness may be relatively satisfactory to both participants, certain balances facilitate the continued and healthy development of the participants.
Optimal balance	Although contextual factors may limit that which is possible, health-facilitating systems are usually characterized by high levels of both connection and separateness.

This apparent paradox, that a relationship can be both connected and separate, is important in the therapeutic relationship. The therapist must somehow be both close to and distant from the client. The 'balance of power' must meet the needs of the client for safety, closeness and separateness.

Therapists must neither submerge their personality in an attempt to validate that of the client, nor use the relationship to meet their own needs. However, there is also the implication that a health-facilitating relationship may benefit both parties to it. A therapist should not be damaged by a therapeutic relationship, any more than the client should be.

No wonder that the therapeutic relationship can be a delicate and difficult plant to nurture.

Lewis notes how little we know about the nature of such relationships:

Although we have evidence that adult relationships transform lives we know little about how such healing relationships come about and what their dynamics might be... it appears that some relationships may be brought about through mechanisms of emotional support and affirmation (empathy, warmth and genuineness) and others through providing a specific relationship ingredient that is needed. At this stage of our knowledge, however, we do not know whether the crucial factors are to be found in the personalities of individuals, the structure of transforming relationships or both.

CLIENT-CENTRED APPROACHES

The style of relationship adopted by occupational therapists has been influenced by humanistic psychology and philosophy. This approach is based on an intrinsically optimistic view of human beings.

Primary assumptions of this approach include:

Valuing personal experience; since no one else can experience it, no one should attempt to influence another's choices or interpretations of reality.

The individual must be considered as a whole in the context of his physical and social reality.

An individual has the right to personal choice (and to all other human rights).

The goal of the individual is to function as a free, self-directing, honest person whose life is meaningful and satisfying.

The individual is capable of directing his own life and should therefore direct his own learning or therapy as far as may be possible.

An individual is innately capable of positive development.

Hagedorn (1997)

Therapists have tended to interpret this frame of reference within the partnership model of interaction, rather than the more strongly person-centred counselling model where the therapist largely seeks to reflect back the client's own feelings and wishes.

A dynamic and interactive partnership is an essential feature of the participatory nature of occupational therapy. The therapist seeks, within the framework of a supportive and facilitating relationship, to pass the power to the client to enable the client to achieve personal goals.

This is made explicit in the Canadian Client-Centred Model of Practice which is strongly focused on a set of values and beliefs (Canadian Association of Occupational Therapists 1997). These include the following statements about the person, and about the nature of client-centred practice:

About the person

We believe that:

> humans are occupational beings
> every person is unique
> every person has intrinsic dignity and worth
> every person can make choices about life
> every person has some capacity for self-determination
> every person has some ability to participate in occupations
> every person has some potential to change
> persons are social and spiritual beings
> persons have diverse abilities for participating in occupations
> persons shape and are shaped by their environment

About client-centred practice

We believe that:

> clients have experiences and knowledge about their occupations
> clients are active partners in the occupational therapy process
> risk-taking is necessary for positive change
> client-centred practice of occupational therapy focuses on enabling occupation.

COPE is based on a similar set of values, but is, perhaps, less strongly client-centred, in that therapist and client are equal partners and share the process of evaluation and goal setting, whereas in the Canadian Model the client directs these processes.

RISK-TAKING

The statement that 'risk-taking is necessary for positive change' is both provocative and important.

The statement is based first on fundamental assumptions accepted by occupational therapists that normal living is intrinsically risky and that people have a right (within certain limits) to be at risk. Attempts to protect clients from all possible risk lead inevitably to unacceptable use of restraint and limitations of freedom.

Second, change may involve acceptance of risk. 'Nothing venture, nothing win' is a good axiom for a therapist. Occupational therapy often means helping the client to push past the boundaries which confine the client's life within 'safe' but restricting limits.

Risk-taking occurs within relationships. Trust, confiding, personal disclosure, expression of vulnerability, acceptance of closeness are all risky. A helping relationship can be threatening. While the client may apparently be more likely to feel threatened, and to need support, it is a mistake to ignore the threats to the therapist.

More practical risk-taking occurs frequently in the process of therapy. When a client takes the first steps across a room without a walking aid, or pours hot water from a kettle, there is risk. The therapist judges risks of this kind continually. The therapist must not endanger the client, but cannot achieve progress if the client is 'wrapped in cotton wool'.

Part of the art of building a therapeutic relationship is the development of the client's confidence so that risky things may be attempted. This confidence is derived from a complex mixture of belief in the therapist and belief in self. As the authors of the Canadian Model point out, this acceptance of risk also entails acceptance of the possibility of failure, and the need to support the client through this.

A third form of risk-taking happens when the client insists on doing something (or refusing to do something) in a manner which the therapist considers to be overstepping the acceptable boundaries of risk.

A key to handling risky situations is to use the therapeutic relationship to explore and discuss risk in a practical manner, evaluating the potential for harm, and seeking to reduce it if possible.

Thus, the therapist cannot insist that the unsteady client who is liable to fall must install a grab rail; the therapist can explore the risk of tripping or slipping, the advantages of a rail in reducing risk, and ways of coping if a fall should happen.

Dealing with risk involves a balancing act in which individual freedom and choice have to be weighed against the possibility of harm.

The therapist may find ethical and professional conflicts between accepting risk and reporting risky situations to others difficult to deal with.

It is not, however, acceptable to leave a person in some kind of serious risk situation without alerting others to this, even if nothing can be done about it, for this places the therapist at risk of being negligent.

DEVELOPING A THERAPEUTIC RELATIONSHIP

Like any other continuing relationship, a therapeutic relationship has to evolve over a period of time. During this time the relationship will probably pass through various stages moving along continums from distance to closeness, distrust to trust, formality to informality, depending on the circumstances.

Both partners in the relationship need to contribute to it, to bring their own experience and knowledge and to feel that these are valued.

The art of developing a relationship is extremely difficult to convey. It is partly a matter of personality, partly of social and communication skills, partly related to experience, and partly a result of highly effective interactive reasoning.

Equally challenging is the art of bringing the relationship to a mutually satisfactory close, avoiding problems of dependency or loss.

INTERACTIVE REASONING

Interactive reasoning is a process whereby the therapist simultaneously interacts and monitors the interaction, shaping it as it evolves, responding spontaneously to events and reactions of the person.

Recent studies of interactive reasoning illuminate the complexity of the process of developing and sustaining a therapeutic relationship and suggest some of the skills which are needed.

Fleming (1994) draws from the literature nine purposes of interactive reasoning which may be summarized as:

- to engage the person in the treatment session
- to know the person as a person
- to understand disability from the patient's point of view
- to 'individualize' treatment (make a closer match between treatment goals and strategies for a particular person)
- to communicate a sense of acceptance, trust or hope
- to use humour to relieve tension
- to construct a shared language of actions and meanings
- to determine if the treatment session is going well
- to show interest in the person and the person's concerns.

Munroe (1992) found that therapists in community practice used technical, procedural and interactive reasoning, and that of these, interactive reasoning was the most commonly used mode.

We have seen how therapeutic use of self is 'planned' in the sense that the therapist has some preconceived notion of how the therapist wishes a relationship to evolve, and the outcomes of this. However, it is impossible to interact with another person in a totally 'pre-planned' fashion. This would make the interaction seem stilted and artificial like a tightly scripted interview.

Mattingly & Fleming (1994) show that competence in interactive reasoning takes time to develop; novices have difficulty with simultaneously 'doing and modifying doing', but experienced practitioners do this automatically as an integrated part of practice.

This ability has led Mattingly & Fleming to propose the concept of 'three track reasoning' during which the therapist simultaneously carries out an intervention and interaction while monitoring the results and planning the next move. This complex mode of reasoning was also found by Ryan (1992).

Mattingly & Fleming also noted that therapists with quite different personalities showed a common ability to be very flexible in style of interaction, 'fine-tuning' as they went, moving fluidly from one style to another if required, maximizing every therapeutic opportunity.

They contrast the different 'languages' used by therapists as 'chart talk' (the kind of clinical/medical language used when communicating with other professionals or giving a report) and 'story talk' the informal language of narrative and personal experience used when speaking to a patient 'as a person'.

It seems likely that the ability to 'switch modes' and use an appropriate method of communication depends on cue acquisition, cognitive processing, and a very flexible set of verbal and non-verbal responses.

More research into these skills is needed, but it is useful to explore some of the cues and responses involved, and this will be covered in the next chapter.

AVOIDING THE PITFALLS

Interactive reasoning is also needed when monitoring less obvious elements in an interaction.

These may relate to implied prejudices, attitudes or values (on both sides).

It may also be necessary to be aware of the classic dynamics of therapeutic relationships, which may result in defence mechanisms or negative emotional coping strategies intruding into the relationship (again, on both sides).

While it is useful to become aware of mechanisms which may affect a relationship, the therapist needs to guard against lapsing into 'analyst-speak' ('he's in denial'; 'she's projecting') as a substitute for genuine reflection on, or analysis of, a relationship, especially one which is not going as well as one might wish.

Use of an experienced supervisor becomes essential when working in situations where relationships may easily become highly charged or where stressful material is uncovered.

Dyadic interaction: styles and skills

DYADIC INTERACTION

Much of the therapist's time is spent interacting with another person in one-to-one situations. Interactions happen between therapist and client, and between therapist and other professionals or other people connected with a client.

While the personal skills of the therapist may be used at full stretch on occasion, much interaction is relatively straightforward. This does not mean that it is casual or unskilled.

Dyadic interactions vary in duration, intention and intensity. They range from a casual, brief social contact to an extended period of focused interaction during which a therapeutic relationship evolves.

Different situations demand differing styles of interaction and different communication skills. In each case, the nature of the interaction must match the situation. Part of the art of therapeutic use of self lies in judging the right mode of interaction for each occasion.

Humans, as social animals, automatically make these judgements all the time. We do not communicate in the same way with our boss, friend, child, lover, colleague or client, or the person we bump into in the super-market. We show these people different aspects of ourselves, often using different forms of speech. In a therapeutic context, we may need to make these decisions a little more consciously and work a little harder to 'get it right'.

Common situations in which dyadic interactions take place are:

- during an interview
- during assessment of a patient
- during treatment of a patient
- when teaching
- during counselling
- in social settings
- when liaising with another health care professional
- when using the telephone.

CUES TO INTERACTIONS

We learn to interpret expression, gesture, body language and verbal communication from an early age. It is said that the first 5 seconds of a meeting between strangers is taken up by a rapid appraisal of the situation, gathering cues to intentions, roles and the correct social responses.

Therapists who show mastery in developing adaptive therapeutic relationships are usually people who have refined this ability rapidly to observe and interpret cues to a fine art.

Cues may be non-verbal, verbal or behavioural. Cues are also provided by the content of the environment and the context or situation.

NON-VERBAL CUES

Non verbal cues include posture, eye contact, expression, gesture and emotional behaviours.

As humans we learn to respond to gesture, expression and tone of voice long before we have learned to understand language. These primitive methods of communication remain important and powerful.

Because non-verbal communication precedes language, it is also the mode of communication to which people revert under extreme stress, or when damage causes regression to an earlier developmental level.

Responses to non-verbal cues

Therapists often mirror non-verbal cues, or respond to them with non-verbal behaviour of their own such as safe touch or empathetic expression as a means of maintaining communication at an appropriate level.

It is important that non-verbal 'language' is consistent with the situation and with what is being said.

Touch can be an important means of providing reassurance, but it needs to be used with discretion. In most situations, touching another person with your hand should be brief, and directed towards 'safe' body areas such as the hand or shoulder. Sometimes a brief squeeze or hug is appropriate. Prolonged hand-holding, strokes, cuddles and hugs are unwise.

VERBAL CUES

The information content of speech is very variable. Sometimes a lot of relevant information is given in a short time. Much more often, as can be seen if ordinary conversations are taped, bits of information come out, interspersed with apparently irrelevant comments, asides, stops and starts, deviations from the theme and returns to it.

Sounds indicative of pain, fatigue, boredom, frustration or confusion may also be made.

It seems that therapists have a well-developed ability to 'sift' this information and to select relevant from irrelevant items (Mattingly & Fleming 1994). However, this is not a simple matter of doggedly pursuing a subject and disregarding whatever else the patient may say. That could easily become inquisitorial. Therapists also pay attention to the 'subtext' of interaction. This includes both what is said, and what remains unsaid.

In ordinary social 'chat', people exchange the trivial details of their lives. They talk about shopping, holidays, families, events, likes and dislikes and opinions. The therapist uses this kind of non-threatening information-giving to provide a safe and familiar kind of social milieu in which to build rapport and develop a rounded picture of the client. Information about interests, attitudes and anxieties can be gathered. Equally, without undue disclosure, the therapist may respond with personal information of a similar kind, which may help to build a web of shared experiences.

Responses to verbal cues

Therapists respond to verbal cues in many ways:

- listening
- making a neutral non-verbal response
- mirroring content
- questioning; seeking information
- affirming
- valuing
- encouraging
- challenging
- comforting or reassuring
- using humour
- explaining or clarifying
- giving information
- suggesting action
- proposing a solution
- asking about wants or needs.

The therapist may decide to pursue a subject, or to pull away from it, to terminate or change an intervention or to take some other action.

It is remarkable that this amount of mental processing occurs so rapidly, and, usually, accurately, while a seamless flow of conversation is maintained.

BEHAVIOURAL CUES

Behaviour is anything a person does. It therefore combines actions, interactions and reactions. Behavioural cues affect relationships. Cues may be produced by constructive, neutral or destructive behaviour, and by lack of expected behaviour.

Simple behavioural cues

Simple behavioural cues often indicate attitudes and emotions, and can be valuable to the therapist in giving an indication of how the client is feeling.

Behaviour is learnt, and it is possible to learn to give unhelpful or inaccurate cues to interaction. For this reason, the significance of behavioural cues needs to be interpreted with care.

For example, in 'pain behaviour', which is a characteristic feature of chronic pain syndrome, the client may wince, grunt, adopt a noticeably awkward posture, make some kind of comment to draw attention to the pain, ostentatiously use a stick, splint or bandage, or take medication in an obvious manner.

These are normal behaviours learnt in response to pain which also act as a 'signal' to others that the sufferer is in discomfort, or needs sympathy. In chronic pain syndrome, they can become habitual and unhelpful.

While a few individuals may use these signals in a deliberate or manipulative manner, the client is more often unaware of using this type of behaviour or of its effect on relationships with others, which is often counterproductive.

Similarly, a person with a physical disability may learn protective behaviours such as 'nursing' a hand, or keeping weight off a leg which continue beyond the point when they are useful.

Occupational behaviour as a cue to interaction

Therapists are particularly concerned with the nature of occupational behaviour. One of the foundation assumptions of occupational therapy is that communication between people and the nature of relationships can be impeded or enhanced through shared occupational performance.

The therapist can use performance demand to enhance communication, by using an environment and activity which will promote social interaction, sharing information, problem-solving, expression of emotion, or whatever is seen as useful to the intervention.

ENVIRONMENTAL CUES

The demand of the environment is equally important, especially if the therapist wishes to facilitate the client's disclosure of personal matters.

A formal or highly clinical environment may constrain a relationship within the limiting boundaries of professional 'chart talk'.

An environment which is relaxed and informal may be too unstructured to facilitate focused attention on a specific topic.

The correct amount of light, the right position of chairs, tables and the therapist can greatly enhance communication.

These considerations are dealt with in more detail in Chapter 14.

BASIC COMMUNICATION SKILLS

Any person who works closely with others requires good communication skills: non-verbal, verbal, and written. Communication skills are triggered by the cues described above. For an occupational therapist the ability to communicate with clarity and in a variety of styles is fundamental; a poor communicator will fail as a therapist.

Therapists are well aware of the need to teach communication skills to clients, but they are not always so good at following basic rules of good communication themselves.

VERBAL COMMUNICATION

Verbal communication depends on providing information, listening to replies, and taking turns to speak. These are excellent examples of apparently simple skills being complex when one comes to analyse them.

Basic considerations include:

- the person being addressed
- the environment
- the speaker
- the context
- the content.

The person being addressed

When communicating with other professionals or with relatives or carers, the therapist needs to consider the needs and expectations of the listener and must use an appropriate style and language.

When communicating with clients, as well as the usual considerations of culture, age, role, and emotional state, it is important to consider less obvious aspects affecting communication.

Visual or auditory difficulties, perceptual or cognitive deficits, speech problems and speaking a language other than English all affect the ability of the individual to hear and respond.

The therapist must rapidly identify any problem and take action to compensate for this.

The environment

The place must be suited to the type, purpose and content of what is communicated (see Ch. 34).

In a more formal setting, the relationship of speaker and client to desk, table or chairs is also very important in setting the tone of the interchange.

The position of the therapist in relation to the source of light is important; light should illuminate the face of the speaker so that expression and lip movements can clearly be seen. Light which comes from behind obscures the face and may dazzle the client.

Distractions, visual and auditory, need to be minimized. If necessary, aids to communication such as writing material, magnifying aids or hearing aids, or translated phrases, should be available.

The speaker

It is essential that the therapist adopts the most appropriate position, posture and language for the situation. For example, when speaking briefly to a person in a wheelchair, a therapist will usually squat or kneel so that the therapist's face is level with that of the client. This prevents bad posture for both speakers and ensures that the therapist is communicating on an equal basis with the client. The therapist must not invade the client's space or territory (for example, sitting uninvited on a bed, or moving too close to someone standing).

Tone of voice is important. A monotonous delivery or mumble will fail to communicate effectively. Tone should reflect content, and also be aimed at provoking a response. A useful technique is deliberately to raise the tone of voice at regular intervals; television and radio presenters do this much of the time to add colour and emphasis to their delivery.

Avoid talking too much; allow the other person to have a turn and listen actively. Do not 'jump in' with a ready reply. Pauses are also important as emphasis, and to give time for assimilation of information.

Eye contact helps to engage the listener and indicates attention to what the client says.

The context

The context of the communication governs its style, length and purpose. It is essential to judge this match correctly as a mismatch (for example, being too informal; taking too long when the other person is in a hurry) condemns the exchange to failure.

The content

In most interactions, something is to be communicated. If this is an instruction, the speaker must be particularly careful to impart precise meaning.

It is important to choose language which is age-appropriate. It is for too easy, in an effort to explain simply, to 'dumb down' language and content in a condescending or patronizing manner. (A personal 'pet hate' when communicating with adults, is the use of the word 'little' as in 'I'd just like to have a little chat' or 'Let's go for a little walk'.)

Resist the temptation to 'know it all'. It is better to say 'I do not know, but I will find out' than to give erroneous information.

Devise and practise tactful methods of bringing an over-long conversation or discussion to a close

USING THE TELEPHONE

Since the telephone is such an integral part of life, it may seem strange to include notes on using it. However, it is alarming how often the basic rules for answering the phone, taking messages or contacting others are ignored, a fact which has prompted many health service employers to send their staff on 'customer care' courses to remind them of good practice.

When answering the phone, it is essential to:

- give your name and position
- ask for the other person's name and position
- write down any message; date it and sign it. Use a clean message pad (and ensure it gets to the right person, fast)
- obtain a phone number or address if a response is needed
- give your phone number or professional address
- avoid giving any confidential information unless you are totally certain that the caller is entitled to receive it (bogus callers do exist). If you do give sensitive information you must follow local policies (some employers prohibit giving any such information by phone)
- master the local system for transfering calls, holding, bleeping and using the 'secrecy' button.

When making a call, similar principles apply. Keep your communications clear and to the point; check that any message you want to give has been taken down; double check numbers for returning the call.

COUNSELLING

Counselling seems to have become an indispensable aid to modern life. Unfortunately, the term is much misused. Even more unfortunate is the variation in expertise in 'counsellors'. In the UK, a counsellor like a 'therapist' needs no more than the title and a suitable advertisement to be able to practise.

Counsellors include well-qualified professionals who have had a graduate training with an additional, comprehensive, carefully supervised diploma in counselling and, at the other extreme, the person who went on a 2- or 3-day counselling course (or read a book!).

Originally, 'to counsel' meant to give wise advice. It is important to recognize that in most forms of counselling giving advice, in the old sense of 'telling someone what to do', is usually avoided.

Counselling is an interaction between two people in which the counsellor acts as a facilitator to draw out from the client personal thoughts, feelings and perceptions about a situation. By exploring these, the client is encouraged to review meanings, explore options, and come to some conclusion about the future.

There are different forms of counselling based on differing psychotherapeutic theories and practices. Therapists who wish to develop skills as counsellors need to have additional post-basic training.

Basic counselling skills are, however, of value in many settings, and do form part of an occupational therapist's therapeutic use of self. In fact, these skills are used every time a therapist sits down with a client to discuss the goals of therapy and possible actions, particularly when a client-centred approach is in use.

It is essential to recognize the boundary between this type of informal use of counselling skills, and formal counselling. If an interaction is moving into 'deep waters' which are beyond the competence (or available time) of the therapist to deal with, the client must be tactfully advised to seek qualified help and assisted to do so if necessary.

BASIC COUNSELLING SKILLS
Active listening

The occupational therapist may well be the first person to have had time to listen to what the client wants to say and to allow space for the client to say it.

Active listening involves monitoring what is being said, remembering important points, and judging when, or if, to respond.

Active listening is accepting and non-judgemental. Perhaps the most important skill is the suppression of one's personal agenda and the desire to leap into the conversation with comments, solutions or advice. It is essential to avoid the trap of immediately relating the problem to one's personal experience. Silence may be more helpful than comment.

It may be necessary to facilitate the client to continue by an encouraging, attentive 'mmm' or 'uh-huh'. The listener must cultivate stillness and a listening body language, providing good eye contact, while avoiding fixing the client with a penetrating stare.

It is important, however, to remain peripherally aware of one's surroundings in relation to what is being said. Sometimes it may be better to move to a more private area to preserve confidentiality, even if it means breaking the flow.

Similarly, if time is genuinely limited or it is plain that the client has issues which need more detailed exploration, it may be necessary to draw the session tactfully to a close with a promise of another if the client would like this. Even if under pressure of time, it is important not to give the client the impression that you are eager to go, since this may well cut off the desire to communicate.

Active listening is part of 'getting clients to tell their story': 'storytelling' is being explored by occupational scientists and practitioners as a valuable therapeutic tool (see Mattingly & Fleming 1994, Kielhofner 1995).

Reflecting

A frequently used counselling technique is verbally to reflect back to the client something which the client has said. This needs to be done with discretion, and not simply parrot fashion.

In counselling, the purpose of reflection is to draw the client's attention to something. This may be the recognition of personal meaning, or an emotion, or the significance of an experience.

Reflection is also used to mirror feelings or thoughts which appear as a subtext in the conversation. For example, if a woman constantly refers to the death of her husband, even though this happened 5 years ago, the therapist might say 'The loss of your husband still seems very fresh to you.' or 'It sounds as if you still miss your husband very much.' It is important, however, not to slip too far into 'counselling mode' unless the setting and circumstances are truly apropriate.

It takes much practice to acquire this skill at more than basic level, and it is better not to attempt it unless one feels reasonably secure in doing so.

It is probably easier to restrict reflection to clarification of statements by making comments which pick up either an obvious subtext such as 'It sounds as though you are really angry about this' or actual words 'You feel trapped?'

Moving towards action

Occupational therapy is essentially a process of active engagement and problem-solving. Some forms of counselling are not really compatible with this approach.

Having given sufficient time, possibly on more than one occasion, to explore the client's perceptions of a situation, the therapist will want to facilitate some kind of action from the client.

This process of facilitation has to achieve a difficult balancing act between 'telling the client what to do' and allowing the client to drift along without any real change or outcome. Occupational therapists often take a problem-based approach.

The therapist has to encourage the client to:

- formulate a statement of the problem
- recognize whether or not the client wants to act (and if there is potential for change, or whether action must be by personal adaptation rather than practical problem-solving)
- summarize the available options for action
- decide on priorities and set goals
- formulate an action plan.

It is essential that these stages are carried out by the client, in the client's', own words, but the therapist can provide information, and help the client to 'see the wood for the trees' by listening and reflecting.

It may rapidly become obvious that this approach is inappropriate or that the client requires much more time and more skilled help than the therapist can provide, and in this case the possibility of referral to a well-qualified counsellor needs to considered.

INTERACTION DURING TREATMENT

As reported in detail by Mattingly & Fleming (1994), therapists continually interact with their patients during one-to-one treatment sessions.

These interactions take the form of brief comments, questions, responses, informal 'chat' and snippets of information woven into the process of occupational performance or during gaps or rests.

Mattingly & Fleming propose that these informal interactions are a valuable, and under-rated, part of therapy. They give many examples from transcripts of therapists' conversations with patients which illustrate that such interactions have many functions, for example:

- maintaining rapport and emphasizing the individuality of the client:
  - asking about things client has recently done
  - asking about friends, pets or family
  - talking about recent sporting events
  - discussing topics of mutual interest

- teaching:
  - explaining what is to be done, why and how
  - motivating effort
  - prompting, shaping and reinforcing behaviour
  - giving praise or a social reward

- providing therapy:
  - keeping the session 'on track', i.e. focused on goals
  - checking progress, and making the patient aware of it
  - reminding of precautions or indicating hazards
  - relating treatment to goals or 'real-life' situations
  - distracting from effort or discomfort
  - monitoring comfort, checking for distress
  - testing for client's reactions or perceptions
  - provoking a change of mood, especially laughter
  - reassuring
  - building confidence.

ACQUIRING GOOD INTERACTIVE SKILLS

Students need to observe experienced therapists at work in order to analyse the content and purpose of interaction.

It also helps to listen out for the 'clanger' – the wrong thing said at the wrong time – and to try to understand what went wrong.

The student must acquire the ability to think over interactions, re-examine them critically in order to extract information and continually assess personal performance. Above all, the student needs to seek and be receptive to constructive comment from others.

14

Interviewing

INTERVIEWING STYLES

Interviewing is widely used by a variety of people. Health service workers, police, journalists, salespeople, researchers and managers all conduct interviews. With this variation in setting and context there are, naturally, numerous styles and techniques for conducting interviews some of which are totally inappropriate for occupational therapists.

Interviews may be formal or informal, and structured, semi-structured or unstructured. Approaches range from friendly and disarming, to stress-provoking, adversarial and confrontational.

Whatever the style, the fundamental purpose of an interview is for one person to obtain information from another.

OCCUPATIONAL THERAPY INTERVIEWS

In this chapter, we are concerned with interviews as used by occupational therapists with their clients, or client's relatives or carers. The most important interview is usually the *initial interview* which is the first contact of the therapist with the client. The style of this interview sets the tone for the entire intervention.

During the initial interview, the therapist seeks information on which to base the intervention and begins the process of evaluation. The client provides information and may also seek it. A dialogue develops.

Neistadt (1998) lists the purposes of interviewing as: understanding the client's story; building the therapeutic alliance; gathering information; observing behaviour; clarifying your role in the client's treatment (or intervention); establishing priorities for intervention.

As therapy proceeds, an interview may serve to explore or discuss progress, set aims, define and solve problems, or terminate intervention.

STRUCTURES FOR AN OCCUPATIONAL THERAPY INTERVIEW

STRUCTURED INTERVIEW

In a *structured* interview, the format is fixed and must be followed to the letter using set questions in a designated order. Standardized assessments often use a structured interview format.

Information is always recorded at the time, either on a form, or using a tape-recorder.

SEMI-STRUCTURED INTERVIEW

In occupational therapy, an interview is usually *semi-structured*. This means that there is a purpose to the questions which may follow a predetermined format, although not necessarily a set sequence. The therapist may choose the way questions are worded, and vary the timing and content as required.

The information collected is usually written down, either at the time, or later, often using some kind of checklist, chart or form as an aid to questioning and recording. This is useful, especially for inexperienced therapists, and as a means of keeping 'on track' but rigid adherence to a formula can limit the scope of the interview.

The experienced therapist often has a mental 'script' – more probably a whole series of scripts – which the therapist can use to elicit information.

As the client responds, a new script may be selected in order to pursue useful information, or verify an assumption. This use of scripts is largely automatic (although it involves rapid interactive reasoning); the therapist often 'changes script' in response to a situation without being consciously aware of doing so.

The therapist simultaneously seeks information, evaluates it, makes matches with known patterns, or identifies gaps, and then seeks more information. The therapist must judge when to pursue information, when to pull back, when to change tack, and, very importantly, when to bring the interview to a close.

This skill can only be developed with time and much practice; the novice therapist is likely to follow a more stereotyped formula.

UNSTRUCTURED INTERVIEW

In an *unstructured* interview, there is a general purpose but no predetermined set of questions or topics. The interviewer facilitates the discussion with some 'trigger' question and then explores topics which occur as the conversation progresses. The interviewer may record the whole interview for later analysis, or may jot down notes either at the time or later.

THE SEMI-STRUCTURED OCCUPATIONAL THERAPY INTERVIEW

DURATION OF THE INTERVIEW

The duration of an interview is variable. It is probably not possible to get useful information in less than 10 minutes. On the other hand, an interview which lasts more than an hour is likely to become very tiring, repetitive and unproductive. It may be necessary to gently bring the interview back on track if 'red herrings' begin to intrude.

It is often helpful to make it clear to the client at the beginning how long you can spend with the client; and, if necessary, this may form an explicit contract.

SETTING UP THE INTERVIEW ENVIRONMENT

Having the right environment is crucial for a successful interview. Ways of setting out an environment for an interview are described in

Chapter 34. The environment determines whether the interview is formal or informal. A formal environment tends to make for a structured interview, whereas informal surroundings facilitate a less structured approach.

A formal interview is usually conducted in a private room where the interviewer will probably sit at a desk or table with the interviewee positioned on the other side of it, or at some distance from the interviewer.

An informal interview may happen almost anywhere, within the limits of maintaining confidentiality and minimizing disturbance or distraction. The interviewer usually tries to be adjacent to the interviewee and to minimize barriers between them.

Initial interviews are usually semi-structured and take place in a quiet, private, but informal area.

PREPARATION FOR THE INTERVIEW

The therapist needs to have a clear idea of the purpose, style and format of the interview before it begins. A certain amount of preliminary briefing is desirable as an interview which is conducted 'cold' is less likely to be satisfactory.

STAGES IN A SEMI-STRUCTURED INITIAL INTERVIEW

An interview needs to be prefaced with a short period of social interaction to set the client at ease after which the interview usually follows a pattern.

The interview begins with an introduction and explanation either of what the client wants from the therapist and/or of what the occupational therapist is concerned with and why the interview is required. An explanation of what occupational therapy involves and how the client may benefit from it is usually required. The client should be informed about confidentiality and told whether or not what the client says will be written down.

A businesslike 'question and answer session' follows, during which information is exchanged and explored.

Usually, the interview finishes with a summary of what has been covered, possibly recalling the main issues and clarifying goals or actions if these have been identified. It is important that the client is left with a clear understanding of what the next step will be and who is responsible for taking any action. If required, a date for another meeting should be set.

Once the necessary information has been exchanged, a winding down and closing section is needed to end the interview, perhaps lightened with some social interaction.

INTERVIEWING SKILLS

The foundation skills for conducting an interview are the basic communication skills required for any dyadic interaction. Neistadt (1998) lists: preparing, questioning, responding, attending and observing; listening. The most important of these are active listening and accurate, structured observation (see Ch. 18).

In addition, a number of specific competencies are needed, including:

- prompting and facilitating information-giving
- keeping the interview 'on track'
- recording information.

PROMPTING AND FACILITATING INFORMATION-GIVING

Evaluating the client's communication skills

It is, of course, necessary to discover at an early stage whether the client is able to understand what is being said and whether the client is likely to be able to answer questions reliably.

An unobtrusive way to discover if the client can hear and understand you, and whether the client is well orientated is to apparently check a piece of routine personal information, giving an incorrect item as you do so (for example, the wrong house number or street name). Most people will quickly correct the error; if it is not spotted, the therapist is prompted to investigate further.

Asking for the facts

Much of an initial interview is likely to be concerned with obtaining basic information about the client by going through the usual routine of name, age, address, type of home, occupation and recent history.

The therapist should make every effort to have obtained all available information from existing sources before the interview. This can then be checked and expanded rather than repeated. It is intensely irritating to the client to have a series of professionals asking the same set of questions over and over again, and it also gives the impression (all too often correct!) that those concerned do not communicate.

It is helpful to start by explaining to the client why additional information is needed. Questions should be brief and to the point, but asked in a relaxed manner which avoids any impression of 'interrogation'.

To keep you, and the client, on track, it may help if information is repeated after it is given, or as it is recorded, which can serve both as a confirmation that you have heard it correctly and as a lead into the next question.

Thus the client says 'I live in a bungalow' and the therapist repeats while writing the answer down 'A bungalow, right... have you been there long?' Over-use of this technique is tedious, however, and should be avoided.

Obtaining a history

The therapist may be interested in the client's recent or past medical history, but is more likely to be interested in the 'occupational history' or 'life story' of the client.

Usually, questions of the 'who, what, where, how, how often, when,' type are enough to elicit a history. The therapist will probably need to explore some answers, seeking clarification or more information. Prompts such as 'That's interesting', 'Tell me more about...' and 'And after that?' can be used to steer the conversation in the desired direction. Sensitivity and tact are needed to discuss private and personal matters.

In complex cases, there is unlikely to be time during a first interview to take a comprehensive history so if this is needed another interview can be arranged for the purpose. This also allows some time for development of rapport and trust. Although health-care settings promote disclosure, it is unlikely that a client will be willing to confide in someone the client has only just met.

Closed questions and open questions

There are different ways of posing interview questions. *Closed* questions seek definite, factual information or positive or negative answers. *Open* questions elicit subjective material such as feelings, opinions or values.

Open questions are more difficult to frame because of the problems which can be caused by phrasing the question in a way which makes a particular response more likely, or 'puts words into' the respondent's mouth.

The phenomenon of the 'leading question' is well recognized in courts of law, where a judge must be vigilant in preventing a barrister from phrasing a question in a way which ensures that a particular response is produced. (For example 'Was that when the accused hit you?' rather than 'What happened next?')

In high profile cases of 'satanic' child abuse in the UK in the early 1990s, there was much criticism of the way in which children were interviewed and asked leading questions.

Thus, in an occupational therapy interview, 'How does that make you feel?' is an open question which permits all responses. 'Does that make you feel angry or sad?' directs the respondent away from other possible feelings.

As the interview develops, the therapist may become aware of themes in the conversation which may need to be explored later, or which give an insight into circumstances in the client's life. These can be returned to on a subsequent occasion.

KEEPING 'ON TRACK'

It sometimes begins to feel as if there are only two kinds of clients, those who hardly say anything, from whom information has to be prised a piece at a time, and those who, once started, never stop.

To some extent, the therapist has to accept that clients will (or will not) tell their stories in their own way, be it fast or slow, to the point or rambling. If there is time, it is better to listen to the client and to conform to the client's style, rather than being over-directive, but unfortunately time is not always available.

'Starting and stopping' clients in a tactful manner takes a good deal of practice. It does help to explain the purpose of the interview and to give some indication of the time available at the start. It is then more acceptable to gently terminate a long description and bring matters 'back to business'.

RECORDING INFORMATION

Memory is fallible, and although therapists can, with practice, develop a remarkable facility for recalling conversations and mentally 'replaying' them, it is usually necessary to record the information gained, either at the time, or shortly afterwards. Take time to explain to the client what you need to record and why, and, if necessary, who should have access to it.

When taking notes of an interview, it may be helpful to distinguish between the subjective material (personal feelings, opinions or experiences) and objective material (facts) which have been obtained. It is also important to separate interview material (what was said) from observations by the therapist (what happened, what was seen) and interpretations of that material (what it may mean).

DISCLOSURE OF INFORMATION

All information given to the therapist during an interview is confidential and the explicit agreement of the client must be obtained if it is to be given to others. If the therapist is working as a team member, it is helpful to explain to the client at the outset that the information given will be shared with team members, and to check that this is acceptable in specific instances.

For example, if the client tells the therapist about some symptom or circumstance which the doctor ought to know about, the therapist might say 'I think Dr Blank should know about this. Is it all right if I tell him?' or alternatively, 'I really think you should tell Dr Blank about this at the next ward round, or would you rather that I did?'

During an interview, a client may occasionally disclose to the therapist confidential information which is of a sensitive nature or indicative of some kind of risk which cannot be ignored, for example, a confession of having done something illegal, or the intention to harm self or others.

This can place the therapist in an acute, ethical dilemma. There are usually local policies about disclosure and confidentiality and the therapist working in areas of practice where this is likely to be a problem needs to know how to handle the situation. To prevent conflict between confidentiality and legitimate disclosure, the client must 'know the rules' before the interview starts.

DEALING WITH VERBAL AGGRESSION

Aggressive behaviour is intended to alarm, to exert control or to draw attention. There are many reasons for clients to become aggressive during an interview and the therapist needs to understand the psychological mechanisms which underlie aggressive behaviour and the best ways of dealing with aggression.

Like all others forms of behaviour, aggression is a learnt response. Some people behave aggressively much of the time, even when they are not particularly angry. These clients may benefit from an anger management course which teaches them to recognize how unproductive anger is, and to use coping strategies to reduce confrontation.

Aggression tends to provoke a 'fight or flight' response in others; personal responses vary, and therapists may need to learn coping strategies in order to control their own reactions in difficult situations. Aggressive clients are now so common that many health care facilities provide courses for staff in how to deal with them.

The therapist needs to be able to distinguish between aggression which is fundamentally rational, in that it can be tracked back to a real external cause, and that which is irrational, stemming from some kind of psychological disorder or delusion, or the effects of a drug or alcohol.

Irrational aggression requires skilful handling. Therapists who work in units where aggressive or violent behaviour may be anticipated require special training in appropriate management techniques.

In a normal interview setting, anger is usually provoked by a situation which the client perceives as unjust, threatening, or in some way infringing the client's rights.

In this situation, prevention is the best strategy; it is usually possible to see that a client is becoming angry and to steer away from this, unless for some therapeutic reason it will be helpful to look at the situation. In that case it may be better to attempt to discover the underlying problem before emotions get out of hand. Anger often arises because of lack of information and misunderstandings. Good eye contact and taking time to give simple explanations may be all that is needed.

Aggressive behaviour with a fundamentally rational basis can usually be defused by a calm and assertive response. Clients need to 'have their say'. The therapist should listen attentively but noncommittally avoid making either emotional or verbal responses until the outburst is over.

While the client is angry, it is wise to avoid disputing facts or perceptions, or becoming defensive (which will almost certainly fuel an argument), or giving apologies, or attempting to 'smooth things over' (which is likely to be interpreted as condescending or patronizing). It is also essential not to promise action unless it will be taken.

If possible, once the client has 'exploded', a problem-solving approach should be adopted, recognizing the anger, identifying exactly what the problem is, what the client wants to do about it, and what action can be taken, either by the therapist or someone else. If nothing can be done, this should be stated explicitly, giving the reasons.

If the time is not right for problem-solving, it is better to acknowledge that fact but to leave the client with the offer of looking at the situation again if the client wishes. It is important for the client to know that 'the door is open'.

While the therapist does need to have a high tolerance for angry behaviour, the therapist is entitled to respect and conventional politeness. If a client repeatedly offers verbal abuse, the therapist needs to make it clear that being subjected to this is not part of the 'therapeutic alliance'. If the client really wants the therapist's assistance, some degree of mutual respect is required and a contract to this effect may need to be made if intervention is to continue (O'Neil 1995a,b).

15 Working with groups

DIFFERENT TYPES OF GROUP WORK

The term 'group work' is often associated with mental health settings, although groups can be used with clients with a variety of needs. There are several types of group, each with a different structure, purpose and process.

All group work requires advanced use of interactive skills and therapeutic use of self.

PSYCHOTHERAPY GROUP

Groups of this kind are used to enable the client to explore personal feelings, reactions, experiences, conflicts or self-perceptions in a safe and supportive environment.

A psychotherapeutic group may or may not have a specific 'task', and may sometimes use projective media such as drama or art; more often these groups are primarily verbal.

These 'talking therapy groups' need to be distinguished from occupational therapy activity groups, educational groups, and also from more general diversional, social or recreational groups which have no specific therapeutic purpose.

Group work is widely accepted as a powerful therapeutic tool in mental health settings. A functioning group is far more than the sum of its parts and the dynamics of group behaviour are extremely complex. The occupational therapist requires additional training before leading or facilitating a psychotherapy group.

There are many styles of therapeutic group work – for example, analytical, cognitive, client-centred, developmental – and various group leadership styles and techniques. Numerous books have been written about group theory, group processes and the specific skills needed to manage or facilitate group work. These skills are not, however, uniquely 'OT skills'. They are employed by a range of health care professionals.

In view of the numerous specialist texts already available these will not be dealt with in detail in this book. An overview of occupational therapy theory and practice in group work and creative therapy is given in Willson (1996) and Creek (1997). Other references are given at the end of this chapter.

EDUCATIONAL GROUP

The main purpose of an educational group is, naturally, to teach something to the participants. This may be some aspect of daily living, a health-related topic, or a specific set of skills such as anxiety management or relaxation.

Distinctions between educational groups and activity groups do tend to blur; it is a matter of where the emphasis is placed when the aim of the group is specified.

In an educational group, the emphasis is on 'knowing more' or 'knowing how and why', or on practising some new skill, whereas in an activity group the emphasis is on 'being involved in doing something'. Adult educational groups are described in Chapter 16.

DIVERSIONAL OR RECREATIONAL GROUP

A diversional or recreational group may be organized by a member of staff, a volunteer or the clients. In a group of this kind there is no subtext. The aim is simply to participate in and enjoy the activity.

This may well be 'therapeutic' in the general sense, but it does not require an occupational therapist to run this kind of group, simply a person who is a reliable organizer with a lot of common sense and the skills to 'get the group going'.

This kind of group may engage participants in hobbies, creative activities, special interests such as gardening or music, or games, sports or recreational activities.

ACTIVITY GROUP

In an *activity group*, the therapist seeks to involve a number of people simultaneously in one or more productive, creative or social tasks or activities for a specific therapeutic purpose.

An activity group can be used with clients in a mental health setting, with older people, people with physical disabilities, or people with learning disabilities.

To manage an activity group the occupational therapist must unite all of the primary core skills of practice, assessment, environmental adaptation, occupational adaptation and therapeutic use of self.

ASPECTS OF AN ACTIVITY GROUP

An activity group has three aspects: purpose, process and product.

The *purpose* of the group is its overt reason for existence; this is explicitly therapeutic. The clients should normally be aware of the general purpose, although this is sometimes 'buried' as a subtext within a more general statement of what the group is going to do.

Process includes the experience of the group session, the interactions, actions, and reactions of members with each other and with the therapist in the course of engagement in the activity. It is through the process of engagement in the group that individuals work towards therapeutic objectives.

Product is the overt and observable outcome. Products may include things which are made, but also include completed shared experiences, decisions or solutions to problems.

The therapist may wish to focus on purpose, process or on product, or may decide to combine aspects of the three. The degree to which the clients and the therapist share awareness of these focuses is likely to differ, especially at the beginning of a group.

The presence of a therapeutic subtext of which participants are unaware may sometimes be necessary if the group is to be effective. For example, while most group activities intrinsically have a high demand for social and communication skills, it may well be inhibiting for a group member to be told 'This group is to help you to communicate better with others'. It may be better for that person to enjoy the social aspects of the group, and then later be encouraged to see how it helped to improve personal skills.

GROUP STRUCTURES

Any situation where three or more people are involved in an activity may be regarded as 'group work'; a group does, however, need a viable number to function.

There appears to be a kind of 'critical mass' for a group, which varies somewhat depending on the nature of the activity. Too small a number of participants may make them feel over-exposed and vulnerable; dominant individuals can take over or participants may fail to operate as a group. On the other hand, large groups can become hard to manage, and the opportunity for specific therapeutic work is reduced.

Therapeutic activity groups typically occur on a regular basis over a period of time. This permits relationships and roles to develop and allows for development of the activity as well.

Groups may be ongoing, with new members coming and old ones leaving, or be set to run for a predetermined number of sessions. Continuing groups allow for development and progression, both in terms of interpersonal dynamics and the challenges of the activity. As with psychotherapy groups, membership may be open to allcomers, or closed, involving a defined number of participants who all attend for a designated number of sessions.

TYPES OF ACTIVITY GROUPS

Mixed group

A mixed group consists of individuals who have differing needs and goals but who, for practical or therapeutic reasons, are brought together as a group. The needs of the group are usually compatible, but they are viewed as individuals who happen to occupy the same space for the duration of the group.

Members of the group will engage in various tasks of benefit to themselves, which relate to an individual goal, in the company of others who are similarly engaged. Each group member may work on a different project, or on part of a shared project. The group contributes advantages of scale, effectiveness or social contact which benefit all participants but it does not really function as a group in the accepted sense.

This kind of group is a useful way of introducing people to working with others before they are ready to participate in a more integrated type of group.

Productive or creative task-orientated groups, project groups and social groups can all be structured for mixed ability clients.

Homogenous group

This is a group of people who have similar goals and needs. They are brought together explicitly to share a set of activities or experiences. The needs of the individual are, in this setting, somewhat subordinate to the needs of the group.

In a homogenous group, the 'subtext' may be much more important than the text. What is happening is likely to be a vehicle for shared learning of some kind, or the exploration of themes, meaning or experiences, rather than an end in itself.

This subtlety of intention may or may not be explicit for group members, but it will certainly be explicit in the mind of the therapist, who will design the activities and environment to contribute to the intended goal.

Client-led activity group

In both of the above groups, the degree to which the therapist or the participants take charge of the organization of the activity is variable, and depends on the needs and aims of the group.

In some settings, however, clients may be encouraged to select and run their own activities or events without the intervention of the therapist. Usually, these are of a social, recreational or creative nature.

The therapist acts as facilitator and resource person, and the participants run the activity. The therapist may, or may not, be invited to attend or participate.

Some client-led groups are run 'just for fun'. There is absolutely nothing wrong with this, and there will be some peripheral 'therapeutic' gains along the way. It would be a somewhat grim unit which focused on 'therapy' 24 hours a day. (They do exist, and they are very exhausting for all concerned.)

At other times, the therapist works to 'engineer' the client-led group because of gains for the participants in terms of personal organization, leadership skills, communication and self-esteem.

MOSEY'S CLASSIFICATION OF ACTIVITY GROUPS

Ann Cronin Mosey gives a very comprehensive account of group dynamics, group skills and types of group (Mosey 1986). She proposes that, in the context of mental health practice, there are six major categories of activity groups, some of which can be subdivided.

Linking with her models of practice, Mosey takes a developmental perspective, designing groups for patients with differing levels of interpersonal and communication skills.

Mosey differentiates between activity groups and verbal therapy groups by the emphasis placed on the components; in the activity group, the activity is central, the group is concerned with the 'here and now' and the focus is narrow. In the verbal group, there may be no focus on activity, the group is concerned with 'then and there' and has a more general focus. This is, perhaps, a generalization, but the immediacy of experience in an activity group is certainly a key feature.

She describes various types of activity groups (Box 15.1; descriptions in quotation marks are taken from Mosey's text).

Allen (1985) also describes a developmental approach to organizing activity groups using craft-work, based on her theories about cognitive function in people with mental disorders or dementia. Allen's approach is based on very careful analysis of task and environment and will be referred to in other Sections.

Box 15.1	Types of activity group
Evaluative group	To assess aspects of client performance or ability to function in a group setting.
Task-oriented group	'Designed to help members to become aware of their needs, values, ideas and feelings as they influence action.'
Developmental group	Meeting the needs of clients at different developmental levels of social skill (six types are described).
Thematic group	'Focus on gaining knowledge, skills and attitudes necessary for mastery of performance components and specific occupational performances.'
Topical group	'A discussion group that focuses on participation in activities which take place outside the group' – this may involve anticipated activities or those which are currently taking place.
Instrumental group	Meeting health needs and maintaining function and well-being.

Both Mosey and Allen emphasize the importance of detailed planning and structuring of activity groups in order to achieve specific aims for group members.

ACTIVITY GROUPS IN RELATION TO OCCUPATIONAL LEVELS

Developmental level

At this level, the group activity is designed, modified and led by the therapist. Group choices are limited to within carefully controlled parameters which meet therapeutic requirements and reflect the abilities of those involved to make choices.

The therapist is mainly concerned with the development of skills. A group setting is often chosen to promote social and communication skills, but the whole spectrum of physical and cognitive skills may also be practised.

As already noted, the therapist needs to spend considerable time analysing the task sequence demand and the environmental demand, and presenting tasks in a manner which will best promote learning and motivate participation.

Ideally, a developmental group should be small, no more than four to eight people, depending on level of ability and number of staff available. Clients often need close supervision and one-to-one attention to get the most from the group.

Effective level

Most of the groups which have been described above fit best into this level where a rich experience of participation can be provided.

At this level, situational meanings, complex relationships and realistic problem-solving come into play.

Practical aspects of organizing activity groups are described in Chapter 34.

'FLOW' AND 'JAMMING' AS A GROUP EXPERIENCE

Groups, especially in mental health practice, often seem aimed at promoting self-disclosure and examination of personal experiences. These things are, of course, valuable. They also tend to be threatening and uncomfortable.

An activity may provide a means of prompting such disclosure in a more relaxed and comfortable setting but occupational therapists recognize that shared engagement in activity *without* disclosure can also be valuable.

'Flow' is the expression used by Csikzentmihali to describe the kind of focused engagement in which a person becomes totally absorbed in an occupation and loses awareness of self and the passage of time. Flow is deeply satisfying and rewarding. It occurs when the challenges of the occupation are sufficient to stimulate response, but not so great that they become stressful.

Flow is usually described as an individual, perhaps solitary experience, because awareness of others is limited by the total absorption in doing and being. However, some of the elements of flow can be experienced during group activity when the whole group is engaged in what is going on to the extent that they are unaware of external surroundings and events.

The ultimate expression of flow as a group experience has been called 'jamming' – a term derived from jazz musicians who come together to play in a spontaneous manner. Jamming is:

> fluid behavioural co-ordination that occurs without detailed knowledge of personality. Satisfaction comes simply from acting together. It is unhindered by expectations of self revelation. Meaning is co-constructed in social interaction. Personal control is surrendered in the experience of doing. Jamming creates a transcendent experience between people who would not normally communicate with each other.
>
> *Clark (1997)*

Activities which promote jamming are typically highly structured, governed by rules and depend on physical skill, so that little or no personal information needs to be exchanged. Anyone can join in.

Musical performances, mime, games and sports, and some forms of non-verbal creative activities may promote jamming, but it is a rare and elusive experience which is very difficult to create deliberately and artificially.

A group which has had a jamming session tends to form a strong bond as a result, even when the members are very disparate. It may be that people who combine to deal with a disaster, such as digging survivors from a crash or earthquake, develop a sense of comradeship through an extreme (and, in this case, traumatic) version of jamming.

These theories are being explored as part of the developing area of enquiry of occupational science. They are useful in giving a basis for the long-held assumption that group activities which bring people together in a shared, enjoyable, absorbing, experience are valuable in a special way which relates to the nature of the experience, rather than because of the content, product, or overt learning which may take place.

BASIC SKILLS FOR RUNNING ACTIVITY GROUPS

In addition to knowledge of group theory and the usual repertoire of personal communication skills, the therapist needs the following specific skills:

- a repertoire of skills in a variety of creative, recreational or social activities
- organization and planning
- a repertoire of leadership styles
- the ability to motivate participation and 'sell' the activity
- the ability to monitor the activity as it happens in order to exploit opportunities to increase therapeutic benefit
- the ability to judge how best to involve each individual as a member of the group
- the ability to foster group cohesion and to get the group to 'work'.

A REPERTOIRE OF PERSONAL SKILLS

In order to engage others in an activity, one needs to know how to do it, at least at a basic level. Although it is not necessary to be 'an expert', therapists cannot undertake the essential activity analysis and therapeutic adaptation, or teach clients how to do an unfamiliar task, without knowing how to do it themselves.

It is possible to compensate for lack of knowledge by employing a specialist to do the teaching, but the therapist still needs to understand and analyse what is going on.

ORGANIZATION AND PLANNING

A therapeutic activity group does not 'just happen'. The amount of planning and organization required is usually considerable and even if the practicalities can be delegated, the therapist must keep in control in order to ensure that the therapeutic objectives are achieved. Some of the aspects which need to be considered are described in Chapter 34.

A REPERTOIRE OF LEADERSHIP STYLES

Many texts deal with group leadership styles. In the context of an activity group, the therapist is normally the organizer or provider and acts as 'resource person' as the activity takes place.

The group may need a directive style in which the therapist 'takes charge' and takes total responsibility for the activity, or the therapist may act as facilitator, enabling clients to do what is needed to move the activity along.

Quite often the therapist needs to move imperceptibly from being directive to passing control to the clients.

THE ABILITY TO MOTIVATE PARTICIPATION

The degree of motivation with which clients will approach a new activity is very variable.

Any unfamiliar environment in which one must encounter a number of new people provokes a degree of anxiety in all but the most self-assured. Add to that uncertain expectations of what one is to be asked to do and whether one will be able to do it, and it is unsurprising that many clients' attitudes to an activity group are less than enthusiastic.

The therapist needs to get past these barriers in order to promote engagement. There are a number of ways of doing this, some overt, others subtle.

Frequently, the therapist must be prepared to 'put on an act' in order to gain attention and engender enthusiasm. Personal enthusiasm is catching; even if the activity is not a personal favourite, acting as if it is often convinces others to give it a try.

THE ABILITY TO EXPLOIT THERAPEUTIC OPPORTUNITIES

The activity has a therapeutic aim, for the group as a whole and for individuals within it.

The therapist must pay continuous focused attention to what is going on in order to 'seize the moment' and take advantage of it. Each experience or event, whether positive or negative, may have potential to be exploited for therapeutic gain. Sometimes this is done overtly, at other times it must be achieved more subtly, but it must take place, otherwise the activity group will become a pleasant, but unspecific, diversion.

In order to achieve this aim, the therapist may, for example:

- draw attention to an event, either at the time or when reflecting on the process
- create or exploit opportunities to practise previously specified skills or to provide information
- make connections between events and the successful use of skill or knowledge
- ask 'loaded' questions in order to prompt a desired response
- praise behaviour which provides a good role model
- ask the group to say what worked and why, or how something could have been done differently to produce a better result
- use difficulties as a basis for group problem-solving
- Draw attention to group achievements.

It is important for the therapist to remain honest and authentic in this process; it is not therapeutic to 'over-engineer' the group, or to pretend to the group that things have been successful when they have not.

THE ABILITY TO INVOLVE EACH INDIVIDUAL

Individuals have many roles or functions in group settings. The therapist may want to provide the opportunity for someone to lead, or follow, initiate, problem-solve, 'gate-keep', share or co-operate.

There may be individual aims such as 'improve verbal communication'; 'increase attention span'; 'encourage client to walk unaided'.

Task analysis of the activity will show the therapist which stages will offer most scope for practising these skills. The therapist will try to ensure the appropriate client performs the relevant part of the task.

THE ABILITY TO FOSTER GROUP COHESION

If one is fortunate, a group can 'gel' very quickly; the simple fact of bringing people together to work on a shared project rapidly produces a sense of group identity and common purpose. This is one of the chief benefits of using an activity as a focus for the group.

Most groups take a while to form and to establish a group culture and some common expectations, and time must be allowed for this. The process of co-operatively planning an activity facilitates the transition from this stage to one where the group begins to work together.

Fostering group identity in the early stages can be assisted by social introductions, provision of a welcoming, safe atmosphere, and use of simple 'warm-ups' to get things going.

It is well-known, however, that groups go through stages (variously described by theorists) before they 'perform' and some groups get 'stuck' at an early stage and never get to the point of becoming a functioning group.

In the context of a particular group this may or may not matter. If it is important that the group does move on, the therapist must analyse why it is stuck and see if anything can be done to provoke movement.

Given that many clients who attend occupational therapy groups do so precisely because they do not have good group skills, it is a tribute to therapists that activity groups do work more often than not.

TEAMWORK

A team is a group. This fact ought to be self-evident, yet, oddly, therapists and other health professionals who have excellent group skills when it comes to dealing with clients often fail to transfer these into use when working within a team.

Effective teamwork requires good management and leadership, and an understanding of the roles of team members. The theory and skills of team building are more often dealt with in management textbooks than in those on therapy.

For example, Mullins (1993) provides a comprehensive description of the eseential issues concerning the nature of groups, group processes and behaviour and the function of leaders. Every therapist should understand these issues as they influence both managerial and clinical aspects of practice.

Reasons why teams succeed or fail are complex. They stem from organizational issues, such as failure to understand the structure, function and aims of the team, leadership problems, personality issues, and the built-in 'traps' of team dynamics and group decision-taking.

One of the most frequent causes of conflict or ineffective team work is that no-one took the time to detach the team from its immediate concerns for long enough to establish common goals, understandings and theoretical framework for practice.

People from different professions bring a richness of knowledge and experience to teamwork which can be invaluable; they also bring the potential for misunderstandings, incompatible approaches or expectations and conflicts over roles.

'Time out' for team building is not a luxury. Management teams now recognize this and spend 'away days' on team building and defining mutual aims and styles of working. Clinical teams should be offered the chance to do the same.

FURTHER READING

Bernard P 1996 Acquiring interpersonal skills: a handbook of experiential learning for health professionals, 2nd edn. Chapman and Hall, London

Cole M B 1998 Group dynamics in occupational therapy: the theoretical basis and practical application of group treatment, 2nd edn. Slack, NJ

Finlay L 1997 The practice of psychosocial occupational therapy, 2nd edn. Stanley Thomas, Cheltenham

Wondrake R 1998 Interpersonal skills for nurses and health care professionals. Blackwell Science, Oxford

16 Teaching

THEORIES OF LEARNING

Much of what an occupational therapist does involves helping an individual to learn. In order to do this, the therapist must understand the processes by which people learn, and the best means of enabling them to do so.

'Learning' has been variously defined and learning theory is complex. As summarized in Chapter 10, there are several models to explain learning: developmental, behavioural, cognitive, social, person-centred. Humans learn in many ways and develop individual styles of learning. The therapist should have a good understanding of these models and their approaches.

Learning theories provide different explanations of the degree to which a person can be 'made to learn', and the manner in which the teacher can act to assist learning to happen. This ranges from the inevitability of behavioural conditioning, through the experiential interactions between person and environment, to the humanistic theories concerning learning as a self-directed process of personal development and the making of meaning.

In the context of therapy, learning may mean:

- gaining information or understanding
- acquiring skill
- changing the way things are valued
- problem-solving.

The speed of learning is also highly variable. Sometimes there is an instantaneous insightful 'click' as something is understood. More often, especially in the case of skill acquisition, but also where attitudinal or cognitive change is taking place, there is a step-like progression until eventually the learning curve flattens out. While learning requires a degree of challenge, pushing clients to learn faster than is comfortable for them is not usually effective.

TEXT AND SUBTEXT: TEACHING AND THE FUNDAMENTAL ASSUMPTIONS OF PRACTICE

The fact that people 'learn through doing' is a foundation assumption in occupational therapy. Even more fundamental is the assumption that a thing may be learnt or experienced through the medium of doing something else which is not necessarily directly connected with it.

Occupational therapists do teach skills in a straightforward way for the obvious reasons. A man needs to learn to cook in order to survive on his own in the community. A woman needs to improve her skills of time-keeping and personal organization in order to gain a job. These things can be directly taught and practised.

But the occupational therapist may use creative, technical or craft skills for a great variety of reasons. The therapist may 'teach' cooking – involving the client in a cooking session, providing hints and information, assisting with problem-solving – as a means of assessing cognitive abilities, fostering creativity, promoting social interaction, improving self-esteem, or recapitulating an aspect of nurturing.

For the therapist, therefore, engagement in an activity has both 'main text' – the obvious, surface content of the task and situation – and 'subtext' – the subterranean elements. This 'submerged part of the iceberg' is often of more importance to the therapist than the visible part, a fact which has led to numerous misunderstandings by casual observers of a therapeutic situation. Analysis of subtext is one of the main aims of occupational analysis.

The subtext in a situation – the part the therapist is interested in as therapy – may be just one part of the task in which the client is engaged.

For example, in physical, remedial settings it may be a movement, or a position, or the length of time spent in active engagement.

On the other hand, it may be the press of the whole situation, the performance demand of tasks and environment, which is important because engagement will result in opportunities for learning. In this context, learning may include improving understanding, gaining insight, exploration of meanings or personal development of some kind.

As a teacher of a skill, therefore, the therapist needs to be aware of where to place the emphasis. The client may be learning the skill for its own sake, perhaps in a situation where the client must achieve a certain standard of competence. Alternatively, the skill may be simply a means to an end and standards can be more flexible; it is enough to be able to participate.

TEACHING AS A COMMUNICATION PROCESS

Teaching is essentially a communication process. The relationship of teacher and student is an aspect of the therapeutic relationship and requires the use of interpersonal skills.

Some people appear to be 'born teachers'. They have the capacity to impart enthusiasm for a topic and to inspire a desire to learn. This gift seems to be an aspect of personality as much as it is a result of skill, but techniques of teaching also have to be mastered, and this requires practice.

During therapy with an individual, teaching is mainly informal, but this does not mean that it is unstructured or casual. Sometimes, formal teaching methods are needed for individuals or groups.

A teacher, like a therapist, is a reflective practitioner who must be a manager of knowledge, a manager of the environment and a manager of personal attributes and responses (Van Manan 1995).

Just as therapists need to be versatile and adaptive in their styles of communication so they need to be versatile and flexible in their styles of teaching. They also need to be consistent within the chosen style because 'mixed messages' tend to inhibit learning.

TEACHER-CENTRED VERSUS STUDENT-CENTRED APPROACHES

One important difference in style is that between 'teacher-centred' and 'student-centred' techniques. In teacher-centred settings, the teacher is 'in control'. The teacher sets the learning objectives and methods of assessment and uses formal, didactic methods such as lectures, demonstrations and 'talk and chalk' teaching. The student is a recipient of the knowledge or skill imparted by the teacher.

Formal teaching of this kind is effective in imparting information or demonstrating a skill in a relatively short time, but learning may not be long-lasting or thorough unless the information is put into practice and integrated into the learner's daily life.

In student-centred learning, the learner is self-motivated; the student sets the goals and the means of assessing learning. The student decides what is to be learnt and then selects methods by which this will take place. The student is active in pursuit of information. The teacher acts as resource person and facilitator, responding to student needs and pointing the student in the right direction to meet these. Because self-directed learning is by definition meaningful and relevant to the learner, adults are said to learn best using this style, and what is learnt tends to persist, but the process may be slow.

These different approaches have advantages and disadvantages and suit different situations. Both are useful in the right setting. It is possible to combine elements from both styles if this is done with care.

In the next part of this chapter, some basic teaching techniques will be described.

SETTING LEARNING OBJECTIVES

It is not possible to teach unless one is clear from the start what is to be taught, and what the results of learning should be. As a teacher, the therapist needs to set learning objectives. There are various forms for writing these. The way the objective is written should reflect the degree to which the therapist negotiates with the student in setting the objective, and also to the complexity of the item to be learnt.

BEHAVIOURAL LEARNING OBJECTIVES

This form of objective originates in behavioural modification as practised by clinical psychologists. Behavioural objectives relate to performance of simple skills at the acquisional or constructive levels. There is little or no subtext in this situation. The objective is to master the skill to a defined level of competence.

The first stage in setting such objectives is educational task analysis. The task is broken down into observable behavioural components. This approach is particularly useful in educational programmes for people with severe learning disabilities or brain damage.

For example, the ability to eat a mouthful of food requires the following sequence of task stages:

- recognize that a meal is to be eaten
- identify food on plate
- grasp utensil
- get a portion of food onto utensil
- transfer food to mouth
- chew and swallow food.

Each of these stages can be broken down into task segments, for example:

- identify food on plate
  - locate plate on surface in front of eater
  - look at food on plate
  - recognize food as something to be eaten
  - identify part of food to eat first.

Behavioural learning objectives translate these stages into targets for learning which state what is to be learnt, the conditions for learning and the outcome by which successful learning can be measured.

Thus, some learning objectives for the task stage 'identify food on plate' might include:

- The plate will be placed in front of the student. The student will be given the verbal prompt 'Here is your lunch.'

- The student will visually scan the table surface to locate the plate.
- The student will give the plate and its contents focused attention for at least 3 seconds.

This very detailed form of objective setting is useful in sequencing the acquisition of skills, and can be used in backward chaining, where the teaching of the task is taken from the point of completion back to the starting point.

In the above example, this might mean starting by placing a mouthful of food in the learner's mouth and ensuring correct mastication and swallowing; once mastered, the student could grasp a ready-filled spoon and take this to the mouth, and carry out the other steps back down the chain of actions.

This is a very effective system of teaching simple task performance. Rewards can be included, such as verbal praise, or some enjoyed sound or object.

ADVANCED BEHAVIOURAL OBJECTIVES

In occupational therapy, behavioural objectives are more usually used in modified form for task performance at constructive level and can be used as objectives for therapy. These are often phrased as simple performance and outcome statements. As before, the circumstances of performance may be specified:

'Mr Smith will put on his underwear without assistance or prompts, taking no longer than 10 minutes to do so.'

'Miss Jones will stay inside the supermarket for 10 minutes, purchasing three items from her shopping list. She will then sit outside on a bench and practise relaxation techniques for 5 minutes.'

Objectives of this kind can be discussed with, and negotiated with, the client. They ensure that everyone concerned understands what is to be done, and knows when it has been achieved. The therapist can then decide, with the client, what has to be learnt or practised in order to perform the task.

So, Mr Smith may need a demonstration of a dressing technique, and then a period of practice

at this. Miss Jones may need to understand the nature of the stress response, and be taught a simple relaxation technique. Once again, there is little subtext.

COMPETENCIES

At the effective level, performance becomes integrated and the learner needs to demonstrate appropriate knowledge skills and attitudes.

To demonstrate competence, the student should be able to undertake an activity to a specified level of success on several occasions and, if applicable, in different situations. Performance need not be perfect, but the student may need to show the ability, predict, avoid, spot and remedy errors or problems.

The type of performance, or the way knowledge has been acquired may need to be formally tested. A driving test is a good example of assessment of this type. The learner is asked to demonstrate skill in realistic conditions and is then asked a set of questions about theoretical aspects, or potentially risky situations.

STUDENT-CENTRED OBJECTIVES

Student-centred learning should not be seen as an aimless pursuit of some rather vague form of knowledge or skill. Like any other form of learning, it works best when the student is absolutely clear about what is to be learned, why and how.

The difference is that students have specified these aims for themselves, with help from the therapist to clarify goals and methods if required.

So, for example, a disabled man decides that he would like to learn to use a word processor. The therapist may discuss this with him and talk through various strategies to start him off.

The student might decide to get someone to demonstrate a word processor to him, phone several local colleges to see what courses are available, or send off for information about word processors and programmes which are specially suited to his needs. The therapist might provide him with a resource file giving relevant information so that he can pursue these goals.

The student may or may not decide to record his goals in a formal manner. The therapist, however, will need to record the goals as part of the file notes, so that the therapist can help to keep the learning process on track.

PREPARATION OF A LEARNING ENVIRONMENT

A learning environment needs to press for learning. This may seem self-evident, but it is not so easy to achieve. Demand results from a mixture of appropriate resources and opportunities, together with a set of explicit or implicit expectations to which the environment and its users should provide cues.

In a formal classroom setting, the demand is obvious: the seating arrangement, the teaching aids, the cultural understanding of what a classroom is for and the rules of behaviour within a classroom all contribute.

However, it is plain from the experience of mainstream education that providing the right environment facilitates but does not automatically cue learning behaviours. Learning also depends on a complex set of interactions between learners, between learner and teacher, and between learner and the item to be learnt.

It is very difficult to get the balance between these factors right. An environment which presses too hard for conformity may in fact produce rebellion. A rich but unstructured environment may overstimulate and confuse some people.

There are a number of keys to effective learning. The most essential is relevance and meaning in the situation which promote good motivation on the part of the learner; people rarely learn things well which seem irrelevant to their lives.

Adequate resources and opportunities for safe exploration are also desirable. The initial stages of learning can provoke feelings of insecurity, anxiety and uncertainty so 'psychological comfort' is important. At the same time, there needs to be some sense of challenge within the safe parameters of the setting.

Many of these factors ultimately depend on the skill of the teacher. Even in very student-centred settings, the human resources of the teacher, and other students, is of more importance than the environment. A 'poor' learning environment can be compensated for by an able teacher, but a 'good' environment is of little use if the teacher fails to communicate or fails to inspire the desire to learn.

In occupational therapy, much learning takes place in protected environments such as a therapy department. This is useful at early stages in the learning process, but the therapist may need to ensure that the learner is able to operate successfully in normal, less predictable environments. If the learning cannot be transferred to a variety of settings, it remains only partially useful.

DEMONSTRATION

Demonstration is an essential technique for the therapist. There are numerous occasions when some task or activity or piece of equipment must be demonstrated to someone. It takes planning and practice to give a good demonstration.

HOW TO GIVE AN EFFECTIVE DEMONSTRATION

Preparation

Preparation is the most important part of a demonstration, and time must be allotted for this.

1. Analyse the task to be demonstrated, breaking it into stages. Each stage should be of a convenient length and have, as far as possible, a logical beginning and end.

2. Assemble all materials, tools and equipment.

3. Plan the demonstration. Work out for each stage what you will say, what you will do, or what you will ask the learner to do. Build in time for questions, practice, or repetition if required. Consider the way you will position yourself in relation to the learner, and the best position for your materials. Take account of lighting, and plan to reduce distractions. You may decide to have everything on view to

begin with, or to keep things needed for a later stage in reserve to avoid confusion.

4. Ensure that the nature of the demonstration will be understood. The learner needs to have an overview of what is to be done before the demonstration begins. The adage 'Tell them what you are going to tell them, tell them, and tell them what you have told them' is founded on sound learning principles. Have samples of task stages and products if this will help; 'here is one I made earlier' helps to give substance to otherwise abstract descriptions.

   Consider whether or not to show a finished product: while it may be helpful to show what it looks like, an overly perfect sample may put students off as their initial efforts may suffer by comparison.

5. Written instructions, diagrams or handouts may help. Ensure these are produced to a good standard of presentation and design, with attention to problems of language, or visual deficits which your learner may have.

6. If you have not got extensive personal experience of the task to be demonstrated, you must practise. Even if you are very familiar with the task, a practice demonstration to someone who does not know how to do it will rapidly indicate if you have left something out, or need to modify your plan in some way.

Conducting the demonstration

If your preparation has been sufficient, you should have little trouble with the actual demonstration. What you need to pay attention to is the reaction of the learner. You may need to modify your explanations, the tone of your voice, speed up or slow down, or allow more or less time for questions and hands-on practice.

Assessing whether learning has taken place

You can do this by asking questions, getting the learner to repeat the demonstration at the time, and by giving the learner subsequent opportunities to put learning into practice, with prompts, cues and shaping from you if required.

TEACHING A SKILL TO AN INDIVIDUAL

Demonstration often plays a part in teaching a skill, but in the context of occupational therapy, teaching of skills is usually a more informal process which happens as part of a therapy session.

As already noted, when teaching a creative or productive skill there may be both text and subtext. The therapist may need to move from 'teaching' to 'treating' and back again in response to the needs of the patient and the way the session develops.

The boundaries between teaching and therapy tend to blur at this point. The therapist will 'teach' in the sense of demonstrating, giving information, prompting, cueing, shaping and reinforcing performance, enhancing awareness of elements which contribute to the subtext, all as part of the total intervention. Later on the therapist may coach the client to polish and improve performance.

'Prompting, cueing, shaping and reinforcing' are terms drawn from behavioural teaching, but therapists tend to use these techniques in many situations in the early stages of teaching a skill.

To prompt is to give a verbal suggestion or reminder. Prompts can be direct, such as a reminder of the next action, or indirect. Indirect prompts are aimed at getting learners to remember for themselves what happens next, on the basis of past learning. 'Do you remember what happens next?' 'How did we do it last time?' 'What do you need now?' are examples of indirect prompts. Actively recalling information is more effective in promoting learning than simply being told the information.

A cue is something in the environment or situation which triggers a response. The cue might be provided by the therapist's expression or position, or by having tools or materials within sight.

Shaping. When a skill is being learnt, performance starts off by being approximate, and gradually gets closer to what is required until finally the skill is perfected. During the 'experimental' stage, the therapist may shape performance by giving verbal feedback, drawing attention to the elements which most closely resemble what is wanted. This is usually done by providing praise, and pointing out what needs to happen to make performance even better.

Reinforcement is provided when a reward is given for successful performance. The reward is usually praise, but sometimes a rest, or a drink may be used. Therapists are naturally affirmative people who give a lot of praise and positive feedback in the course of their interactions with a client. Care must be taken to use rewards appropriately and not too much. Continual praise or praise for something which both therapist and learner know does not merit it is always inadvisable.

Coaching is used to improve performance when the basics have been mastered. The therapist offers suggestions or advice as the learner works, gives specific forms of practice to improve subskills, or else may take time to reflect on a period of work with the learner, pointing out or discussing how performance might be improved.

EXPERIENTIAL LEARNING

Complex situations require an individual to learn and integrate many skills at once. The individual cannot easily break these skills up into simple 'learning packages'. Learning has to happen experientially; the learner must explore, discover, learn by a mixture of trial and error and problem-solving. The individual needs to discover what works and what does not; the individual may need to make mistakes as part of the learning process.

In this situation, the therapist needs to construct a situation in which learning can take place. The therapist may or may not be present, but will probably not intervene (unless something goes badly wrong).

In order to gain from the experience, however, the learner may need help from the therapist to make sense of it. The learner may need to discover what has been learned, and may need

help to reflect on the situation, especially if it could have been handled differently. This is especially true when it is the subtext which is important.

Here, the therapist tries to hold up a mirror to reflect the situation, so that the patient can learn from it. The therapist may discuss what happened, point out events and get the patient to review what happened, conduct a problem-solving exercise to explore different solutions or actions, and discuss how to approach the situation next time. Examining thoughts and feelings might be as important as actions.

ADULT EDUCATION IN A GROUP SETTING

In adult education, the emphasis is on involvement of the participants with the educators as equals in the learning situation. Adults have a great deal of personal experience to contribute and the teacher needs to facilitate sharing and mutual support.

Therapists are increasingly involved in health promotion with groups of adults which is conducted using an educational approach. Examples might include sessions on the benefits of a healthy lifestyle, information about a specific condition and techniques for managing this, or guidance on retirement or the use of hobbies in leisure time. These settings require the therapist to adopt an adult education approach.

Some forms of group education are carried out by a team of which the therapist is a member. Pain management and stress management are examples.

The preceding notes on preparation and having clear educational aims are equally relevant, especially when working as part of a team where the contributions of each member must be complementary to the others.

It is important to ensure that educational groups remain *educational* and do not become *therapy*. Boundaries between reasonable disclosure of personal experience and the kind of disclosure or exploration which may happen in therapeutic group work must be maintained.

Some of the group facilitation techniques used in group therapy can be useful in adult education, but these must be used with discretion.

SELECTION OF PARTICIPANTS

Education of adults in a group does impose some limitations on membership of the group. Participants need to be selected with clear, preferably written, criteria in mind. They need to be very well briefed on the purpose of the sessions and the practical requirements and commitment required. Where possible, they should be encouraged to 'opt in', rather than being 'sent to the group'.

Some disabilities or communication problems do make it difficult for the individual to participate in the session, and may create problems for the teacher. This is particularly true when the individual will be 'the odd one out'; where the problem affects all members, the teaching techniques can be adapted to take account of this.

These problems include: learning difficulties, visual or hearing loss, poor literacy, imperfect comprehension of English, and a mental disorder with overt behavioural components.

If a candidate for a group is excluded because of one of these problems, efforts should be made to provide the information by another means. This might be on a one-to-one basis, or by providing the individual with a personal helper who can compensate for the problem, for example, by translating or signing. It is especially important to ensure that ethnic minorities are not excluded simply because they do not speak English.

PROVIDING THE RIGHT ENVIRONMENT

For a group to be able to work, the room must be reasonably quiet and free from distraction, and access by others should be restricted for the duration of the session. Physical comfort, (heating, lighting, seating, ventilation) needs to be considered, with special provision for any participant with a physical disability.

Access to a toilet and to refreshments if the session lasts more than an hour is also essential. The usual educational equipment – overhead projector, video, flip chart, white board – should be available.

The provision of an environment which is clearly educational and suitable for adults is important. The therapist must work hard to maintain an identity as a teacher and not a therapist.

Anything which divides the learners from the teacher should be avoided. Therefore, it is preferable for the setting to be non-clinical. Chairs should be in a circle, not in rows. The teaching therapist should be part of the group, not 'centre stage'. It is preferable for the therapist to wear ordinary clothes, not uniform.

GROUP TEACHING TECHNIQUES

Adult education typically takes place in the form of 'a course' run for a small group over a number of sessions.

There should be a curriculum and learning objectives. Teaching methods may be outlined. Learners should have a clear understanding of why they are attending the course, and any 'ground rules' for attendance.

Sessions need to be split up to maintain attention, but content should not become disconnected. A course programme is useful for both therapist and participants, but there should be flexibility to vary this if necessary as adults often produce ideas and issues which need exploration at the time, rather than later. The exact sequence and detailed content of information-giving depends on how the course progresses.

The teacher needs to establish an equal footing with the learners, whose views and contributions are overtly sought and valued. The role of the teacher is to act as a resource person who facilitates learning. The teacher must avoid appearing as a didactic expert who 'knows it all'.

Occupational therapists working with adults need to pay special attention to the age-appropriateness of both environment and educational techniques. If these produce a demand reminiscent of childhood education, the student is likely to respond 'childishly'.

The teacher must use adult words (even if these must be kept simple), adult materials (*not* 'play school' ones), and must relate to participants as adults, seeking and valuing their own experiences and contributions, and avoiding patronizingly 'dumbing down', complex topics.

The differences can be quite subtle. For example, the word 'homework' is often used to indicate tasks which the learner should do between one session and the next; homework is, however, generally accepted as something which children do. Adult students have tasks, projects or assignments.

The teacher proposes questions or problems rather than offering solutions. During group discussion, learners are challenged to provide their own ideas, and the teacher then 'fills the gaps'. If questions or problems are posed by students the teacher seeks the opinion of the group before offering a personal solution.

Like any other group of strangers who come together for the first time, the participants need time to get to know each other and the teacher. Introductions should be made, using any of the 'icebreaking' techniques appropriate to adult education. It may be useful to go through course content and to get a view of the interests, expectations and goals of the participants. Emergency safety procedures can be dealt with.

It is common to use small-group work in syndicates, 'gaming', problem-solving and brainstorming exercises as teaching media. (There are textbooks on how to use these.) Students may be asked to prepare handouts, or be encouraged to discover and present information to others.

Alternatively, the group can be split into smaller units of two or three people who are given a task. Tasks might include discussion of a point, identifying issues of interest, sharing experience, providing solutions to a problem, making a poster or handout, and other 'workshop'-style activities.

Conventional teaching or demonstrating may form part of the sessions but it is important to use a variety of techniques and to involve participants actively.

If a therapist is familier with more formal teacher-centred methods, or with teaching in clinical settings, adult education techniques can feel unstructured and uncomfortable. In fact, the therapist needs to be well-prepared with a range of options for each session or potential responses to likely situations; however, whether or not these are used, and in what sequence, depends on what happens and how the learners respond.

EVALUATION

Thought should be given to how the session or course will end, and whether there is any kind of assessment or evaluation.

Assessment can be informal, for example as a quiz, or it may be more formal. A useful technique is to construct a questionnaire covering knowledge of the topics to be covered which can be given to participants at the beginning of the course and again at the end to see if there is a difference.

A simple multiple choice test could be used. Participants might be asked to prepare a short summary of some aspect of the topic to share with others.

Evaluation forms for completion by participants are useful. The form may ask the participant to rate how well various topics have been covered, and to rate the facilities and the performance of teachers. Forms can be anonymously completed if preferred. The group may be asked to discuss the session and say what they found useful, or what has changed for them since the course began.

17

Professional education

LIFELONG LEARNING

It is the responsibility of all occupational therapists to ensure that they are suitably trained and educated to practise and that they remain up to date. A commitment to 'lifelong learning' is essential now that the pace of change in health care is so rapid. Therapists also need to participate in the education of their own and other professions. Therefore, although at first sight it may appear that professional education has little to do with 'therapeutic use of self', in the sense of maintaining and using 'self as therapist', it seems legitimate to include these things as core competencies.

Professional education may include:

- informal sharing of ideas and techniques with others
- reflection on practice
- development of new techniques
- keeping up to date with research and other developments
- formal presentation of new information or research
- education of students
- explaining occupational therapy to others.

Many of the techniques needed in professional education are based on the student-centred, adult education model previously described for use with clients.

A full discussion of professional education is beyond the scope of this book, but some practical techniques are described.

INFORMAL EDUCATION

Informal education may happen spontaneously, but is usually more effective when planned. It is informal in that it typically takes place at work, with small groups, and follows the adult education model. Organization may be the responsibility of one person, or a group, or may rotate each time an event is planned.

Informal education has the advantage of being relatively inexpensive, except in terms of staff time, relevant to local needs and readily accessible.

Informal education sessions work best when there is some kind of focus or structure. Examples include: topic presentation; case presentation; journal club; reflective discussion.

TOPIC PRESENTATION

A typical format might be for a therapist to be allocated (or to select) a topic of interest to others. The therapist then prepares and presents a '10-minute talk' on the subject (or perhaps a demonstration of a skill), following which the rest of the group can ask questions and discuss the topic.

Apart from offering useful information in a convenient chunk without disrupting work schedules, this format has the advantage of helping to prepare staff to give more formal short presentations at meetings or conferences.

CASE PRESENTATION

A single case study, or a group of case studies, is presented to the group. The presenter needs to be clear and specific, and to structure the presentation so as to highlight relevant or interesting aspects. It is usually necessary to avoid giving personal details in order to preserve confidentiality. The permission of the client may need to be obtained. If in doubt, the local policy on case presentations should be checked.

After the presentation, the case can be discussed by others, and discussion may take various forms. It might include problem-solving, identification of good practice, sharing of techniques, or discussion of potential research topics.

JOURNAL CLUB

A journal club may be for a single profession or multidisciplinary. Usually each member of the group in turn reviews a set selection of journals and presents either an overview of current topics or recent research findings, or a more detailed summary and critical review of a particular article.

It can be hard to maintain enthusiasm and focus in a group of this kind; one solution is to link reading to a defined topic of interest to the group, or to development of evidence of effectiveness.

REFLECTIVE DISCUSSION

The aim of this approach is to share and discuss some aspect of practice in order to illuminate understanding of it. Busy therapists typically lack time to actually talk about what they are doing, yet this is an important way to develop and improve practice.

The discussion does need some structure; it should aim to capture common themes, attitudes or approaches, or to highlight differences or problems, and then discuss these and what they mean in the context of local practice with a view to action.

FORMAL EDUCATION

Formal education is structured, carefully planned, and may be conducted away from the workplace. Provision should be related to individual learning needs, and these in turn must be linked to job requirements.

RUNNING A SHORT COURSE OR STUDY DAY

The work involved in running a short course must not be underestimated. It takes time, resources and administrative assistance. Apart from the educational aspects such as setting aims and objectives, planning content, and booking speakers, there are numerous managerial processes which the therapist must either tackle alone or delegate. These include costing the course, advertising, finding a venue, and perhaps accommodation for delegates, dealing with applications, arranging refreshments, sorting out travel or parking problems, obtaining equipment, and numerous other practicalities.

The novice course arranger is advised to go to find someone who has plenty of experience and who can guide the novice through the process and assist in avoiding pitfalls.

RUNNING A WORKSHOP

A workshop is an interactive learning situation where participants share information, perform tasks, and then summarize and share the results with others. Workshops are frequently used for professional education.

The workshop is usually facilitated by a nominated person. Workshops are sometimes very freely structured, but this can result in a 'talking shop' with indefinite outcome.

It is more productive, especially if time is short, to have preset topics or questions for discussion. A commonly used format is for small groups to work on the topics individually. The groups can either all tackle the same topic, or be given different ones. After a reasonable (but not too lengthy) period of time, each group is asked to nominate a member to summarize findings and present these to the others. Flip chart 'posters' or lists of points may be produced.

Once all the reports have been made, the facilitator stimulates a discussion, and may draw together a 'master summary' of all the different points.

A workshop can last for 1 hour or up to 3, although longer workshops usually have several tasks and are somewhat tiring.

NOMINAL GROUP TECHNIQUE

This technique is useful as a workshop exercise. It was developed as a method of group problem-solving by Delbeq & Van de Ven (1971).

It is designed for use with large groups to obtain a rapid consensus view of a range of opinions on a topic without providing the opportunity for articulate or opinionated people, or those with vested interests, to dominate or influence the discussion. The results can be used as a basis for discussion, setting priorities or decision-making.

The technique has five phases:

- problem exploration
- knowledge exploration
- priority development
- programme development
- programme evaluation.

The original version was designed as a model (the Program Planning Model (PMP)) for interdisciplinary consultation which took place over an extended period. In the version of which I have experience, the process is somewhat accelerated and concentrates on the first three phases. The foundation exercise of problem exploration and prioritizing can be completed in about an hour and a half.

The session is managed by a facilitator who should be impartial and uninvolved in any outcome. In the first stage, individuals are asked to brainstorm a list of all the points or items which they consider important. The facilitator explains that most problems have both emotional and organizational aspects. Each person is given a card with the headings 'personal feelings' and 'organizational difficulties' on each side. (If the issue is fundamentally uncontentious, the 'feelings' issues can be omitted to save time, but exploration of these is often very useful since most of the barriers to change originate here.)

Once individual lists are produced, which only takes 5 to 10 minutes, participants get together in threes or fours to amalgamate their lists. It may be helpful, if the group is composed of different professions or grades of staff, to separate the small groups of participants according to these divisions. One person undertakes the task of capturing all the ideas so far expressed. This person asks each member of the group in turn to read out one item, and continues with this until all have been recorded. At this stage, two rules apply: no discussion, and nothing is to be left off the list. Similar ideas can be 'clumped' but not amalgamated. Organizational difficulties are dealt with first and then feelings.

In the extended version of the exercise, or if the group is very large (say 50 or more), the groups are given half-an-hour to discuss the items. At the end of this period, each person is asked to vote privately, by number (that is, by giving the top priority a score of five, and so on down the list), on the five items considered most important on each list. The results of this exercise are obtained by the recorder, who, by a process of simple arithmetic, arrives at a priority order for the popularity or priority given to the items on the list, the highest scoring items having the most priority.

The results of each group's prioritizing exercise is then communicated to the facilitator. The results are discussed by the group.

Alternatively, if the group is of a more manageable number, this exercise can be done by the whole group. The recorder from each group (a junior staff member is suggested) reads out the list. The facilitator ensures that all the ideas are gathered and written on a large board or flip chart. Individuals once again make their own lists, taking the items on the main list and putting them into their personal order of priority with a numerical score. Finally, each person is asked to read out the personal rating for each item. The numbers are written on the board, and when all have given their ratings, the numbers are added up by the facilitator. (It is worth noting that what is *not* listed can sometimes be as revealing as what is.)

What happens next depends on the available time and the complexity of the problems being explored. If it is a relatively simple matter of deciding on priorities for, say, spending a training budget, the exercise should have produced the answer and action can be taken.

If, however, the problems are complex and it is necessary to address the feelings expressed as well as organizational issues, the facilitator asks the groups to vote for representatives who can take the process forward to the other phases, exploring knowledge, generating solutions, agreeing ultimate priorities and taking action. Anyone who intends to use the longer version of the technique should refer to the original paper which gives detailed instructions on how to do this.

LECTURING

A lecture is a formal event in which the lecturer imparts information or ideas to an audience. The therapist may lecture to clients, relatives, people in the community or professional colleagues.

A lecture is not usually participatory, although questions may be asked of the lecturer at intervals or at the end. Lecturing styles vary from the dry and didactic to the amusing and entertaining. Good lecturers need to be good actors, capable of effective use of voice, posture and eye-contact, and able to convey interest and enthusiasm.

The approach may vary a little with the nature of the audience, but the principles remain the same. Lecturing, like demonstrating, depends on preparation.

PREPARING A LECTURE
Research

The first stage is research: the lecturer needs a sound understanding of the subject. (One of the most effective methods of self-directed learning is to give a lecture on an unfamiliar topic!) Even if the lecturer is familiar with the subject, it is good practice to check up on recent developments or look up references.

Writing

The next stage is writing. If the lecture is to be published as a paper, it will have to be formally written, and in this case full references are essential. It is useful to ask a mentor to read and criticize the paper. The requirements of the journal in which it is to be published should be borne in mind.

A formal paper may be read as written, although this may sound dry and pedantic.

Alternatively, the lecturer may use the paper as a basis for a 'performed' version.

A less formal lecture can be written down verbatim, or recorded on tape as a starting point for constructing the lecture. The lecturer then uses the written version to prepare an outline script, summarizing the essential points using headings, or cue cards with key words and phrases, headline points or cue-words to help to keep the talk on track.

Only very confident, fluent and experienced lecturers can deliver a good lecture with no script at all.

Visual aids

Slides, overhead projector transparencies, prepared posters or flip chart diagrams give life to a verbal presentation, improve audience attention and enhance understanding. Video can be used, but it is not easy for an amateur to prepare good teaching material.

All visual aids must be carefully designed, and the amount and layout of information are very important. Nowadays standards of presentation, especially at professional conferences, are very high and shoddy presentations are embarrassingly obvious. Hand-written items are only acceptable in very informal settings.

Slides need careful preparation and enough time must be allocated for this work (allowing time also for things to go wrong!). Computer-generated colour slides are now easy to obtain and look very professional. One's own photographs can be useful, but must be of good quality. They also need to be planned to integrate with the lecture. Occasional use of an amusing or odd visual image as a 'wake up' slide is effective, but this technique can be overdone.

Overheads can be made from text produced on a word processor and can include diagrams which should, if possible, be professionally drawn. It is permissible to photocopy limited amounts of information from a book for educational purposes but borrowed material must always be attributed with a full reference.

Text on each slide or overhead should be limited, and the size of print must be large enough for easy reading. It is worth remembering that the human brain is only capable of effectively processing around five pieces of information at a time; fewer may be better. Use of colour can enhance the overhead. Other visual aids or objects need equally careful preparation.

REHEARSAL

The lecturer needs to practise use of technical equipment, and must take care to stand in the right place so as not to obstruct the audience's view of the screen.

Elementary lecturing faults such as speaking to the projector screen instead of the audience must be avoided. It helps to have printed copies of overheads in front of one to avoid the temptation to read from the screen.

A personal style will develop in time, but pay attention to honest and impartial feedback, and try to avoid irritating verbal or physical mannerisms (e.g. 'ums and errs', repetitive phrases such as 'you see' or 'OK', continual fingering of a button).

Timing of the lecture is particularly important. Good timing comes with experience. A lecture should be rehearsed and timed several times if necessary. Take a watch with you as some venues lack a clock or the clock cannot be seen from the platform.

CHECK THE EQUIPMENT AND VENUE

If lecturing in an unfamiliar place, check ahead of time that all necessary visual aids, equipment and microphone will be available. Check for lectern, table, chairs or any other necessary items.

Find out the layout of the area, and whether you will need to rearrange it, or get someone to do this in advance. It may be useful to check whether there is a coloured background behind the lecturing position so that you can check that your clothes do not clash, or cause you to vanish into the background.

It is wise to take your own additional supply of overhead markers, dry markers, cloth to wipe board, and any other essential small item which is likely to be missing when you arrive.

Arrive early and check everything. Switch on equipment, find switches and introduce yourself to any technicians. Microphones need to be tried out.

Also, find out the location of lavatories and emergency exits; check if you are to give out this information before you start or whether someone else will.

PRESENTATION

A lecture is essentially a performance. All novice lecturers are nervous; the skill lies in appearing confident. This is partly achieved by good preparation and rehearsal, and partly by using confident body language and voice which not only puts the audience at ease, but also helps to convince you that you are comfortable.

A short spell of relaxation breathing does help to calm nerves. A pause to sip a glass of water can be a good way of getting back on track if 'nerves' are taking over.

During the presentation, the lecturer must judge pace, check that content is as it should be, and keep an eye on the time. It may be necessary to curtail the presentation if it is running over time or if the audience seems to be losing attention. Allow time for questions and facilitate these if necessary.

Good lecturing style is best acquired by watching other lecturers and trying to copy techniques and 'tricks' which work and avoid those which do not.

Assessment of individual potential, ability and needs

SECTION CONTENTS

18

Introduction to assessment of individual potential, ability and needs

ASSESSMENT

In occupational therapy to assess means to judge, measure, quantify or describe some aspect of occupational performance, or the foundation skills required in order to perform, and to form some conclusions based on this data. The latter process is referred to as evaluation.

Individuals are complex; it follows that assessment of the individual is also a complex matter. Assessments range from the specific to the general, from single items to holistic reviews of function and patterns of performance. The process of assessment is further complicated by conflicting theories and models, and the numerous techniques which must be mastered to assess effectively.

Unlike other core processes, where information is often sparse and scattered, the process of assessment suffers from an information overload. Assessment methodology is, perhaps, the most discussed and documented aspect of occupational therapy. The problem is not lack of literature and research, but that there is altogether too much. New assessments are continually being produced; technical aspects of test construction are described; journals and textbooks are awash with details of evaluative techniques related to every possible specialism. The reader is rapidly submerged by data.

In this chapter, some of the issues and controversies over assessment will be summarized, together with some of the basic principles and foundation skills.

In the rest of Section 3, assessment will be described in relation to the occupational levels: developmental, effective and organizational.

The reader needs to be aware, however, that any author tackling this topic is chasing a moving target. It is extremely difficult to keep up to date with developments and it is necessary for therapists to ensure that they keep up with current texts and data bases relevant to their area of practice.

WHY ASSESS?

Assessment has to be undertaken for a reason. It is a means to an end, not an end in itself. There is very little point in 'assessing' unless the material will be used and some useful action or intervention will follow.

The reasons for assessment are various, and sometimes become entangled in a way which blurs the issues. Assessment takes place at different stages in the occupational therapy process and at different occupational levels. It also takes place in different settings - hospital, clinic and home - and in the context of different medical specialisms or service cultures.

In each case there may be different aims for the assessment process, and a need for different methods or assessment tools. If the purpose of assessment is not crystal clear, the process cannot be effective.

Assessment may be used as a management tool, as a clinical tool, or to determine the wishes and needs of the client and to ascertain the client's ultimate satisfaction with the therapeutic process.

As Austin & Clark (1993) point out, the concerns of managers, clinicians and patients are not necessarily the same, which implies that the assessment measures may also be different.

ASSESSMENT AS A MANAGEMENT TOOL

The crucial questions about any form of intervention are 'Has it made a difference?' 'Is it worth doing?' and 'Has it been done well? A means of measuring the degree to which an intervention has achieved its aims within given quality standards or criteria of efficiency and effectiveness is called an *outcome measure*.

Austin & Clark (1993) list the following purposes of outcome measures:

- to show that intervention is appropriate and effective
- to indicate areas where service development might be required or additional resources deployed
- to enable changes that lead to improvement in consumer satisfaction
- to show that a contracted service has been provided

- to indicate the effective use of health resources.

It is plain from this list that an outcome measure is a management tool as much (or more) than it is a therapeutic one, and this can cause problems for therapists, especially if pressed by managers to use measures which are not compatible with, or valid measures of, the process of occupational therapy.

This section deals with assessment primarily as a clinical tool of use to client and therapist, rather than as a tool for managers.

Some occupational therapy assessments can also be used as outcome measures, but these need to be carefully designed for the purpose (see Jeffrey 1993, Fricke 1993). Recent attempts to combine clinical assessment with a standard outcome measure include the Canadian Occupational Performance Measure (Law et al 1994). Some of the issues which arise from attempts to demonstrate the positive effect of occupational therapy on function and well-being are discussed by Farrar Edwards (1997).

ASSESSMENT: THE CLIENT'S PERSPECTIVE

The client wants to have the assurance that the therapist is efficiently and considerately providing relevant and meaningful services which will meet a personal need or goal.

Given the active investment of time and effort required in order to participate in occupational therapy, the client also needs to feel that progress is being made and the client's time is not being wasted.

What the client does not want is the feeling of being 'a bug on a pin' to be poked, examined, tested and put under the microscope, whether the client wishes or not. Equally unwelcome is the feeling of having to 'pass an examination' set by some kind of authority figure who will use the results in a way which the client cannot predict or control. The therapist (and I have met some) who talks of 'doing an assessment on her' (i.e. the client) has missed the point.

Client engagement in the process of self-assessment, identification of goals and measurement of progress is crucial. It can also reasonably be argued that, ultimately, the client is the only person who is really in a position to evaluate whether therapy has been effective in improving function or promoting well-being.

ASSESSMENT AS A CLINICAL TOOL

From the therapist's perspective, assessment is primarily a clinical tool which provides information to guide the processes of therapy.

According to Laver-Ingram (1997: citing Rogers & Holm 1989) the purposes of assessments have been classified as:

Predictive	Giving a guide to the expected level of future occupational performance.
Discriminative	Using norms to measure and compare performances for the purpose of diagnosis, placement and determining the level of function in comparison to that of the normative group.
Descriptive	Describing the current functional status of the client.
Evaluative	An assessment which is sufficiently sensitive to be capable of detecting clinical change when used sequentially.

EXAMPLES OF AIMS OF ASSESSMENT RELEVANT TO THE THERAPIST

- To determine the potential for or level of skill
- To determine whether functional performance is effective, competent or appropriate
- To obtain an occupational history and profile of an individual
- To provide a baseline for intervention
- To measure progress during intervention
- To measure the effectiveness of intervention
- To measure risk
- To ascertain readiness for discharge from care
- To ascertain need for support services or resources in the community

- To find out the client's views of a situation.

It is plain that these aims have different purposes, operate at different levels and require different assessment tools and methods.

Assessment in relation to occupational levels

Laver-Ingram (1997) relates levels of assessment to the five level hierarchy of dysfunction developed by the National Centre for Medicine Rehabilitation Research (NCMRR 1993) and gives examples of assessment domains at each level (Table 18.1). Ottenbacher & Christiansen (1997) provide a similar analysis.

One of the fundamental problems of assessment is that, as one moves up through the occupational levels, it becomes more and more difficult to measure change.

At the developmental level, a reductionist, 'bottom up' approach involving specific, therapist-led assessment is quite appropriate. At this level, it is possible to say specifically 'Last week the client did that; this week he can do more' and to quantify the difference. Knowledge can be tested in terms of 'this is known; that is not'.

At the effective level, where performance is integrated and situational, some aspects of competence can be assessed, although with limitations which have been described in Chapter 7.

By the time one reaches the organizational level, it becomes very difficult to find ways of measuring change in the totality of human performances. This is why much assessment is conducted lower down the occupational levels.

As one moves up the occupational levels, it also becomes increasingly important to take a 'top down' approach which involves the client and to move towards client-centred assessment methods.

Recognition of the different aims, scope of assessment and expected outcomes at each level helps to structure and simplify selection of appropriate assessments.

WHO ASSESSES?

This is a key issue in current practice. In the traditional rehabilitation approach, the therapist is responsible for assessment. The therapist selects the method, conducts the assessment by objective observation, measurement or other tests, and tells the client the outcome. The client, while expected to co-operate actively with the assessment process, is a relatively passive contributor to the results and consequent judgements, and the client's subjective views often do not enter into the assessment process.

In client-centred practice, the therapist and client jointly conduct the assessment process,

Table 18.1 Assessment domains in relation to NCMRR levels of disability (adapted from Laver-Ingram 1997)

	Level of dysfunction Patho-physiology Impairment		Functional limitation	Disability	Societal limitation
Examples of assessment domains	Specific deficits, e.g. agnosia, apraxia, spasticity, loss of sensation, pain	Skill components sensori-motor cognitive–perceptual interpersonal	Skills	Self-care activities; work and productive activities; leisure	Roles and performance within physical and social environment
	Proto-occupational *COPE Levels of occupation*	Aquisitional	Constructive	Effective	Organizational

with the client as a very active, or leading, partner. Self-assessment by the client, and close consideration of the subjective views and feelings of the client are an integral part of the process.

Although the therapist may interpret the results, decisions about consequent action are evolved by discussion with the client, who is again expected to contribute actively to this process.

Working within a client-centred model constrains the degree to which the therapist can treat the client as the object or subject of a clinical assessment process. Clinically based assessments may be inappropriate in some settings (e.g. in the client's own home), or must be modified in presentation for use within the framework of the client-centred approach.

While it is plain that these two approaches are substantially different and in many ways incompatible, it is not a question of either being 'right' or 'wrong' but of selecting the appropriate assessment methods for each situation and the relevant occupational level.

WHEN TO ASSESS?

The short answer is 'when it is necessary' – but how does one evaluate necessity?

Assessment is an adjunct to clinical reasoning and decision-making. It provides the data on the basis of which hypotheses can be tested, predictions made and decisions taken.

The test is whether the assessment really does contribute something extra to the process. All too often the results of an assessment simply confirm something which the therapist already knows from observation or experience. It may be reassuring to have such confirmation, or data may be required in order to provide firm 'evidence'. However, in purely practical terms, when treatment time is usually limited, it is redundant to 'assess for assessment's sake', especially if it takes half an hour to provide information which you had already gained through rapid but structured observation, based on good clinical knowledge and experience.

Over-dependence on formal assessment purely as a means of demonstrating some kind of

professional 'respectability' to others, devalues professional expertise and judgment and risks reducing the process of evaluation to a set of technical procedures.

That being said, assessment remains the foundation of the occupational therapy process. It may be a one-off procedure, to provide a snapshot in time, or it may be conducted sequentially over a period of time in order to demonstrate change. Continuous, informal evaluation of progress may be augmented by intermittent formal assessment to 'benchmark' change.

As well as taking time, some assessments have specific requirements for equipment, space, or replicability of situation. These practical requirements also require consideration. The assessment must not only be necessary, but also practical, possible, replicable and valid.

WHICH ASSESSMENT?

There are hundreds of potential assessment tools and methods. If one extends the search to assessments produced by doctors, psychologists or other health professions, the list may well run into thousands. However, there is no easy guide to finding the right one. Although lists of assessments are published, there is (at the time of writing) no single comprehensive database to guide the search. All too often it means trawling through the literature.

Even when a suitable assessment is located, unless it can readily be purchased, it can be hard to obtain a copy. Copyright rules limit the scope for reproduction. Research articles refer to assessments, but rarely give details of use, or copies of forms or protocols. It is also quite difficult for a novice assessor to evaluate critically technical aspects of test design or scoring.

It is perhaps unsurprising that therapists, faced with these problems, still resort to designing their own 'ad hoc' assessments, of variable standards. There is, however, no excuse for inventing a second rate assessment simply because one cannot be bothered to find one which is already available.

It is, however, legitimate to design a new assessment if there really is nothing suitable.

This may happen in research settings, or in client-centred practice where fewer assessments are available.

If the therapist is clear in advance about approach, aims, and required outcomes, it makes selection easier.

Sources of information on assessment are given at the end of this chapter and in the Appendix.

WHAT DO OCCUPATIONAL THERAPISTS ASSESS?

In general, they focus on the knowledge, attitudes/values and skills of individuals in the context of their environment and their occupational needs and goals, with a view to evaluating whether performance is competent (see following chapters).

WHERE DOES ASSESSMENT TAKE PLACE?

Assessment in clinical settings

Much assessment takes place in a hospital ward or occupational therapy department or other clinical setting. Inevitably, this process is heavily influenced by the medical rehabilitation model, or, in mental health settings, by medical or psychological models.

The basic sequence of events and aims is much the same in any setting, although methods and assessment tools will vary.

Assessment in relation to stages in the occupational therapy process in a clinical setting

It can be seen from this summary that different things happen at each stage. In the initial stage, the emphasis is on *description*, exploring issues and gathering *baseline* information so that the situation is sufficiently understood. This is frequently done by means of interview, but some formal assessment may be used to aid goal-setting. However, the time available for information-gathering is often limited and the therapist

Initial assessment	To gather relevant information on which to base intervention. To explore issues of concern to the client. To determine treatment goals.
Assessment during intervention	To obtain more detailed information concerning abilities and needs. To plan therapy or intervention. To set a baseline for measurement of progress. To evaluate and measure subsequent change. To predict outcomes.
Assessment prior to discharge	To evaluate performance in relation to an individual's roles, patterns of required occupational performance and the used environment. To predict and evaluate risk. To predict and evaluate the need for environmental support or adaptation.

may be restricted by working within a very specific approach which limits the scope of information-gathering.

During the intervention stage, the assessor needs to observe, measure, judge and record. This implies a more structured approach. On the basis of this evaluation predictions can be made about progress or likely outcomes, and intervention can be modified accordingly. The *effectiveness* of the therapy can be measured.

In the final stage, the therapist becomes concerned with resettlement and may take a more holistic view of the capacity of the individual to cope in the community. Again, prediction, is important.

The process of information-gathering and evaluation serves to move the focus of enquiry from the past, through the present and into the future.

ASSESSMENT METHODS AND TOOLS

There are many different techniques used in assessment and various types of assessment; informal, formal, unstructured, structured and standardized. These are described in most occupational therapy textbooks where further details can be found. Some examples are given in Box 18.1.

Quantitative assessment measures something in terms of quantity, or quality, which is usually scored or expressed numerically.

Qualitative assessment is concerned with subjective aspects of personal experience and perceptions, and tends to be descriptive.

Box 18.1 Assessment methods and tools

Information-gathering	Collection of relevant data from written sources and interviews with the client or others. Information is summarized and recorded before evaluation.
Checklists	A checklist is an aid to recording information and observations. The checklist is not in itself an assessment; the procedure and method of evaluation of the collected data constitutes the assessment.
Assessment of performance components	Specific skills (motor, sensory, cognitive, perceptual, social) are measured. Tests are designed to discriminate between and measure different performance components.
Functional assessment	The client is asked to perform a task (usually self-care or work). The performance is recorded and compared to norms or criteria.
Assessment of occupational performance	A holistic approach is adopted in which past and present patterns of performance are identified and analysed in relation to work, leisure and self-care.

Box 18.2 Criteria for selection of assessments in clinical settings

Reliability	Consistent and repeatable results.
Validity	Construct validity; content validity criterion validity. A valid test accurately measures the item, and gives a precise, predictive score.
Test responsiveness	The test must detect change at the appropriate level to provide meaningful clinical data.
Practicality	Can be used with available resources, level of knowledge and competence.

These attributes of clinical assessments (together with examples of assessments) have been discussed in detail in many occupational therapy texts and will not be described further. Readers can refer to Hagedorn (1995a), Foster (1996), Ottenbacher & Christiansen (1997) and Polgar (1998); the last provides a useful guide to critiquing assessments.

Another, pragmatic, approach to clinical assessment is to view it as a continuum which moves the individual from 'sick person' (where there is the expectation of a passive and compliant attitude to therapy in which the therapist is the dominant partner) through to 'well person' who is capable of expressing choice and making informed decisions. This continuum suggests that assessments in the early stages of an intervention may be more structured and therapist-led, and that methods can move gradually towards a more client-centred approach as the individual recovers and is better able to participate.

ISSUES WHEN SELECTING CLINICAL ASSESSMENT

As previously noted, medical and psychological assessment methods and principles generally apply in clinical settings. This means taking a scientific and usually reductionist, approach. Assessments need to meet a set of criteria (Box 18.2).

ASSESSMENT IN COMMUNITY SETTINGS

When dealing with a client in the home, the therapist is working with the client as advisor, resource person or facilitator. The therapist probably does not provide 'therapy' as such. The therapist may not wear uniform and is working in a domestic setting which has both practical and cultural constraints on the therapeutic relationship and on what form of assessment can be carried out.

For this reason, the approach in a community setting is likely to be client-centred and 'needs led'. Client and therapist co-operate in the process of assessment, evaluation and goal-setting. However, the methods used, and the way in which 'client-centred' is interpreted vary widely.

In some cases, the process remains directed by the therapist to a large extent, with some nominal attention to involvement of the client. In other cases, the client is overtly enabled and empowered to take control of the assessment and intervention process.

CLIENT-CENTRED ASSESSMENT

In the past decade, there has been a reaction against, and questioning of, the 'medical model' approach to occupational therapy. This has included a critical appraisal of assessments derived from medical, psychological or rehabilitation approaches.

The result is the development of an increasing number of assessments which are, more or less, client-centred. This usually means that the client is involved in self-assessment, aided by some kind of form or checklist.

The most significant example is the Canadian Occupational Performance Measure (COPM) (Law et al 1994). This tool is unique in being both client-centred *and* scored in a manner which enables outcomes to be measured.

The designers of this assessment reviewed and rejected numerous existing assessments before developing their own. In many cases, assessments have evolved directly from, or in the context of, an existing model. In the case of the COPM, this process has been reversed. Development of an assessment tool has led to the development of the client-centred Canadian Occupational Performance Model (Canadian Association of Occupational Therapists 1997).

Other client-centred assessments have been developed for use within the model of human occupation.

FOUNDATION SKILLS

The foundation skills for assessment are:

- observation
- measurement
- recording
- evaluating results.

OBSERVATION

Observation is the key skill when assessing a client. Although most humans are naturally observant, this does not make them good observers; indeed studies of individuals' powers of observation and ability to recall what they have seen (for example during a crime) tend to show that untrained observers can be highly inaccurate, and are influenced by events both during and after the incident being observed.

Accurate and objective observation is a precise, focused and structured process which can only be acquired with practice. Observation for assessment purposes has an objective. *Something* is to be observed. This means that observation must be a selective process during which the observer homes in on the required information and discards material which is irrelevant. Part of the skill lies in deciding what is, or is not significant in what has been observed. Precision and accuracy are essential.

Although observation is a descriptive process, in most cases the results of the observation need to be recorded with simplicity and brevity. (There are exceptions; some qualitative, ethnographic techniques require a detailed, 'blow-by-blow' account.) Observation should provide precise answers to questions such as:

- What happened: what did you see –
  people; tasks; content of the environment?
- What behaviours or performances occurred?
- In describing these:
  for how long?
  how often?
  when?
  was it consistent?
  was it effective?

what level of competence was shown?
how did the person (others) react?

● What is the content and context of the environment?

● What demands do the task and environment impose? Is the client able to meet these?

If observation of performance is to be repeated, it is important to decide in advance whether the circumstances and conditions should be exactly replicated on each occasion, or whether changes can be made.

Unless the observer is concealed (for example behind a one-way mirror, or watching a video screen), the observer will inevitably influence what he is observing. This has been proved by several well-known studies. The observer may be a participant (which is less threatening, but makes observation more difficult), or a neutral, non-participant who acts as a 'fly on the wall' (which is quite threatening, but more accurate). There are several other roles for observers described in the literature.

In occupational therapy, observations often take place during treatment sessions. It is then particularly important for the therapist to take account of personal input; it is usual to assist, prompt or cue performance. These interventions affect performance and need to be observed, recorded and their effect on performance evaluated.

Measurement

Measurement of the individual

The therapist may need to record measurement of some part of the client's body or movements. The techniques for using tape measures, goniometers, dynamometers and other physiological measurement devices have to be mastered.

If sequential measurements are to be taken, efforts should be made to minimize the differences between one occasion and the next. This is not as easy as it sounds; for example, if a goniometer is not positioned in precisely the same place each time, the reading can be altered by several degrees.

Measurement also involves precise use of psychometric rating scales or scoring systems on standardized tests.

In an educational approach, measurement may include assessment of the level of knowledge or skill, compared to specified standards.

Measurement of the environment

Aspects of the environment – heights of furniture, length of walking aid, space to manoeuvre a wheelchair – may also need to be measured.

RECORDING

The results of observation need to have some permanent record. This is usually written, perhaps using a checklist or form of some kind to structure the content. Alternatively, sound recordings or video recordings can be used.

Recording, like observation, takes practice. Apart from practicalities such as neatness, legible writing and generally professional presentation, there are some fundamental principles (Box 18.3)

Box 18.3 Fundamental principles of recording	
Attribution	Records must contain the name of the person being observed and also the name and signature of the observer.
Date	All records must be dated. It may be useful to add the time in some circumstances.
Clarity and brevity	The record must be concise, and yet so clearly presented that someone reading the notes who was not present can understand exactly what happened.
State facts	Facts should be stated: that is, observations of what happened which are, as far as is possible, objective and unbiased. Assumptions about what might have happened but was not seen should be avoided or clearly separated from actual observations. Subjective and objective information should also be separated. Personal opinions about the character of a client must be avoided.

EVALUATION

Evaluation of assessment data presents one of the biggest challenges to clinical reasoning. There is the data – often too much of it – but what does it all *mean*?

If using a standardized test, there may be guidelines on interpretation; more often, though, the therapist must rely on clinical knowledge and experience.

The most common error in evaluation is to attempt to make assumptions or conclusions which are wider or more generalized than can be supported by the data. Unless the test has been validated as predictive, the therapist should avoid making firm predictions, especially when based on limited observations.

Explicit statements of results or facts are preferable; it is possible to say what the client can and cannot do on a certain occasion. What this indicates about future performance is usually a matter of probabilities. There are techniques for quantifying probability but these tend to involve more time and mathematical aptitude than the average therapist possesses.

While it is essential for the therapist to ensure good practice in assessment procedures, and to be able to demonstrate these if challenged, when communicating results to others the therapist needs to be aware that what they usually want is simply the conclusions.

SOURCES OF INFORMATION ON ASSESSMENT (SEE ALSO APPENDIX)

Assessment in occupational therapy (theory, methods, techniques, tools)

Assessment (Creek J) in: Creek J (ed) 1997 Occupational therapy and mental health, 2nd edn. Churchill Livingstone, Edinburgh

Assessment (Foster M) in: Turner A, Foster M, Johnson SE (eds) 1996 Occupational therapy and physical dysfunction: principles, skills and practice, 4th edn. Churchill Livingstone, Edinburgh

Occupational performance assessment (Ottenbacher KJ & Christiansen C) in: Christiansen C Baum C (eds) 1997 Occupational therapy, enabling function and wellbeing, 2nd edn. Slack, New Jersey

Occupational therapy evaluation (Unit VI) in: Neistadt ME, Crepeau EB (eds) 1998 Willard and Spackman's occupational therapy, 9th edn. Lippincott, Philadelphia.

19

Assessment at the developmental level

DEVELOPMENTAL LEVEL

As described in Chapter 5, the developmental level is divided into three sections: the proto-occupational level, the acquisitional level and the constructive level. The boundary between each level is not well defined as development of simple occupational performances is a continuous process in which each stage merges imperceptibly into the next in a seamless transition. Assessment can take place at each of these levels, and is often conducted within the framework of a specific frame of reference, appropriate to a particular specialism or field of work.

The developmental level is especially significant to the occupational therapist because it is where the individual's potential for performance, and the skill components of occupational performance, are generated and assembled.

Inevitably, especially at the proto-occupational and acquisitional levels, assessment tends to be somewhat reductive, a 'bottom up' approach, evaluating separate skills and small pieces of performance, rather than integrated performances. For this reason, it is necessary for the therapist continually to relate and associate findings in a holistic manner in relation to the wider context of the goals and needs of the client.

ASSESSMENT AT THE PROTO-OCCUPATIONAL LEVEL

At the proto-occupational level, performance is very limited. Basic physiological processes, movements and automatic, or simple, actions, interactions and reactions are all that occur. These do not combine to form sequences of purposeful or productive occupational behaviour, although very simple behaviours may be produced at the point where performance is moving into the acquisitional level.

At this primitive level, the therapist is concerned with evaluating the potential for performance rather than performance itself. The question is not 'what can this person do?' but rather 'what might the person be capable of doing?'

This area of assessment is highly important when working with children (a specialist area not covered by this book), but it is also needed when working with adult clients who have profound learning difficulties, brain damage, an acutely withdrawn psychotic state, or any other condition which has resulted in a regression to the lowest level.

ASSESSING THE POTENTIAL FOR ACTION

At the proto-occupational level, the therapist needs to understand the potential for movement, and something about the quality and characteristics of any movement which is present.

Assessment techniques at this level tend to be of two kinds, either 'hands on' measurements (such as using a goniometer to measure joint range, or manually testing muscle strength or the degree of tone), or observations of simple movements.

Action requires co-ordinated, targeted movement. Both sensorimotor and neurodevelopmental aspects have to be considered. Areas to be assessed might include:

- the presence or absence of abnormal patterns of movement or muscle tone
- the ability to produce reflex movements such as blinking or moving away from a painful stimulus
- posture and postural reflexes and awareness of the position of the body in space
- the ability to produce movements of limbs and body, including joint range and muscle strength

- the ability to grip, hold and release
- the ability to control movement to achieve a goal
- the ability to perform functional movements, e.g. roll, crawl, sit, stand, step, reach.

ASSESSING THE POTENTIAL TO REACT TO EXTERNAL STIMULI

Perception of stimuli such as pain, heat, touch, vibration, sound, light, smells and tastes are basic requirements for awareness of the environment. Once these sensations have been recognized, there also needs to be an appropriate response. Examples of areas to assess may include:

- avoidance reactions – e.g. moving away from unpleasant stimulus or bright light or reacting to loud sound. Making a negative affective response – crying, grimacing vocalizing
- positive, seeking reactions – e.g. looking, holding, stroking, exploring, expressing pleasure
- specific responses to sensory stimuli – e.g. to deep or light touch; brushing, tapping, textures, sounds, objects, scents, tastes which are liked or disliked
- degree to which individual actively explores and responds to sensory components of the environment.

ASSESSING THE POTENTIAL TO INTERACT WITH PEOPLE OR OBJECTS

Interactions with others include emotional reactions, touch, vocalizations, gestures or signs, recognition of others and appropriate responses to input from another person, and attempts to communicate own needs and preferences.

Interactions with objects include paying attention to them, handling, manipulation, exploration, recognition of objects as significant and attempts to associate one object with another. Examples of assessment areas include:

Interactions with others
- appropriate affective reactions as indicated by expressions and behaviours

- ability to distinguish between people and other objects
- recognition of other person, and of familiar people
- ability to understand basic communication from others
- ability to initiate simple communication with others.

Interactions with objects
- ability to pay attention to objects
- ability to recognize and distinguish between objects
- ability to interact with objects by moving or handling them
- expression of preferences or dislikes of objects
- behaviour showing comprehension of the function of familiar objects
- recognition and avoidance of objects which are potentially uncomfortable or dangerous, e.g. too hot, sharp, hard
- show awareness and a repertoire of simple behaviours appropriate to a range of normal circumstances.

PUBLISHED ASSESSMENTS AT THE PROTO-OCCUPATIONAL LEVEL

It is important to distinguish between tests of *function* which operate at higher levels, and tests of basic skill components. At the bottom of the proto-occupational level, tests should isolate specific skills in a manner which is outside of the context of occupational performance although capable of being related to it (e.g. psychometric tests, neurological assessments).

As one moves up towards the acquisitional level, assessment usually has a more obvious functional relationship. This may include use of very simple performance components (e.g. naming, recognizing, holding, placing, moving) as required by perceptual tests, mobility tests and cognitive tests.

Informal tests, based on structured observation recorded on a checklist, can often be of value as a screening tool, but lack the quantitative elements which are usually provided by published, standardized tests.

Many of the published tests at this level are validated for use with children, but not with adults. Others are designed for use by psychologists or other health professions and the occupational therapist may require special training to use some of these. (References are provided in the Appendix)

ASSESSMENT AT THE ACQUISITIONAL LEVEL

At this level, assessment moves from providing evidence of potential ability and development of skill components, to evaluation of the start of functional use of these abilities in order to explore and interact with the environment.

Examples include physical performance components which are required for simple personal tasks such as eating or dressing; simple social and communication skills; basic cognitive perceptual processing, such as recognizing an object and understanding its use; and the ability to solve very simple problems such as opening a box to obtain an item.

As most task-based assessments combine tests of performance at both acquisitional and constructive level, references to these assessments are provided in the next section. Examples of some simple tests of skill components are listed below.

EXAMPLES OF TESTS AND MEASUREMENT OF SPECIFIC SKILL COMPONENTS AT THE PROTO-OCCUPATIONAL AND ACQUISITIONAL LEVELS

Movement

- Berg Balance Scale (Berg et al 1995)
- Tinetti Balance & Gait Evaluation (Tinetti 1995).

Cognitive–perceptual tests (some movement components)

- Rivermead Perceptual Assessment Battery (PAB) (Whiting et al 1985)
- Chessington Occupational Therapy Neurological Assessment Battery (COTNAB) (Tyerman et al 1986).

Test of cognition/confusion

- Clifton Assessment Procedures for the Elderly (CAPE) (Pattie & Gilleard 1979)
- Middlesex Elderly Assessment of Mental State (MEAMS) (Golding 1989)
- Mini Mental State Evaluation (Folstein et al 1975).

Numerous examples of other specific tests are given by Kohlmeyer (1998) in her chapter entitled 'Assessment of performance components' which also provides a clear description of manual testing techniques such as measuring joint range and muscle strength.

Other sources of information on assessment at the proto-occupational and acquisitional levels include:

Christiansen & Baum (1997), e.g. pp. 243-246: balance assessments, dexterity assessments; selected co-ordination assessments, stroke motor function assessments; p. 295: comprehensive and specialized neuropsychological assessments.

Foster (1996) p. 173: onward: physical measurement.

ASSESSMENT AT THE CONSTRUCTIVE LEVEL

By the time an individual reaches this stage in the development of occupational performance, skill components have been mastered and integrated to enable task performance to be undertaken.

The individual now has the ability to do many things: by re-assembling foundation skill components in response to task demand, new skills are learnt and performance is practised and perfected. A person can, for example, remember the sequence of task stages required for putting on a garment, eating a meal and combing the hair.

At the top end of this level, as it merges into the effective level, simple self-care tasks such as basic meal preparation, or housework tasks are added to the repertoire together with social and recreational or creative activities. At this point, basic, culturally appropriate education should have further enlarged individuals' view of the world, their information about it and techniques for dealing with it. Basic literacy and numeracy should have been acquired and put into use.

In addition, as interaction between person, task and environment develops, individuals begin to perceive themselves as actors in the world. They can make choices, express preferences, take decisions about what to do or not do, decide who they like and who they do not, and make relationships accordingly. They may begin to differentiate between types of occupational performance, work, leisure or self-care.

Assessment at this level is typically based on observation of functional performance of simple, personal, daily living tasks, or of other constructive or productive tasks which enable aspects of performance, such as information-processing or problem-solving to be assessed. Construction of functional assessments requires good use of task analysis (see Section 4).

FUNCTIONAL ASSESSMENT OF PERSONAL ACTIVITIES OF DAILY LIVING

There are numerous functional assessments, designed by doctors, nurses, therapists and psychologists. A number have been criticized and evaluated by therapists, and many have been found wanting in some respect (e.g. see Eakin 1989a, 1989b, Law & Letts 1993, Unsworth 1993). Opinions differ about which are 'the best', but a number of standard assessments are widely used and have reasonable validity.

Apart from deficits in technical aspects of test construction, one of the main weaknesses of assessments used at this level is that they tend to consider performance in 'can do/can't do' terms; 'shades of grey' are often not allowed for. They take little account of the way in which the circumstances or environment of task performance may affect outcomes. Social and interactive skills are often omitted, especially when working in a physical setting.

It is important, if using a standardized test, to ensure that it is validated for the type of client with whom you wish to use it. It is also essential to stick to protocols, procedures and scoring systems, without attempting to alter these, since to do so will invalidate the test.

Many assessments of functional performance deal with both personal activities of daily living (PADL) and the performance of domestic or instrumental activities of daily living (IADL). In the context of the COPE taxonomy, these operate at the effective level and are considered in the next chapter.

TESTS OF FUNCTION

Tests of function dealing with PADL include:

Barthel ADL Index (BI) (Mahoney & Barthel 1965)

This assessment is still widely used; it is scored, standardized, and is regarded by some as a 'gold standard' for evaluation. It has the advantages of simplicity, brevity and ease of use. However, the chief disadvantage is that, although it is useful for rapid screening of a population in an institutional setting, it does not have very good responsiveness to measurement of small but significant changes. It is best used as a 'large sieve' to separate people who perform well from those who do not. Some variations on the BI are available, notably the one produced by Shah (Murdock 1992 and Shah & Cooper 1993).

Functional Independence Measure (FIM) (UDSMR 1993)

The FIM is widely used, and preferred by many therapists. It is standardized, scored, and covers a useful, but not over-extensive, range of 18 critical tasks.

It takes somewhat longer than the BI to administer, and requires more training and experience to develop a consistent interpretation of the scoring system. There are two versions of the score, 4-point and 7-point, and the latter is better at detecting change.

This test also has the advantage of taking account of the type and amount of assistance required to perform a task.

Assessment of Motor and Process Skills (AMPS) (Fisher 1994)

The AMPS uses 56 calibrated instrumental tasks in order to rate performance of 16 motor skills and 20 process skills (see also, Ch. 24, p. 188).

The assessment spans the range of skill use from the acquisitional level to a point somewhere at the lower end of the effective level. While IADL tasks are performed (whereas the majority of functional assessments at this level focus on PADL), this is done in isolation and out of context. The tasks are not combined, or sequenced into more complicated activities and processes as they would be higher up the effective level. Tasks have to be performed in a structured manner which does not allow for the effects of the environment in 'real-life' situations.

Initial screening is done by an interview, but the client is subsequently asked to perform a selection of tasks, usually within a simulated environment. Scores are then translated into an interval scale, which can be adjusted for rater leniency and task difficulty.

The scoring system is well researched, and validated. The results not only indicate the quality of performance but can also be used predictively.

The AMPS has been extensively researched. Use of the AMPS requires special training and accreditation to ensure inter-rater reliability is maintained.

Other tests

Similar tests which give information about cognitive, perceptual, sensory and motor function include:

- Structured Observational Test of Function (SOTOF) (Laver & Powell 1995)
- Arndottir OT–ADL Neurobehavioural Evaluation (A–ONE) (Arndottir 1990)
- Functional Skills programme for the Neurologically Impaired Client (Warmbolt

1996) (includes tracking system to evaluate progress in subskills).

Allen Cognitive Level Test (ACL) (Allen 1985)

This assessment was designed for use with clients having cognitive damage owing to mental health problems, dementia or acquired brain damage.

Allen's assessment spans the whole potential range of human performance from the protooccupational (level 1) to the organizational (level 6).

Using careful observation of structured simple tasks and activities, the therapist can rate the client's performance as occurring at one of six cognitive levels (for comparison of COPE levels and ACL refer to Table 5.1, p. 31).

Allen's cognitive disability model is based on the assumption that working to improve clients' skills is often ineffective when there is cognitive damage. The results of the assessment enable the therapist to adapt the task and the environment in order to maximize functional use of abilities.

Other performance-based tests of cognitive function include:

- Bristol Activities of Daily Living Scale (Bucks et al 1996)

- Kitchen Task Assessment (KTA) (Baum & Edwards 1993).

ASSESSMENT OF BASIC SOCIAL SKILLS

It is difficult to find standardized assessments of basic adult social and communication skills in the occupational therapy literature. This may be because assessments in this area seem to be developed mainly by psychologists, or remedial teachers and these can be found in assessment catalogues. Language assessments are used by speech and language therapists.

Occupational therapists concerned with social skills appear to either use the former tests (some of which are mentioned in the references previously cited) or use unstandardized tests based on structured observation.

EXAMPLES OF ASSESMENTS

- Functional Needs Assessment Treatment Guide (Dombrowski & Kane 1997) includes evaluation of verbal communication, self-care, community skills and prevocational skills
- Assessment of Communication and Interaction Skills (ACIS) (version 4.0) (Forsyth et al 1998).

Assessment at the effective level

In normal life, adult occupational performance is complex, well integrated and covers a wide repertoire of skills in activities associated with self-care, work and leisure.

Performance at this level has to be evaluated holistically with regard to the context and environment. The reductive approaches which are helpful when assessing and analysing at the developmental level may now become constraints. Equally, the more complex and integrated the performance becomes, the more difficult it is to apply reductive methods of assessment. It is not sufficient simply to determine whether a client *can or cannot perform*. It is also necessary to explore areas such as safety, satisfaction with performance, motivation to perform, social and practical resources to support performance, the way performance changes in response to environmental conditions, and quality of life issues.

At the same time, the adult who can perform at this level is capable of much more active involvement in the whole process of therapy, and the decisions about aims and interventions. An active, collaborative, client-centred, partnership approach is needed, rather than the more directive approach which may be required at lower levels when the client may be less able to participate.

There is, however, as previously noted, a tension between the need for accurate clinical assessment and the desire to take a client-centred approach. The degree to which the approach can be wholeheartedly client-centred may depend on the environment of practice. Clinical environments will press for a more structured and clinical approach to assessment; work in the community presses towards being more client-centred. In addition, there is a gradual transition from use of therapist-based methods to client-centred approaches as one moves from the bottom to the top of the effective level.

The PEOP family of occupational performance models is particularly useful at the effective level as the models emphasize both the necessity of being client-centred, and the importance of taking a holistic approach to the assessment of competent, adaptive, occupational performance which takes account of both objective and subjective aspects. This is important when working in community settings.

However, the practicalities of working within specialisms may still confine the therapist's range of assessments to particular aspects of human function. A frame of reference may be used to provide a more limited and better focused interpretation of the interactions between the person, the occupation and the environment (COPE). This has been illustrated by Table 2.1 in Chapter 2. The approaches which are most relevant at the effective level include:

- functional activities approach
- cognitive/cognitive–behavioural approaches
- group work (social skills) approach
- educational approach.

Examples of assessment used in some of these approaches will be given in this chapter; numerous others can be found by reference to occupational therapy textbooks and journals.

The biomechanical/mobility approach, graded activities approach, neurodevelopmental approach, cognitive – perceptual approach, and social skills training approach are applicable for use in therapeutic settings at the developmental level but are not suited to use at the effective level because they deal with isolated skill components and task performances.

METHODS OF ASSESSMENT

The therapist may base assessment on a single method, but more usually combines several methods to produce a rounded view. These include:

Self-assessment	The client rates own performance and evaluates degree of competence in relation to personal perceptions of needs and goals.
Interview	Asking the client about personal abilities and problems provides a simple method of screening out areas which do not need assessment and focusing on those which do. However, the client's perceptions, while important, may not reflect actual performance.
Structured observation	The client performs tasks and activities while being observed by the therapist. The stages of each task may be listed and separately evaluated. Results are recorded on a checklist and may be quantified. When well conducted, this method yields valuable information, but it may be hard to replicate assessment conditions precisely on subsequent occasions unless the test includes specific performance conditions.
Performance tests	A performance test is based on evaluation of performance in relation to standards, criteria or norms. Results can usually be quantified and may be predictive.

ASSESSMENT OF FUNCTIONAL ACTIVITIES

Competence in a repertoire of activities of daily living, (personal care, instrumental activities, work activities and leisure activities) is essential for independent living.

The client must either be able to perform the required activities or be able to organize resources so that these are performed by others.

Performance of daily living activities can be evaluated by reference to a number of parameters (Rogers & Holm 1998). These authors list the following as important:

Value	The value which the client places on the ability to perform the activity.
Independence	Being able to perform without help.
Safety	The degree of risk during performance.
Quality	The quality of performance in relation to the goal or outcomes of the activity. This includes efficiency and adequacy/ acceptability.

These parameters have been developed into a structure for organization of data acquisition, recording and interpretation.

EXAMPLES OF ASSESSMENTS OF PERSONAL AND INSTRUMENTAL ACTIVITIES OF DAILY LIVING

There is a bewildering number of available functional assessments and it is only possible to mention a few as examples of different approaches and methods.

Satisfaction with Performance Scaled Questionnaire (SPSQ) (Yerxa et al 1988)

This questionnaire is completed by the client. It rates 24 home management skills and 22 social/community skills using a 5-point scale related to client satisfaction over the past 6 months.

Community Dependency Index (CDI) (Eakin & Baird 1995)

This assessment is designed for use in a client's own home, in order to provide information which enables the community occupational therapist to have an outcome measure before and after intervention. It assists in identifying the category of handicap and the need for resources to support community living. It can also provide management information.

The test is based on structured observation of performance of 10 personal care tasks in the home environment, including basic mobility. The test is standardized and scored and the approach appears somewhat reductive. However, it is included at the effective level because it does take account of factors in the home environment.

Subsequent research comparing the CDI with the BI (Ward et al 1998) found that the test was 'equally sensitive to change in time (compared to the BI) but tended to give lower scores'. The researchers hypothesized that this might be due to the better ability of the CDI to take account of adaptive change (compensations for disability made by the client in the home environment).

Assessment of Living Skills and Resources (ALSAR) (Williams et al 1991)

The tool was developed for use with older people in the community. It deals with 11 'complex, self-maintenance tasks essential for a safe, satisfying and independent lifestyle' (Williams et al 1991).

It takes the form of a structured interview in which the client is asked to rate each activity for the current level of independence and also the presence or absence of resources for performance. Each reply therefore has two scores, for independence and for resources. The scores are combined and analysed by the therapist to produce a risk rating 'R'.

The inclusion of access to resources – practical and social – is a particularly useful feature of this assessment, as it makes the link between independence and the environment.

Another unusual feature is that the ability to successfully procure help from others in order to be independent is also taken into account. For example, the client may be unable to cook, but competently organizes the delivery of prepared meals.

Safety Assessment of Function and the Environment for Rehabilitation (SAFER Tool) (Letts et al 1998)

The tool was developed specifically to take account of the problem that assessment of the home environment is frequently based only on observation of the physical structure and content of the home. The SAFER attempts to take account of the way in which the user interacts with the environment during task performance.

Assessment takes place in the client's home and is scored. It can be used as a questionnaire or as a basis for structured observation of task performance. The SAFER Tool consists of 97 items arranged in checklist format. It deals with PADL and IADL tasks, mobility and environmental safety issues.

Research indicates good content validity and suggests that inter-rater reliability and validity are acceptable with various client groups. This is a new test and at the time of writing predictive validity, construct validity and the ability to use the tests to measure levels of independence are still being evaluated.

Community Integration Questionnaire (CIQ) (Willier et al 1993)

This has 15 items divided into three domains: home integration, social integration and integration into productive activities.

The questionnaire is usually completed by the client, but can be used as an interview.

The score indicates the level of community involvement.

SF-36 Health Status Questionnaire (Ware et al 1993)/short form SF-36 (Jenkinson et al 1993)

The SF-36 is a highly regarded and well-validated research tool. In the longer version, the client is asked to complete a 113-item questionnaire (alternatively the questionnaire can be administered by the therapist), which includes sections on feelings about current health and well-being, pain, depression/anxiety, the ability to perform a number of self-care tasks and the degree of social contact with others. The responses are scored by the therapist. The scoring system is somewhat complex and time-consuming, but the questionnaire is good at detecting change if used as an outcome measure.

The shorter version includes eight core domains involving 36 items.

ASSESSMENT OF ADVANCED PROCESS SKILLS

Advanced process skills are those which are required to chain and sequence complex activities. They include logical reasoning, problem analysis and problem-solving, planning, prioritizing and organizing resources. The degree to which the client needs to use these skills is related to the client's occupational and social roles and environment.

These skills are difficult to test in isolation or out of context because they require integrated use of many subskills, and adaptive and creative abilities.

The most usual approach is to use some kind of complex activity as a performance assessment. Alternatively, some of the gaming exercises developed for management training can be used.

Allen's cognitive level test will identify clients who are capable of functioning at level 6, which is where high level process skills are employed. It is worth noting that Allen believes that a proportion of the normal population does not function above level 5.

ASSESSMENT AT THE HIGHER END OF THE EFFECTIVE LEVEL

Despite the holistic approach, at the low to mid-point of the effective level the emphasis of assessment tends to be on evaluation of performance of selected PADL and IADL tasks which are essential for physical well-being. Because all humans have similar physical needs it is possible to standardize assessment to a large extent. Individuality is recognized in terms of medical history or social and physical environmental demands. This is a pragmatic approach. It acknowledges that therapeutic time is limited, and targets essentials.

In terms of the parameters of task performance as stated by Rogers & Holm (1998), in the traditional approach to ADL assessment, independence and safety are well covered. Quality is interpreted in terms of efficiency / difficulty / adequacy. It is, however, very likely that little attention will have been given to the values of the client, or to the client's feelings of satisfaction. If one can function competently in performing PADL and IADL at the mid-range of the effective level, one can certainly survive. The quality of that survival may, however, be open to question.

As occupational performance moves upwards towards the organizational level, it becomes richer, more individualized and far more complex. Subjective viewpoints, attitudes, values and quality of life issues become important. At this point, it becomes increasingly difficult to use traditional, standardized assessments because they tend to press both therapist and client to focus on a narrow band of self-care performances.

The therapist now needs client-centred tools and methods which are sufficiently flexible to cope with each individualized situation. The therapist may want to review the whole range of advanced performances including:

- ability to manage self-maintenance and care of others
- ability to meet the demands of work
- ability to engage in leisure occupations
- ability to use high level process skills.

In order to achieve this, the therapist may first need to move assessment up into the organizational level in order to understand the whole range of the client's roles, relationships, and patterns of occupational performance, past and present (see Ch. 21).

Once this information has been acquired, understood and processed by both client and therapist, assessment can be brought back into the effective level to explore specific abilities and needs. This transition from the largely 'bottom up' approach used at lower occupational levels to a 'top down' approach is highly significant. The point at which it occurs has to be a matter for the clinical judgement of the therapist.

Assessment of activities of daily lving has already been described. Assessment of capacity to work, or of the ability to engage in leisure tasks involves a somewhat different set of assessments.

WORK ASSESSMENT

Work assessment is based on finding out what the client's previous work experience consist of, what the client is currently capable of doing, and how these profiles relate to the demand of a current or future form of employment.

OBTAINING A WORK HISTORY

This usually takes place in the form of an interview.

Typical information which may be required for a basic work history includes:

- usual details identifying the client's age, gender, address, marital status and dependents
- details of past work; this might include a review of all previous jobs, or simply a description of the last one
- details of qualifications, special training, or personal skills
- details of educational attainments
- information about personal interests.

The interview may then progress (on the same or subsequent occasions) to exploring some of the issues raised by the history. Depending on the situation of the client, this might include exploration of work patterns (number of jobs, length of time in jobs, time off for illness or unemployment), looking at attitudes to the last job or to work as a whole, exploring skills and interests which might lead towards a new job and identifying training needs.

Analysis of this material leads on to identification of skill assets and deficits, educational needs, cognitive or attitudinal problems and other concerns that may require intervention.

Where indicated, the therapist may set up a simulated work environment in order to assess or observe performance over an extended period of time. There are, however, obvious limitations to the extent to which specialized skills involving professional work, machinery or technical production processes can be simulated.

Standardized vocational questionnaires and aptitude tests are available but occupational therapists do not usually perform detailed vocational aptitude tests or provide advice on careers or training. These are specialist areas in which some therapists have developed expertise, but where referral to an appropriate professional or employment service is usually required.

ASSESSMENTS

The following formats for recording this type of information may be useful:

- Vocational Guidance Form (Appendix VI); Employment Evaluation Application Form; Job Suggestion List (Appendix VII) (Baxter et al 1995)
- Guidelines for Work Interview (Appendix H) (Cynkin & Robinson 1990)
- Worker Role Interview (Velozo et al 1998).

More general information is given in:

- Treatment of Work and Productive Activities: Functional Restoration, An Industrial Rehabilitation Approach (Fenton & Gagnon 1998)
- Working (Foster 1996: 212–220)
- Work Assessment and Programming (Jacobs 1993)
- Understanding the Statistical Concepts of Measures of Work Performance (McFadyen & Pratt 1997).

ASSESSMENT OF THE ABILITY TO PARTICIPATE IN LEISURE ACTIVITIES

Leisure participation depends on a combination of personal preference and motivation and personal attitudes, knowledge, skills and interests, together with the opportunities afforded by the environment.

The therapist may need to assess the knowledge, and attitudes associated with leisure, or some of the specific skills required for leisure participation, and establish the actual level of engagement in leisure activities.

A useful guide to assessment in this area is provided in Leisure Enhancement Through Occupational Therapy (College of Occupational Therapists 1995).

The Actor-Centred Activities Analysis Outline (Appendix J) (Cynkin & Robinson 1990) provides a set of headings which could be adapted to provide a basis for assessment of the skill components required for a specific leisure activity and personal meanings associated with it.

EXAMPLES OF ASSESSMENTS
Engagement in leisure

- Influences on Leisure Questionnaire (Baxter et al 1995: 46)
- Discovering Leisure Patterns (Baxter et al 1995: 21).

Attitudes to leisure

- Discovering Leisure Attitudes Questionnaire (Baxter et al 1995: 16)
- Understanding Leisure (Baxter et al 1995: 37)
- Your Needs – what are you looking for in your leisure experience? (Baxter et al 1995: 43).

CANADIAN OCCUPATIONAL PERFORMANCE MEASURE (COPM)

This measure is based on clients' assessments of their problems, needs and priorities in the areas of productivity, leisure and self-care within their used environment. Details of development, reliability, validity and methods of use are given in the handbook (Law et al 1994).

The assessment takes place in stages. In the first stage, the client is interviewed about occupational performance in order to identify areas which are of concern. The criterion is not whether the therapist, or others, perceive the activities as 'problems', but only whether the client does so. At the end of the first stage, the client will have listed a number of problems which the client wishes to tackle.

In the second stage, the client is asked to rate each of these items on a 10-point scale for importance. Up to five items are then selected for the next stage of evaluation, on the basis of scored priority.

In the third stage, the client rates these items for ease/difficulty of performance, and for satisfaction with performance. Using a simple formula, the therapist can work out the total performance and satisfaction scores. These scores become benchmarks for measurement of change.

If necessary, other assessments may be used to explore the problem area in more detail. Client and therapist then frame goals connected with the problem activities and plan how to achieve these. Intervention continues as required. After a suitable interval, the performance and satisfaction rating are repeated and compared with the original rating. The score provides an outcome measure.

The COPM is appropriate for use at the effective level because it explores all aspects of performance and guides intervention towards the client's own priorities in the client's unique situation, in a way which leads on to active engagement with therapy or problem-solving.

21

Assessment at the organizational level

At the organizational level, individuals have to combine and co-ordinate all the aspects of their life, including roles, relationships and engagement in self-maintenance, productivity and leisure, to achieve a range of competent performances over extended periods of time.

They also require adaptive skills and attitudes, and positive values concerning engagement in occupational and perceptions of themselves as effective 'occupational beings'.

AREAS FOR ASSESSMENT

At this level, the therapist is chiefly concerned with overall patterns of performance, the balance between roles and occupational elements in the life of an individual, and occupational history. Perceptions of personal autonomy, efficacy and abilities and the meanings of occupations and experiences are also considered.

The overall ability of the individual to respond effectively to the unique set of occupational and environmental demands which the individual encounters has to be evaluated.

To obtain a comprehensive picture the therapist must consider both objective and subjective aspects, in relation to past, present and future performance.

PEOP models provide the theoretical framework for assessment at this level, and assessments have been developed for use within various models of human occupation.

In this chapter assessment of the following areas will be reviewed:

- occupational history including occupational patterns and occupational balance
- occupational storytelling
- perceptions of self as an 'occupational being'.

OBTAINING AN OCCUPATIONAL HISTORY

There are two approaches to obtaining an occupational history. First, there is the objective, 'fact-finding' approach which reviews and documents a specific aspect of past occupational experience.

This may include a work history, as described in the last chapter, which is tackled rather as if one was helping the client to prepare a CV (résumé) for a job application. This is usually done in the context of work assessment or retraining. Alternatively, it may focus on leisure occupations and social roles, also in a factual, retrospective, fashion.

Second, there is the comprehensive profiling approach which explores the totality of the client's occupational roles, including patterns of past and current engagement in work, leisure and self-care, and also identifies social roles and relationships and their occupational relevance.

CREATING A PROFILE OF OCCUPATIONAL AND SOCIAL ROLES AND PATTERNS OF PARTICIPATION

Obtaining a profile of the whole pattern of occupational engagement is inevitably a time-consuming process. It may include a work history or leisure analysis as described in the last chapter, but it also involves exploration of other forms of productivity, spirituality, and evaluation of self-concept and social roles and relationships.

Factors to consider may include:

- the scope of the individual's occupations and roles which may be mapped or profiled
- patterns of participation in these, past and present

- evaluation of these patterns, for example to compare current frequency of engagement with that in the past
- identification of personal interests
- exploration of attitudes to productivity, leisure or self-care
- range of social roles and relationships: exploration of how occupations support or fail to support these
- the performance demand of roles and occupations within the used environment
- cultural and religious dimensions of occupations
- the client's locus of control, perceived self-efficacy and related issues.

Assessment tools frequently take the form of self-rated questionnaires. The client may be asked to gather information by keeping a diary or chart of daily activities which in some cases may include noting reactions to these (physical or psychological). The client may map activities or be engaged in various forms of occupational analysis (see Ch. 27).

A number of different assessments is likely to be needed in order to cover the whole scope of the individual's performances.

EXAMPLES OF ASSESSMENTS
Occupational and social roles

- Role Checklist (Oakley et al 1986)
- Life Experiences Checklist (LEC)
- Role adaptation, Bereavement Inventory
- Life Pattern Grid (roles and relationships related to occupations) (Fanning & Fanning in Baxter et al 1995)

Patterns of engagement in occupations

- Idiosyncratic Activities Configuration Questionnaire (Appendix A) (Cynkin & Robinson 1990)
- 'Round the clock' Participation Diary (Baxter et al 1995: 44)
- Getting Leisure in Balance Questionnaire (Baxter et al 1995: 48).

A number of other assessments have been developed for use within the model of human occupation. These include:

- Assessment of Occupational Functioning
- Interest Checklist
- Occupational Case Analysis Interview and Rating Scale
- Occupational Performance History Interview
- Role Checklist
- Self-Assessment of Occupational Functioning
- Worker Role Interview.

These assessments and details of how to obtain them are summarized in:

Kielhofner G 1995 A model of human occupation theory and application, 2nd edn. Williams & Wilkins, Baltmore, Appendix p 232 onwards.

More recent information is available from the College of Occupational Therapists' Assessment database and also in the Appendix.

EVALUATING OCCUPATIONAL BALANCE

The concept of occupational balance is more complex than may first appear. There is an underlying assumption that an individual needs a balance between different areas of engagement (work, leisure, self-care, rest). It has also been suggested that there should be a balance between 'left brain' and 'right brain' activities, and between activities which engage 'head, hands and heart'.

Balance does not, however, mean some neat formula in which so many hours are allocated to each area. Balance has to be interpreted within the overall context of the roles and occupations of individuals, within their used environment. This picture is further complicated by the subjective views of individuals concerning the nature of their occupations. The experience of work or leisure is situational; the same occupation can be interpreted in different ways.

The assessments previously described will provide an occupational profile and a period of diary-keeping will show up obvious patterns.

It is relatively easy to identify people whose lives are badly out of balance: the workaholic; the person who spends half the time in bed and the rest in front of a television; the severely disabled individual whose whole life is taken up by the struggle for personal survival.

It is more difficult to sort out less obvious dysfunctions, particularly as these may be as much attitudinal and cultural as behavioural. For example, a woman may be unable to permit herself any time for personal enjoyment because she feels that it is wrong to take time which ought to be used for her family; the chores must be done, and they must be done to a high standard because she has been brought up to believe that this is what a wife and mother should do.

The therapist has to be sensitive to cultural issues and must avoid inflicting personal values or standards on the client. In general, problems of this kind are best tackled by a cognitive–behavioural approach, using a mixture of practical goal-setting and problem-solving, but also helping the client to re-assess priorities and appraise the basis for the client's beliefs and actions.

EVALUATION OF PERCEPTIONS OF SELF AS AN 'OCCUPATIONAL BEING'

The effects of positive and negative cycles of action and reaction on performance are well known. Effective performance feeds into positive beliefs about the self as a performer who is 'in control', which in turn predispose the individual to competent performance in future. Similarly the experience of the self as a 'failed performer', controlled by external events, inhibits future attempts to perform.

In terms of these mental mechanisms, it hardly matters whether the perception of performance is accurate; it is how clients feel about themselves that makes the difference. The therapist, however, may well be interested to evaluate the degree to which actual performance is accurately perceived by clients.

Perceptions of self are also affected by the content of the environment and the opportunities it affords. If opportunities for performance are reduced, it follows that engagement will be impoverished and the feedback loop that supports a positive self-image cannot operate.

Some mental health problems have a direct link with damaged self-esteem and self-efficacy. Life events also have a significant effect; sudden illness or disability, change in role, loss of a partner or prolonged stress may reduce the ability of the individual to cope effectively. These factors interact in a complex, and not always predictable, manner.

While an assessment may indicate that a problem *exists*, it may not necessarily indicate its *origin*.

EXAMPLES OF ASSESSMENTS OF PERCEIVED SELF-EFFICACY, PERSONAL CAUSATION AND LOCUS OF CONTROL

- Satisfaction with Performance Scaled Questionnaire (Yerxa et al 1988)
- Self-Efficacy Gauge (Gage et al 1994)
- Role Adaptation Bereavement Inventory
- Life Experiences Checklist
- Assessment of Occupational Functioning (Rev 2) (Watts et al 1989)
- Occupational Case Analysis Interview and Rating Scale (Kaplan & Kielhofner 1989).

There are numerous tests of anxiety, depression, personality, stress, locus of control and self-perception designed by psychologists, for example:

- General Health Questionnaire (Goldberg & Williams 1988)
- Multidimensional Health Locus of Control Scale (Wallston et al 1978)
- Recovery Locus of Control Scale (Wallston et al 1978)
- Perceived Stress Scale.

(Therapists need to check whether any training is required in order to use psychological tests.)

A selection can also be found in: Wright S, Johnson M, Weinman J 1995 Measures in health psychology: A user's portfolios. NFER–Nelson, Windsor.

Further information can be found in: McDowell I, Newell C 1996 Measuring health: a guide to rating scales and questionnaires, 2nd edn. Oxford University Press, Oxford.

OCCUPATIONAL STORYTELLING

The concept of 'storytelling' or construction of therapeutic narrative based on occupational experiences is a recent development which has been given impetus by theories proposed by occupational scientists. The technique owes much to social anthropology and is more subjective and ethnographic than other approaches.

It is based on an understanding (proposed by Bruner and others) that humans naturally turn significant life events into narratives in order to construct and understand their meaning. The telling of these stories becomes a vehicle for communicating personal experiences and desires (see Weber 1998). Sometimes stories become ritualized, a symbol for a whole set of concepts held by storytellers about themselves and their world (for a discussion of meaning and occupation, see Hasselkus & Rosa 1997).

Storytelling is not concerned with simply finding out what happened, but rather with discovering what those experiences have meant to individuals, what they reveal about their perceptions of themselves, and how the life story can be used to guide and illuminate the process of therapy. Mattingly (1994) drew attention to the way in which therapists use narrative as an aid to clinical reasoning, both by listening to, and analysing, the patients' narratives, and also by telling their own stories about their clients.

It is important to emphasize that this storytelling remains *occupational* in focus. This is not psychotherapy, but occupational therapy. The therapist is trying to work with the client to understand the client's life story in terms of *what was done*, with a view to moving forward to *what might be done now*.

The techniques are still evolving. The general principles have been summarized by Clark (1993) and Clark et al (1996). These authors distinguish between *occupational storytelling* and *occupational storymaking*.

Occupational storytelling is aimed at building a common horizon of understanding with the client. This involves collaboration in expressing the story, building empathy, inclusion of (and valuing of) the ordinary, listening and reflection.

The therapist facilitates the process of storytelling, evoking and prompting information, and then begins to analyse the significance of what is being said. This active collaboration and engagement between the therapist and client breaks down barriers, and enables both to enter a shared experience. In the powerful example, cited by Clark, of her dialogue with Penelope Richardson, both participants are changed by the experience and gain new insights.

In order to maintain the occupational focus, Clark suggests prompting questions such as 'What sort of things did you like to do in your childhood?' 'What were the themes which guided these occupations?', 'How did you feel when you did them?' and 'Did you keep anything you made?'

OCCUPATIONAL STORYMAKING

As defined by Clark (1993), this is 'the process of creating a story involving the therapist and the survivor (of some adverse life event) that will be enacted in the future and focused on further development of the survivor as an occupational being' (Clark et al 1996).

The preliminary story has informed the shared understanding of the client as an occupational being who has shaped the client's past occupations and been shaped by them. Using this as a springboard, various techniques can be used to enable the process of shaping a new story for the future.

Occupational coaching involves a number of techniques which are aimed at moving the client towards a positive view of how engagement in occupations might assist the client. These include: giving encouragement and making positive remarks; teaching occupational strategies; teaching about occupation's role in recovery; and making and affirming progress.

Other techniques include: evoking insights about problems and solutions; promoting a broader and more balanced view of activities of daily living (not just 'the chores'); handling emotions in occupational contexts; using occupational contexts to promote friendship and intimacy; and recognizing the symbolic dimensions of occupation.

It is plain that these techniques involve a commitment of time over an extended period in order to be effective, and that measurement of progress has to be subjective and qualitative.

Further work on the use of narrative has been undertaking within the framework of the model of human occupation. This has been described by Helfrich & Kielhofner (1994) and by Helfrich, et al (1994).

Occupational analysis and adaptation

SECTION CONTENTS

22

Introduction to occupational analysis and adaptation

OCCUPATIONAL ANALYSIS

WHAT DO WE MEAN BY ANALYSIS?

Analysis is a logical, reductive process in the course of which something is minutely examined and broken down into simpler components.

Analysis contributes to a greater understanding of the whole, and yet the unified entity remains 'greater than the sum of its parts' and needs to be related to a wider context if it is to be fully understood. We need both perspectives in order to understand human occupations.

WHY ANALYSE OCCUPATIONS?

Occupations are our speciality. We seek to promote competent adaptive performance. We want to help to solve performance problems. To do this we must understand how occupations are performed, both as whole and in parts, at different levels of performance and across different timescales.

Therapists need to have a wide range of personal skills upon which to draw for therapeutic media, but no therapist could ever hope to know everything about every human occupation. When a new form of occupation is encountered, it is necessary to have the analytical tools to enable rapid description of it and to discover what demands it places on the participant, and what adaptive potential it may have.

FORMS OF ANALYSIS

Task analysis and activity analysis have been used by therapists for many decades. The terms appear to be used as synonyms, despite the fact that in practice there are different forms of analysis and different objectives when doing it. For convenience, 'occupational analysis' will be used as a generic term in this text.

In view of the fundamental importance of occupational analysis to therapists, it is strange that few texts describe how it is done in detail.

When preparing this section, a review was conducted of around three thousand occupational therapy references drawn from journals and research literature; only a handful were found which related to occupational analysis. This may be because analysis is a practical exercise and it has therefore mainly been taught by example and by experiment.

The forms of analysis described in this section have been developed in an attempt to help students to understand the differing forms and purposes of analysis and the techniques involved.

It is helpful to distinguish between three forms of occupational analysis:

Basic analysis	Describes part of an occupation. The description includes what is done, the order in which it is done, and the essential tools and materials.
Demand analysis	Describes the *demand* which the task or activity places on the participant.
Applied analysis	Considers the potential remedial benefits and application for a specific condition or particular individual and how the task or activity might be adapted to promote or enhance performance.

BASIC ANALYSIS

Basic analysis is conducted in relation to the occupational levels: organizational, effective and developmental.

In order to conduct analysis it is necessary to determine in general terms at which level the selected 'chunk of doing' is to be considered.

The best guide is the timeframe. The therapist is concerned with an *episode* of performance. An episode is simply a period of time with a defined beginning and end during which performance takes place. It may be quite short, or relatively long. Episodes may be linked together over an extended period of time.

As a general rule, when analysing normal performance, the shorter the episode the simpler the nature of the task and the lower the level involved.

Therefore, as a convenient 'rule of thumb', the guidelines in Table 22.1 can be applied:

Table 22.1 Timeframe guidelines for basic analysis

Level	Timescale	Type of performance
Developmental		
Proto-occupational	Up to 1 minute	Performance unit(s)
Acquisitional	Up to 3 minutes	Task stage
Constructive	Up to 10 minutes	Single task or linked simple tasks
Effective	Up to 1 hour	Chained tasks or an activity; simultaneous tasks
	Longer timeframe, not exceeding 1 day	Linked activities or routines
Organizational	Several weeks	A series of activities linked by one product; a recurring, habitual extended routine
	Months or years	Occupations; roles

The set of guidelines in Table 22.1 should not be regarded as a rigid formula but it does provide a starting point. Complex sequences of varied or unrelated activities and tasks are best treated as separate elements for the purposes of basic analysis, although the description of interlocking patterns may be useful.

A second guide is the nature of the performance. At the developmental level, tasks are simple, concrete and self-contained. Performance occurs in short episodes of action, interaction or reaction, or in definable 'chunks'.

At the effective level, tasks link and interweave in a complex manner, and sometimes several different tasks are performed at once. At the organizational level, performance is concerned with planning what is to be done and appreciating the results of participation.

Using these guidelines, it is possible to allocate observed performance to a level quite quickly. For example, to pick up one crocus bulb is a performance unit. Putting a crocus bulb in a hole in the earth is a task stage. Repetition of that task stage across an area of a garden, together with other task stages, such as open bag of crocus bulbs; decide where to plant; dig hole; insert bulb; fill in hole, comprises the task 'planting crocus bulbs'. This might be a self-contained task, or it might be part of an activity 'planting spring bulbs in the garden'. The gardener might decide to include subsidiary tasks such as weeding and forking over the ground at the same time as planting the bulbs.

This activity might in turn be part of an extended chain of linked activities over several weeks, such as 'select and order bulbs from mail order catalogue'; 'go to garden centre to buy bulbs'; 'read garden design book to get ideas for planting scheme' eventually leading to the desired product of the whole sequence, 'walk round garden to enjoy bulbs as they flower in the spring' (a long effective sequence).

The planning which went into this sequence, identifying in advance the activities needed to have bulbs in the spring is organizational. All these activities are part of the occupation of gardening and the occupational role (work or leisure) of 'being a gardener'.

FORMS OF BASIC ANALYSIS

Because the nature of performance changes as the timeframe extends, basic analysis can be considered as comprising a set of related, but different techniques. These techniques are each appropriate at different levels. A summary is shown in Table 22.2.

At the organizational level, *macroanalysis* or *occupational analysis* is used. At the effective level, *mesoanalysis* or *activity analysis* is required.

Macroanalysis and mesoanalysis are holistic and descriptive. The therapist attempts to obtain a broad understanding of the occupation or linked sequences of activities. Activity analysis provides a description of a particular piece of performance in a defined setting, considering both objective and subjective aspects of performance.

At the developmental level, therapists use *microanalysis* or *task analysis*. Both techniques are essentially objective and reductive. The task or task stage is broken into component parts and minutely examined so that a very detailed understanding of performance is obtained.

USE OF BASIC ANALYSIS IN PRACTICE

In practice the therapist is most usually concerned with microanalysis or task analysis of episodes of between 3 and 10 minutes. Longer episodes become so complex to analyse that they inevitably end up being broken down into smaller units. Activity analysis is also useful in clinical

Table 22.2 Summary of forms of basic occupational analysis

Occupational level	Form of analysis	Type of performance analysed
Organizational	Macroanalysis	Occupations
Effective	Mesoanalysis	Associated activities (routines)
	Activity analysis	Activities (chained tasks)
Developmental	Task analysis	Tasks
		Task stages
	Microanalysis	
		Performance components

settings where a rapid review of demand is required. Mesoanalysis is useful in some settings, but it is time-consuming.

Macroanalysis is, perhaps, more a tool for the occupational scientist than the occupational therapist. Occupations and their processes are such large entities that a 'broad brush' approach has to be taken when attempting to describe them.

DEMAND ANALYSIS

Once a task or activity has been fully described, it is possible to analyse the demand it will place on the participant. Demand means the degree to which the participant is challenged to respond. Difficult, stressful or skilful activities which require active, focused participation have high demand. Those which are relatively unskilled and unchallenging, or which are seen as relaxing or restful, have low demand.

Demand analysis, like basic analysis, is focused entirely on the intrinsic nature of the task. It considers 'normal performance', the generally expected parameters when doing a particular task. Assessment of the skills used, or not used, by an *individual* when performing an activity is a different thing, although it often uses the same headings; so is *therapeutic or applied analysis* which relates performance demand to the therapeutic needs or level of ability of an individual.

It is plainly impossible to conduct a task analysis or activity analysis without any reference to the environment, but it helps to separate the two forms of analysis to begin with because they are both complex and detailed. Eventually both must be combined in order to obtain a full understanding of *performance demand*.

When undertaking analysis of demand, the therapist considers *the requirement for performance skills*, in relation to the *context* of performance and the general *content* of the task or activity. He may also consider *educational demand*, which involves identifying the prerequisite combination of knowledge, attitudes, values and skills required to perform the task or activity, or *developmental demand* which explores the developmental level required to perform the task.

APPLIED ANALYSIS

If any of the core competencies can be described as unique, this is surely the one. Other professions (ergonomists, teachers, psychologists, physiotherapists) undertake task analysis of various kinds, but the concept of using engagement in a task to provide specific therapy is originated by occupational therapists.

There are five aims of applied analysis:

- to enable the therapist to select a suitable activity, tasks or task to achieve the aims of intervention
- to offer appropriate choices to a patient or group of patients
- to assist the therapist to set up, organize and sequence the activity or task
- to facilitate teaching and learning
- to enable appropriate therapeutic adaptation of the activity or task which enables or enhances performance or provides performance demand of a specific and relevant nature.

Basic analysis and demand analysis provide the therapist with information about the tasks to be done. Analysis of the environment shows how the content can assist or impede performance. Analysis of individual potential and abilities and the process of goal-setting provide the context in which therapy is to take place. Applied analysis draws on all these sources to match the task to the therapeutic objectives.

APPLIED ANALYSIS AND OCCUPATIONAL LEVELS

Applied analysis is not relevant at the organizational level because occupations cannot be applied as therapy; they are simply too big for practical application.

The therapist cannot analyse the therapeutic value of cooking, except in the most general of terms. When a therapist decides to 'get the client to cook', it means that the therapist will engage the client in one of the innumerable forms of food preparation.

This will happen at the effective level where performance occurs at a particular time, in a specific place, for a definite purpose. Once the 'chunk of doing' has been identified, the therapist can carry out an applied analysis to check that it is relevant and to decide whether it requires adaptation.

At the acquisitional or constructive levels, the therapist may need to analyse the application of a task or even a task stage. At the proto-occupational level, however, applied analysis once more becomes impossible, because a single performance unit is too small to be applied as therapy (although it may be taught).

Table 22.3 Summary of applied analysis and occupational levels

Organizational level	Not appropriate
Effective level	Applied activity analysis
	Applied task analysis
Developmental level	
Constructive level	Applied task analysis
Acquisitional level	
Proto–occupational level	Not appropriate

In the following chapters in Section 4, the techniques of analysis will be described in detail.

ADAPTATION OF OCCUPATIONS

WHAT IS ADAPTATION?

Competent occupational performance occurs when the individual is able to meet the demands of the task, and when the environment contributes in a positive manner to this performance. Dysfunction arises when one of these elements is out of balance with the others.

It follows that the therapist can enable and enhance function by assisting the individual to change in some way, or by altering the content or demand of the task or the environment, or any combination of these components. Although therapists often think in terms of 'adapting occupations', it is important to recognize that this is only one point on the adaptive triangle. Because of the interactive nature of the components of occupational performance, it is difficult to isolate these different forms of adaptation. In practice, they all often happen simultaneously.

In this section, adaptations to tasks, tools and equipment will be reviewed, together with adaptive techniques which can be taught to assist the individual to understand and cope with performance problems. Environmental adaptations will be described in Section 5.

ADAPTATION OF TASKS OR ACTIVITIES

It is possible, using occupational analysis, to describe a 'normal' – usual or accepted – way of performing a structured task or activity. In the context of therapy, it may be necessary to change some aspect of this normal performance. These changes are *adaptations*. The therapist can adapt aspects of process or product using any performance parameter which is capable of manipulation or control.

Changes are made for two main reasons: to enable or enhance performance (*functional adaptation*), or to provide specific therapy or assessment (*therapeutic adaptation*). It is important to be clear from the outset which of these is required because, although methods may be similar, there are important differences.

THERAPEUTIC ADAPTATIONS

Therapeutic adaptation is required to enhance the benefit of engagement in a task in some specified way. This is normally undertaken in the occupational therapy department or clinic in the context of physical or social rehabilitation. Therapy deals with the *causes* of dysfunction.

The aim of therapeutic adaptation is to provide treatment or to assess particular aspects of performance with a view to treatment. While the patient may well be actively involved in this process, it is controlled and led by the therapist.

The aims and techniques of using activities for therapy, especially in physical rehabilitation, have been extensively documented in standard texts on occupational therapy. Most of these describe adaptations of various kinds. Adaptations may be obvious or quite subtle and can involve sequences and methods, grading, altering tools, materials or the environment, or introducing new tools or equipment.

It seems unnecessary to duplicate these texts. However, information on techniques or adaptation tends to be scattered and is often presented in relation to the treatment of particular conditions. It can therefore be difficult to obtain an overview of what is involved. In this section, a summary of basic principles, approaches and techniques is provided.

Being adaptive requires a combination of imagination, inventiveness and lateral thinking. It means not being limited by the usual conventions of performance, or the usual purposes of tools or materials. Making adaptations to tools and equipment requires some personal technical ability, good problem-solving abilities and an understanding of basic mechanics.

FUNCTIONAL ADAPTATION

Functional adaptations are required to enable an individual to do the things the individual wants or needs to do in normal, daily life. This often involves activities of daily living, but it could also apply to work or leisure activities.

A functional adaptation minimizes the external *effects* of disability, but it does not deal with the *internal causes* nor does it seek directly to improve skills and abilities, although removal of barriers to performance and modifying demand may well enhance performance.

This may mean changing aspects of sequence or method, or modifying equipment or the environment, or introducing new equipment or assistive devices.

Functional adaptation is therefore directed explicitly by the goals of the individual. It is frequently needed in the home or the used environment. Techniques of functional adaptation are described in Chapter 31.

The degree to which an individual wants and will use and accept functional adaptations is variable. Some will accept quite elaborate adaptations if these enable them to engage in cherished activities or maintain a degree of independence. Others may prefer to discontinue doing some tasks, or to do them with a struggle, rather than accept changes. It is essential that the client works in partnership with the therapist to identify performance problems, propose solutions and select adaptations.

23

Approaches to occupational analysis and adaptation

Just as an approach can direct, focus or modify assessment or therapy, so it can be used to limit or structure task analysis or activity analysis or set the parameters for therapeutic adaptation.

Crepeau (1998) notes that activity analysis can be task-focused, theory-focused or individual-focused. Theory-focused activity analysis is concerned with the following questions:

- How does this theory define function, dysfunction and change?
- What are the properties of this activity (task) from this perspective?
- How can activities be graded and adapted consistent with this theory?

The use of an approach modifies the basic analytical technique to limit the scope of the analysis, to make it more relevant or to expand some aspect of the information. Most commonly used frames of reference provide an approach to activity analysis and adaptation. A combination of approaches provides a comprehensive understanding. The main approaches to occupational analysis and adaptation used in rehabilitation are shown in Box 23.1.

The analytical techniques used in an approach or an adaptive technique may or may not be explicit. In some cases, there are well defined analytical procedures or checklists; in other approaches, one must use the theoretical basis to provide a guide to enable one to emphasize some aspects while disregarding others.

Box 23.1 Approaches to occupational analysis and adaptation used in rehabilitation

Frame of reference	Approach	Focus
Biomechanical	Exercise physiology	The effects of task performance on the physiology of muscles, joints, or the work of the cardiovascular system
	Kinesiology	Movement elements of the task; force and motion
	Analysis of muscle work	Identifying which groups of muscles or individual muscles are involved in producing a specific action, and specifying the type of muscle work, e.g. static; active; eccentric, concentric
	Analysis of functional movement	Analysis of the general type of movement in relation to its functional purpose
	Graded activity	The elements of performance which may be adapted to provide therapy or facilitate task performance
Ergonomic	Ergonomic	The design of tools or equipment, content of the environment, sequence of task performance, posture or position of participant in relation to efficiency of performance
Neurodevelopmental	Developmental	The relationship of task components to developmental stages or level of skill
	Sensory	Sensory stimulation provided by task or requirements for sensory discrimination
Cognitive	Cognitive–perceptual	Perception; information-processing; problem-solving; need for knowledge
	Cognitive–developmental	Cues provided by task or environment which influence thoughts, feelings and behaviours
	Social/interactive	Aspects of the task or environment which promote communication and social interaction

BIOMECHANICAL APPROACHES

Biomechanical approaches deal with 'the body as a machine'. The therapist is concerned with the analysis of movement. Extensive examples of the application of the biomechanical approach, and associated adaptations are given in Trombley (1989). Task analysis is implicit in much of this material.

EXERCISE PHYSIOLOGY AND KINESIOLOGY

To be truly accurate, this type of analysis requires the use of sensitive physiological measurement equipment and computer analysis which is not normally available to occupational therapists.

In occupational therapy, these approaches are therefore usually restricted to research settings where special equipment and expertise are available. For this reason, these techniques will not be described in detail.

For an example of this type of analysis refer to the chapter on cardiopulmonary rehabilitation in Trombley (1989) where details of the effects of exercise on the cardiovascular system are provided together with a schedule of the approximate metabolic cost of a variety of activities.

Therapists formerly conducted detailed analysis of 'muscle work' (operations of groups of muscles) and range of movement based on observation, measurement, and a very good knowledge of functional anatomy. This type of analysis is still useful in physical rehabilitation settings and is described in Tyldesley (1996). It is particularly valuable in hand therapy and treatment of upper limb dysfunction.

ANALYSIS OF FUNCTIONAL MOVEMENT

Biomechanical analysis in occupational therapy usually takes a more generalized functional approach in which the components of movement are described and rated.

The taxonomy of joint movements may be used, for example: 'elbow extension, mid-range'; 'seated with knees flexed at 90°; 'pinch grip between thumb and first finger'.

The nature of movement may be described by verbs: bending, reaching and lifting.

The quality of movement required may also be described by using adverbs, or by contrasting descriptors such as fast/slow and dexterous/gross movement.

GRADED ACTIVITY APPROACH

Grading is the precise use, during purposeful activity, of factors which contribute to task demand in order to achieve a therapeutic objective.

Grading means that, over a number of treatment sessions, the demand of the task is modified so that required elements of performance (sensori-motor; cognitive–perceptual; interpersonal) are progressively made more challenging (or made easier).

In order to do this, the nature of normal performance must first be understood to see if there is scope for therapeutic application. Once the nature of the task has been described, the therapist can look for ways to change the demand as required.

If a specific performance element is required, the analysis may be restricted to one approach.

ERGONOMIC APPROACH

The ergonomic approach has been influential in occupational therapy.

Pheasant (1986) accepts the traditional definition of ergonomics as 'the scientific study of human beings in relation to their working environments' but states that 'Ergonomists today mostly think of themselves as technologists or engineers rather than scientists.'

Ergonomists have traditionally worked mainly in the context of industry, although research has been done in domestic settings. Ergonomists aim to improve productivity and worker morale while minimizing the adverse effects of task performance, such as fatigue, repetitive strain, stress, boredom and occupational injuries.

Their work is also used to improve worker selection.

Ergonomists have much in common with occupational therapists. They are interested in the nature of work and its effects on the human body and in the capacity of the individual to respond to these demands. Ergonomists consider the nature of the task, the effects of the working environment on performance and the design of tools, machines, work stations, seating and furniture. Data from ergonomic research and anthropometric data are now widely used to improve the design of new products.

Pheasant takes a broad view of the ergonomist's remit which makes the overlap with occupational therapy very obvious.

the concept of work must encompass a wide range of human behaviour – not only on the tasks performed in the occupational context but leisure and domestic activities as well. Similarly our study of the working environment must include not only the physical environment and the objects within it but also psychological factors such as mental workload and the flow of information and social interaction with other human beings.

What then is the difference between an occupational therapist and an ergonomist? The ergonomist is interested primarily in describing 'normal' populations and normal tasks and in applying the results of research to the working population in industrial settings, or in environmental design.

The occupational therapist is more likely to work with an individual, with a view to enabling, enhancing and empowering more competent performance of work, leisure and self-care activities. Put another way, ergonomists are concerned with *occupational performance* while occupational therapists are concerned with *occupational therapy*.

SYSTEMS OF TASK ANALYSIS DEVELOPED FOR USE IN ERGONOMICS

Ergonomists have developed many systems of task analysis in work settings. Since the aims of the ergonomist and occupational therapist are so similar, it is odd that occupational therapists do not, on the whole, use or refer to these systems.

ERGONOMIC WORK ANALYSIS METHOD

This method has been developed by the Institute of Occupational Health in Helsinki in 1987 (Loupajarvi 1990). There is a list of 14 workplace characteristics. These are rated on a five-point scale from 5, indicating unacceptable danger or health risk, to 1, indicating better-than-average circumstances.

GENERAL ERGONOMIC CHECKLIST

The International Ergonomics Association has produced a 'general ergonomic checklist' (Loupajarvi 1990). This has lists of questions under headings.

AET JOB ANALYSIS PROCEDURE

Another highly detailed analysis system was developed in Germany during the 1970s and published by Rohmert & Landau (1983). It has been used to analyse over 4000 different jobs. This system is known as the AET job analysis procedure from the initials of the very lengthy German title.

The complete analysis programme includes 216 characteristics of the task from which a task profile can be drawn up.

OVAKO WORKING POSTURE ANALYSIS SYSTEM (OWAS)

The OWAS was developed by a Finnish steel company (Karhu et al 1977). It is a movement notation system which uses stylized pictograms depicting body postures so that these can be recorded by an observer as the worker engages in the task.

ACTIVITY MATCHING ABILITY SYSTEM (AMAS)

This was developed by the British Steel Corporation as part of an initiative to improve resettlement of disabled workers into suitable jobs. An activity assessment was developed, considering 100 items divided into four sections:

A social aspects
B work environment
C equipment
D work demands.

Although these items were specifically designed for use in the steel industry, the structure is useful for therapists, especially section D.

JOB DEFINITION DATABASES

Definitions of occupations which include more or less detailed descriptions of what is involved are available in the form of dictionaries or databases of job titles and lists of job specifications intended for use in career advice or training.

USE OF THE ERGONOMIC APPROACH IN OCCUPATIONAL THERAPY

An example of the application of this approach is given in a Guide to Employment Assessment and Preparation (College of Occupational Therapist 1992). This draws on information from the Canadian Classification and Dictionary of Occupations to produce a checklist for job specification and demand analysis.

In the USA, therapists are involved in Job Site Analysis (JSA) which is based on ergonomic principles.

ANTHROPOMETRICS

The need to improve designs to match the sizes and shapes of real people in all their diversity has led to much research. This in turn has produced quantities of anthropometric data concerning working heights, postures, loads and positions. Ergonomists use this data to improve design and function.

A general awareness of anthropmetric principles is useful to the therapist in conducting task analysis and environmental analysis. Anthropometric and ergonomic principles are often applied when re-designing the home of a dis-

abled person, when designing a therapy area or workshop, or when adapting a tool or task for therapeutic purposes.

SUMMARY

Techniques of ergonomic analysis of the work environment and task performance are well developed, and typically include:

- description of the physical and social environment in which the worker operates. Analysis of the relationship of the worker to the tools, equipment and layout of workstations or design of machines
- analysis of task content and structure
- analysis of job demand: physical, cognitive, social
- 'time and motion' analysis
- consideration of health and safety factors; risks and hazards; manual handling; potential for occupational injury.

It will be apparent that there is a wealth of ergonomic literature and research. Any therapist who needs to undertake work analysis or who wishes to undertake research into detailed task analysis should refer to this material before resorting to the invention of a personal methodology, or attempting a job analysis which may already have been carried out.

DEVELOPMENTAL APPROACHES

SENSORI-MOTOR APPROACH

This is based on neurodevelopmental theories and techniques of treating neurological dysfunction or developmental delay. The significant aspects of the task are the position adopted by the worker, and the types of movements used.

The therapist needs to select tasks which are compatible with, or capable of adaptation to conform to, theories about posture, bilateral movement, inhibition of increased muscle tone and other neurodevelopmental principles.

SKILL ACQUISITION APPROACH

Basic skills are acquired in a known developmental sequence. One learns to grasp relatively larger objects before one can manage small ones; one can achieve gross, unco-ordinated movements before mastering fine and dexterous ones; one must achieve balance to stand and walk before one can hop, skip or jump. Cognitive and perceptual skills are also acquired in a sequence.

A task may be analysed to ascertain the level of performance in order to determine whether it is suitable for therapy, or education.

COGNITIVE APPROACHES

COGNITIVE–PERCEPTUAL APPROACH

This focuses on analysis of the perceptual and information-processing components of the task. The therapist may, for example, consider aspects such as the visual cues provided by a task sequence or environment, or the degree of abstract conceptualization or decision-making needed during a task stage. Familiarity with the taxonomy used to describe perceptual processes is required to ensure accurate analysis.

COGNITIVE–DEVELOPMENTAL APPROACH

This might be concerned with skill acquisition, or with the analysis of the task in relation to levels of cognitive ability or development, for example, as suggested by the six levels in Allen's cognitive disability model (Allen 1985).

SOCIAL/INTERACTIVE APPROACHES

Here the focus is on the amount of interaction or communication which is required by, or occurs in connection with, task performance. The demand may be analysed in order to adapt the task to enhance or reduce the required interactive or reactive performances.

In the social approach, the potential of the task or activity for use in group work is especially relevant.

EDUCATIONAL APPROACHES

BEHAVIOURAL APPROACH

This involves microanalysis of the task to identify behavioural components (see example in Ch. 16).

KNOWLEDGE, ATTITUDES, VALUES AND SKILLS (KAVS)

This analysis might be used as a precursor to teaching a new activity or task or assessing whether a person is likely to be able to perform it. It helps to identify the prerequisite learning which is implicit in the task demand.

EXAMPLES OF ANALYSIS USING DIFFERENT APPROACHES

In order to demonstrate how each approach gives different information about a task, a simple task will be analysed using a selection of these approaches. First, a basic sequence analysis is required in order to describe the task stages (Box 23.2).

A comparison of the analyses in Box 23.2 clearly illustrates the value of the different approaches. Each provides a different understanding of the task. A comprehensive analysis might combine the functional, educational and ergonomic approaches.

In practice, the therapist would conduct the analysis in relation to an individual and the reality of the situation in which the task is to be performed. This would be done with a view to either assessing the capacity of the individual to do the task, or modifying the environment or task in order to improve performance.

Box 23.2 Basic sequence analysis of simple task

Task
Write a shopping list
Task sequence
1 Sit at table
2 Pick up pen
3 Write list on paper
4 Check list is complete.

Functional approach: analysis of movements and sensory components

Movements

Sit	Maintain upright sitting balance during task
Pick up	Dominant hand, pinch grip, pen grip
Write	Dominant hand, pen grip, co-ordination and control while writing; hand tracks across paper. Non-dominant hand used to stabilize paper (flat on table)
Sensory components	Vision: sufficient to write and check list Touch: pick up and hold pen and stabilize paper Stereognosis: maintain position of hand and smooth flow whilst writing

Cognitive–perceptual approach

Perception	Recognize pen and paper: object recognition Correctly align writing on paper: spatial Perception and visual scanning
Cognition	Word recognition. Recall items for list – medium-term memory; check list – attention; memory

Educational approach

Knowledge	Understands purpose and use of shopping list Knows how to read and write
Attitude	Has positive regard for planning and organization
Values	Legibility; accuracy
Skills	Able to write Able to read Able accurately to note items required and retain as mental list for checking

Ergonomic approach

Check
- table surface smooth and uncluttered
- height of chair in relation to table
- design of chair provides good support for writing posture
- layout of pen and paper: easily reached and visible
- design of pen: facilitates good grip and flow of ink
- sufficient light
- distractions which might impede recall of items

24

Microanalysis

WHY DO WE NEED MICROANALYSIS?

It is necessary for the therapist to understand how small units of performance build into large and complex ones. Because these are the 'building blocks' of performance, a dysfunction at acquisitional level has a disproportionately large effect across the whole range of human performances. The student needs to understand these relationships, even if, as a therapist, the student does not work in an area where microanalysis is relevant.

Therefore, either for research purposes or in order to work with clients experiencing problems at a developmental level, the therapist must know how to conduct detailed analysis of small episodes of performance or short sequences of task stages.

SEQUENTIAL ANALYSIS OF A PERFORMANCE EPISODE

The first stage of microanalysis aims to identify the nature of performance; the analyst asks the question 'What is going on?' The answer is provided by isolating an episode of time (between 1 and 3 minutes) during which a sequence of performance units takes place. An example will help to demonstrate this process.

SEQUENTIAL ANALYSIS: THREADING A NEEDLE

If we start with the assumption that needle, reel of cotton and pair of scissors are already available (finding them constitutes other tasks), then threading a needle appears to be a simple task which has only two stages: cut cotton; thread needle.

If, however, we think in more detail about performing this task, or perhaps imagine how to explain with great precision to someone else how it should be done, then the details above are plainly insufficient.

It may be useful, for example, to specify the starting position of the performer. Let us assume that the performer is seated by a table on which the needle, cotton and scissors are located.

But we still do not know enough if we are to instruct the user how to thread a needle. We need to describe the performance units, the smallest pieces of performance into which a task stage can be divided.

Performance units in task of threading a needle

Note. As this is a bilateral task, the use of hands is indicated by (L) (left) and (R) (right); in this example, it is assumed that the right hand is dominant.

So far this analysis has been an abstract exercise; it is based on my memory of how to thread

Task stage
Cut cotton
Performance units
Pick up cotton reel (L)
Find end of cotton (R)
Hold cotton reel in one hand (L)
Pull thread to unwind a length of cotton (R)
Judge length of cotton against desired length
Retain hold of cotton reel and measured thread (L)
Pick up scissors (R)
Cut cotton to desired length (R)
Put down scissors (R)
Put down cotton reel (L)
Pick up cotton, retain for use (R)

Task stage
Thread needle
Performance units
Pick up needle at mid-point (L)
Hold needle steady in front of user at face
    height (L)
Turn needle so eye is facing user (L)
Pinch and grip thread near tip (R)
Guide thread through eye of needle (R)
Catch and pull thread through eye from other
    side (R)

a needle. It is useful in that it itemizes the sequence of performance units and shows that the task is bilateral.

If one were to video a number of people attempting to thread a needle, some of these performance units would happen every time, and in the same order: one would normally only thread the needle when the cotton has been cut.

However, individual *variation* would also be observed. Some might stand, others sit. Users would be likely to hold the cotton reel in different ways, and to use left or right hand for different parts of the task. Some might choose to break the cotton by hand, or with the teeth, instead of using scissors. The cotton may or may not be knotted after threading. After threading, the needle will be put somewhere safe while the sewing is prepared.

In addition, some users might react to circumstances which occur as the task is being performed. So, for example, if the needle is not threaded after a few attempts, the user might check the available light, examine the cotton end to see if it is frayed; if it is, the user might trim it or suck the end to smooth it out. The needle eye might be checked to ensure it is not blocked. The user might move to a better light, or go to find a pair of spectacles before completing the task.

ANALYSING THE COMPONENTS OF PERFORMANCE: ACTION, INTERACTION AND REACTION (AIR)

After a sequence analysis has been completed, it is possible to use the lowest level of the COPE taxonomy, *actions, interactions and reactions* in order to further describe what is taking place. To avoid continuous repetition, the combined use of actions, interactions and reactions in an episode of performance will be referred to in this chapter by the acronym AIR.

AIR analysis is useful when analysing a task stage, but it becomes even more useful when the performance episode does not fall neatly into the classification of task performance.

As we saw in the short description given in Chapter 5, tasks are not always undertaken as coherent 'chunks'. Several different pieces of performance may nest and enfold in and around the stages in a task. These pieces of performance can be designated as actions, interactions or reactions.

AIR can occur as short, 'free-standing' sets of performance units. Performance of AIR is often spontaneous rather than planned. It can occur in response to cues from the environment, or in connection with 'mini-tasks' which are really too small and transient to be considered as tasks at all.

For example, during a performance episode which occurs while you are engaged in the routine task sequence of 'getting up, using the bathroom, getting dressed, having coffee' you may conduct many small operations such as opening a door, switching on a light, turning off an appliance or machine, opening and closing a container. You may use tools such as a toothbrush, spoon or comb. You may check your watch and speed up your actions if you are late. You may react to incidents and proceed to answer the phone, pick up and open a newly-delivered letter, turn off a dripping tap or pick up a dropped item. You may speak to other family members or a pet.

At work, a person doing a clerical filing task may continue to sort papers and letters, find and open files, file the papers and replace them in the cabinet, while interacting responsively with others such as replying to a question, cracking a joke to a passing colleague or smiling as someone enters a room. The worker may also initiate small interactions, such as asking a question, confirming that something has been done or seeking a new task.

In order to use the AIR taxonomy in microanalysis, it is necessary to have a clear understanding of each term.

COPE TAXONOMY: ACTION, INTERACTION AND REACTION

Action

An action is a physical performance which may or may not be connected to others. Actions are initiated by the individual and are voluntary, purposeful and intentional. Although performance of actions depends mainly on sensori-motor skill components, actions also require integrated use of process skills, cognitive and perceptual.

INTERACTION

An interaction is behaviour which occurs when an individual attempts to relate to, or find out more about, people, organisms or objects in the environment. It originates from *within* the individual and has the purpose of communicating something to someone else, or exploring the surroundings.

There are three types of interaction recognized by psychologists as defined by Atkinson et al (1993):

proactive interaction is the interaction between individuals and their environments that arises because different individuals choose to enter different situations and to shape these situations differently after entering them.

reactive interaction is the interaction between individuals and their environments that arises because different individuals interpret, experience and react to situations in different ways.

evocative interaction is the interaction between individuals and their environments which arises because the behaviour of individuals evokes different responses from others.

In the context of COPE, interaction is only *proactive*, that is, initiated by the performer. Reactive and evocative interactions come within the domain of reactions – produced by the performer in response to the external environment or situation.

Social interaction is a term used to describe behaviours which occur between individuals (dyadic interaction) and groups (group interactions). Again, in the context of COPE, a social interaction would in fact be analysed as comprising a set of actions (initiated by the individual), interactions (initiated by the individual) and reactions (responses to others).

Reaction

A reaction is 'responsive or reciprocal action' (COD). As used within COPE, a reaction is the observable performance or behaviour (reactive interaction; evocative interaction) which occurs in response to people, objects, incidents and events. It is triggered by something *external* to the individual. (A reaction may also occur in response to an internal physical sensation, but in the context of microanalysis we are not normally concerned with this.)

In order to react, the individual must perceive information about a situation, process this, and come up with an appropriate performance response. Therefore, responses such as active listening, watching or observing are *reactive*.

Reactions may be *affective* (emotional in origin), or *cognitive* (arising from perceptions and thought processes) or *social* (prompted by action of another person), but they are always expressed by behaviour of some kind. They are also influenced by values, attitudes and cultural norms.

Affective reactions can be broadly classified as:

Negative   e.g. prompted by anger, fear, anxiety, horror, grief dislike, dissatisfaction, discomfort, boredom

Positive   e.g. pleasure, liking, enjoyment, satisfaction, comfort, pleased surprise, gratitude

Neutral   in which case little or no observable response may be made.

An avoidance (aversive behaviour) reaction is an action which aims to avoid, or remove the individual from, a situation which poses a risk or threat, or which is perceived negatively (e.g. escape, duck, run away, leave the room, discontinue participation).

A seeking reaction (appetitive behaviour) is one which helps the individual to maintain or obtain something which is viewed as positive (for example, continue participation, ask for more, pick up, hold, gather, collect).

Cognitive reactions occur when the individual has perceived a situation as having some meaning which requires immediate action, such as problem-solving.

Social reactions occur when another person speaks or does something to provoke a response.

OVERLAPS BETWEEN ACTIONS, INTERACTIONS AND REACTIONS

Since all human performance is highly integrated, there is clearly an overlap between actions,

interactions and reactions, but broadly speaking actions and interactions are initiated by the individual as an intentional and proactive means of doing or expressing something, whereas reactions (with the exception of those caused by bodily sensations) occur mainly in response to some external factor (human, organic, inorganic) or to an incident or event.

These terms are not intended to be used in an overly rigid manner; it all depends on the context of a specific episode of performance.

AIR ANALYSIS

Let us return to the example of threading a needle to see what happens when we attempt to use the AIR taxonomy. We will assume that some individual variation occurs in this performance sequence.

AIR ANALYSIS: THREADING A NEEDLE

Note. The starting point is sitting.	
Action	Pick up cotton reel
Action	Find end of cotton
Action	Hold cotton reel in one hand
Action	Pull thread to unwind a length of cotton
Interaction	Judge length of cotton against desired length
Action	Retain hold of cotton reel and measured thread
Action	Pick up scissors
Action	Cut cotton to desired length
Action	Put down scissors
Action	Put down cotton reel
Action	Pick up cotton, retain for use
Action	Pick up needle
Interaction	Check if light is sufficient to see eye (it is not)
Reaction	Look for a better light source
Action	Rise from chair
Action	Walk to the window
Action	Turn needle so that eye faces user with light behind it
Action	Hold needle steady in front of user at face height
Action	Pinch and grip thread near tip
Action	Guide thread through eye of needle (fail)
Reaction	Check end of thread
Action	Suck end of thread to make a point
Action	Guide thread through eye of needle (succeed)
Interaction	Catch and pull thread through eye from other side

This analysis is useful in that it shows that the task is mainly composed of a series of actions. These are interspersed with a few reactions required to solve problems encountered during the task, and the recognition of task completion (successful threading through eye). There is little interactive element in this task, except when the user needs to examine the cotton in order to judge if the length is sufficient, and examine the needle in relation to the environment in order to get it into the best position for threading.

With the analysis so far conducted, the therapist only has limited information about the nature of the performance. This is mainly provided by the verbs used to describe what is done; words such as pick up; check; turn, hold, pinch and guide. We could extend this analysis by highlighting these 'doing words':

Action	Pick-up	cotton reel
Action	Find	end of cotton
Action	Hold	cotton reel in one hand
Action	Pull	thread to unwind a length of cotton
Action	Judge	length of cotton
Action	Retain hold	of reel and measured thread
Reaction	Pick up	scissors
Action	Cut	cotton to desired length
Action	Put down	scissors
Action	Put down	cotton reel
Action	Pick up	cotton
Action	pick up	needle
Interaction	Check	if light is sufficient to see eye
Reaction	Look	for a better light source
Action	Rise	from chair
Action	Walk	to the window
Action	Turn	needle so that eye faces user
Action	Hold	needle steady in front of user
Action	Pinch and grip	thread near tip
Action	Guide	thread through eye of needle (fail)
Reaction	Check	end of thread
Action	Suck	end of thread to make a point
Action	Guide	thread through eye of needle (succeed)
Interaction	Catch and pull	thread through eye

USING THE AIR SYSTEM TO ANALYSE SOCIAL INTERACTIONS

It is a relatively simple matter to undertake a microanalysis of a task, or a performance episode, as the stages are usually clearly defined. In the case of an episode of social interaction, however, it can be more difficult to analyse what is going on.

The following dialogue is taken from *Emma* by Jane Austen, with slight abridgement.

'Emma,' said Mr Knightly presently, 'I have a piece of news for you. You like news – and I heard an article on my way hither that I think will interest you.'

'News! Oh yes, I always like news. What is it? Why do you smile so? Where did you hear it? At Randalls?'

He had time only to say: 'No, not at Randalls; I have not been near Randalls' – when the door was thrown open, and Miss Bates and Miss Fairfax walked into the room. Full of thanks and full of news, Miss Bates knew not which to give quickest. Mr Knightly soon saw that he had lost his moment, and that not another syllable of communication could rest with him.

'Oh, my dear sir, how are you this morning? My dear Miss Woodhouse – I come quite overpowered – have you heard the news? Mr Elton is going to be married.'

Emma had not had time even to think of Mr Elton, and she was so completely surprised, that she could not avoid a little start, and a little blush, at the sound.

'There is my news – I thought it would interest you,' said Mr Knightly with a smile, which implied a conviction of some part of what had passed between them.

How might a therapist analyse this exchange? There are three main participants in the dialogue, and a fourth who says nothing, so we need to examine what is happening to each one in turn, and how their actions, interactions and reactions interlock. To do this we can try to select an appropriate verb to indicate what is going on, and then designate the performance using the AIR system (see Box on page 188).

It becomes clear from this analysis that Emma mainly reacts: she is the passive recipient of information during this exchange. Mr Knightly begins by interacting, but then is obliged to

Mr Knightly	Miss Woodhouse	Miss Bates	Miss Fairfax
I Speaks: informs	R Listens: attends R Responds: questions		
R Responds: smiles Responds: answers	R Listens	A Opens A Enters A Walks	A Enters A Walks
R Watches: welcomes R Withdraws	R Watches: welcomes R Listens	R Acknowledges I Comments Asks Informs	R Acknowledges R Listens
R Listens	R Starts: blushes		R Observes
R Confirms Smiles/informs	R Listens	R Listens	R Listens

A = Action; I = Interaction; R = Reaction

become reactive as Miss Bates takes over. The latter is both physically active and interactive: she dominates the exchange. Miss Fairfax, who enters with her, is left no scope for either interaction or positive reaction; she must simply passively watch and listen. As she has no relevance to the story at this point we are not told how she responds, but one may assume some appropriate polite facial expressions.

This type of analysis would be difficult to conduct as the event happened, but could be a valuable way of interpreting a video recording of an interaction between a number of people. This might assist a therapist to understand how interactions take place, or to analyse interactions between clients so that roles and skills could be identified.

FISHER & KIELHOFNER'S TAXONOMY FOR ANALYSIS OF OBSERVED PERFORMANCE

It has already been noted that humans naturally describe what they do by using verbs. While this is generally informative, it could, in the context of analysis, be criticized as imprecise. There are too many words to choose from and meaning may in some cases be open to interpretation.

Fisher & Kielhofner's taxonomy (Fisher & Kielhofner 1995), shown in Box 24.1, is intended for use with the task-based Assessment of Motor and Process Skills (AMPS). Because this offers a different approach to microanalysis, this system will be considered in more detail.

This terminology is not, like most other systems, based on using skill components or descriptors derived from physiology or cognitive psychology such as 'fine motor' or 'figure and ground perception'. Instead the authors use verbs such as chooses, handles, organizes, notices/responds, articulates and expresses. Their headings are: Motor Skills (5 domains, 16 descriptors), Process skills (5 domains, 20 descriptors), Communication/Interaction (4 domains, 18 descriptors), Social Interaction, (4 domains, 25 descriptors). This is a well-integrated, thoroughly researched system in which each piece of observed performance is identified by a distinct term which is clearly defined.

If this is considered in relation to the two examples of microanalysis given above, the similarities of approach are obvious.

The authors distinguish between the use of this skill taxonomy and traditional activity analysis as follows:

Traditional activity analysis is designed to identify the underlying capacities necessary for skilled performance. We instead focus on the observable skills that occur in a given performance.

Readers who wish to use this taxonomy for basic analysis or demand analysis should refer to Chapter 8 of *A Model for Human Occupation*

Box 24.1 Fisher & Kielhofner's skill taxonomy

Motor domains and skills

Posture	Stabilizes, aligns, positions
Mobility	Walks, reaches, bends, co-ordinates, manipulates, flows
Co-ordination	Co-ordinates, manipulates, flows
Strength and effort	Moves, transports, lifts, calibrates, grips
Energy	Endures, paces

Process domains and skills

Energy	Paces, attends
Knowledge	Chooses, uses, handles, heeds, inquires
Temporal organization	Initiates, continues sequences, terminates
Organizing space and objects	Searches/locates, gathers, organizes, restores, navigates
Adaptation	Notices/responds, accommodates, adjusts

Communication/interaction domains and skills

Physicality	Gestures, gazes, approximates, postures, contacts
Language	Articulates, speaks, focuses, emanates, modulates
Relations	Engages, relates, respects, collaborates
Information exchange	Asks, expresses, shares, asserts

Social interaction domains and skills

Acknowledging	Turns, looks, confirms, touches
Sending	Greets, answers, questions, complies, encourages, extends, clarifies, sets limits, thanks, concludes
Timing	Times response, speaks fluently, takes turns, times duration, completes
Co-ordinating	Approaches, places self, assumes position, matches language, discloses, expresses emotion

---

(Kielhofner 1995) where full definitions of these terms are given, and to the research literature concerning the development of AMPS.

This represents an extremely thorough and well-constructed form of analysis which has a good basis in research. It could have potential for use as a means of microanalysis, but it may be too time-consuming for routine clinical application.

DEMAND ANALYSIS

The third form of microanalysis is *demand analyis*, in which performance units are analysed to determine the skill components required of the participant in order to produce competent performance. This is described in Chapter 28.

Basic task analysis

DEFINING A TASK

In the context of basic analysis, a task is composed of a sequence of performances with a clear purpose and product which takes approximately 3 to 10 minutes to complete (shorter performance episodes require microanalysis and longer chains come under activity analysis).

Performance is typically divisible into self-contained stages or events, each of which contributes something towards completion of the task. Apparently longer task sequences either consist of linked tasks (e.g. walk to corner shop; buy newspaper, walk home again) which can be analysed separately, or are formed by an iterative sequence in which the same or very similar tasks are continually repeated (e.g. ironing; mowing the lawn; painting the walls in a room).

Task analysis is focused on what is done, and the circumstances of doing it. It is important to recognize that an interest in describing the nature and quality of performance is a natural human attribute. As we saw in the microanalysis of threading a needle humans not only 'do' they *name what they do*.

The therapist is only attempting a more analytical and structured version of what humans have always done without really thinking about it.

Task analysis is a reductive, atomistic, analytical process which is most applicable to high visibility performance which is relatively simple, structured and sequenced.

LIMITATIONS OF TASK ANALYSIS

Basic task analysis as practised by occupational therapists is in many respects an artificial process. It looks at isolated episodes of performance at the acquisitional and constructive levels. It is concerned with what happens in one setting on one occasion, or with describing 'typical' performance.

Basic task analysis tends to consider the task out of context. Individual choice, personal reactions and situational factors may cause performance to be varied, but these factors and the effects of differing contexts and environments on task performance are considered at the effective level.

The performance components required to undertake the task are not analysed at this stage, because this comes under *demand analysis* which is a precursor to *applied analysis*. Similarly, the abilities of the individual to do the task, or feelings about it are not considered at this point, as these form part of the therapist's assessment of the individual.

Task analysis is not readily applicable to low visibility performance which is holistic, unstructured and highly reactive and responsive. Nor is it applicable to activities which involve highly integrated cognitive processing and physical skill.

For example, it is possible, (although time-consuming) to do a task analysis of playing scales on a piano or driving a car. It is very difficult (if not impossible) to do a satisfactory task analysis of the performance of a concert pianist or a racing driver, where even a small episode of performance is so complex and integrated that it defies reductive description.

To say that the pianist sits at the piano and plays music, or that the racing driver competitively drives a car at high speed round a circuit does not adequately represent what these individuals are doing, or indicate the skills they need to do it. These activities exist in a different dimension of doing to that of the ordinary task.

Task performance is a dominant form of observable human occupational behaviour but it

is plainly not the only form. There are types of performance which do not fit within the definition of 'a task' as 'a piece of work to be done'. These will be described elsewhere in this section.

Despite these limitations, basic task analysis is the foundation for the analysis of more complex sequences of chained tasks and activities.

SIMPLE TASK ANALYSIS

A 'rough and ready' guide to task analysis is summarized in Kipling's advice to young people in his *Just So Stories*: 'I have six honest servants, they taught me all I knew, their names were What and Why and When, and How and Where and Who.'

This system is described by Johnson (1996) as a simple form of activity analysis. The therapist asks six questions (Box 25.1).

Box 25.1 The six questions' system of basic task analysis	
What is to be done?	Task description or name
Who is involved in the task?	One person or several? Any special characteristics
How is the task performed?	Method; sequence; practical requirements such as tools and materials
Where will it take place?	Location
When will it be done?	Time and place and duration
Why is it to be done?	Product and/or purpose)

While useful as a quick screening process, the six questions' system is not sufficiently detailed to give a full appreciation of the nature of the task.

TYPE OF OCCUPATIONAL PERFORMANCE

The task may also be given a contextual designation as work, leisure or self-care:

Self-care tasks	Make a cup of tea
	Take a shower
	Iron a blouse
Work tasks	Telephone client and book an appointment

Stack new stock on shelf
Sew seams on one garment

Leisure tasks   Do a crossword puzzle
Take the dog for a short walk
Embroider part of a tapestry.

Example

So, for example, the task of threading a needle could be analysed as follows:

What   Thread needle

Who   Student

How   1 (preparatory task) Gather materials and tools (needle and cotton; scissors)
2 Cut cotton
3 Thread needle

Where   Bed-sitting room

When   Evening

Why   Preparatory task stage before sewing hem in order to shorten new trousers (self-care task).

COMPONENTS OF DETAILED TASK ANALYSIS

There are two distinct forms of basic task analysis: content analysis and sequence analysis.

As already described, the most obvious form of analysis is to identify what stages the task has and in what order these should be tackled. This is done by *sequence analysis*. This includes analysis of *order* and/or *method*. Order analysis sorts out the task stages and lists them in the sequence in which they occur. The time required for each stage may also be indicated. Method analysis describes how each part of the task is done.

For a therapist the simple sequence of task stages is not enough. It is necessary to understand what is involved in performing the task. For example, why it is to be done and what product the participant will achieve, or what are the practical requirements such as tools and materials. This is done by *content analysis* which describes features of the task.

CONTENT ANALYSIS

This is a more detailed version of the 'what, why, who, where, when, how' formula.

The headings for content analysis are:

- Task title
- Purpose
- Participant
- Practical requirements
- Environment/location
- Standards.

TITLE AND PURPOSE

A task has an intended aim or purpose which can be conveyed by a short description such as 'ironing a blouse'; 'going to the post office'; 'cleaning the car'; 'having a shower'. This title usually describes the type of action and the object acted upon and needs to be simply and clearly stated.

This purpose may be linked to the occupational designation of the task as work, leisure or self-care.

PARTICIPANT

Number of participants

It is necessary to know whether a task can be done by one person, or if it needs more than one. If more than one person is needed, it may be helpful to specify how they will work together.

Participant specification

In order to perform the task, the participant may need particular physical *abilities or skills*, special *knowledge*, or *attitudes*. It is only necessary to give a general indication at this point as further detail is provided by demand analysis. Age and gender may also be relevant.

PRACTICAL REQUIREMENTS

Most tasks have some minimum requirement for tools, objects or materials. They take place in an environment which may need to contain certain objects or artifacts. A task takes a length of time to complete.

The therapist needs to specify all these requirements in order to be sure that they are available and ready for the task to be performed.

ENVIRONMENT

Location

The location in which the task is to be performed should be specified.

Physical content of environment

The environment must contain tools and materials as specified above, and these items may need to be positioned in a certain way in relation to the user. At this point, task analysis overlaps with and merges into environmental analysis (see Ch. 33).

STANDARDS

Standards are not always important in task performance. It may be enough to judge success by whether or not the task purpose or product was completed. When putting on shoes, the measure of success is that the shoes are put on.

Sometimes, however, there are standards to be met which may be set by the participant or by an external observer or assessor.

For example, the main criterion for successful domestic hoovering is that the floor looks clean afterwards; one person may tolerate the odd crumb or thread, a second may be happy if all visible dirt is removed, while another is only satisfied with a spotless carpet and moves all the furniture every time to get at each nook and cranny. In a work-setting, the cleaner may not only have to produce a clean floor, but also have to complete the task in a set length of time.

SEQUENCE ANALYSIS

If the task is very familiar to the analyst, it is possible to recall the sequence in which personal performance of task stages takes place. Although this will give a general idea of the task, it can be surprisingly difficult for the performer to recall all the stages, and some people are better at this than others.

ANALYSIS OF REMEMBERED TASK

For example, the author's mother, when asked to list the steps involved in ironing a blouse spontaneously produced a very comprehensive instant analysis of the task stages, including both high visibility and low visibility items (*Example A*). Her ability to do this may stem from having been taught a precise method for ironing at school in 'domestic science' classes. Her teacher must have done her own 'task analysis' in order to teach the skills and knowledge required for ironing (a good task analysis is an essential prerequisite for teaching a practical technique).

A young woman, produced a similar, slightly less complete list (*Example B*).

REMEMBERED TASK ANALYSIS: IRONING A BLOUSE

Example A

(Items in brackets indicate stages which were omitted or implied.)

1 Get out ironing board (set it up)
2 Get out iron
3 Plug in iron (switch on; dock iron on rest)
4 Get blouse
5 Examine blouse fabric and decide appropriate heat-setting for iron
6 Select correct heat-setting on iron
7 Place blouse on board with the inside of the back uppermost
8 (pick up iron) Iron this portion
9 (dock iron)
10 Change position of blouse to side 1
11 (pick up iron) Iron side one
12 (dock iron)
13 Change position of blouse to side 2
14 (pick up iron) Iron side two
15 (dock iron)

16 Reposition blouse to iron sleeve 1; check that sleeve is positioned so that iron does not make a crease down the outside of sleeve
17 (dock iron)
18 Position blouse to iron sleeve 2 (check as in 16)
19 (pick up iron) Iron sleeve 2
20 (dock iron)
21 Reposition blouse (right way round) to iron collar and reveres if present
22 (pick up iron)
23 Iron collar etc.
24 (dock iron)
25 Remove blouse from board
26 Check that ironing standard is satisfactory.

Ironing is a good example of a task which has repetitive sequences of similar actions. In this analysis, the only significant stages omitted were the need to switch on the iron and to dock the iron on the iron rest in between episodes of ironing. The over-obvious or automated stage is often omitted in a description of a remembered task. (When a novice student is asked to describe how to make a cup of tea, the need to switch on the kettle is often omitted.)

Example B

1 Get out ironing board
2 Get out iron
3 Get item to be ironed
4 Fill steam iron
5 Turn on iron
6 Iron collar of blouse
7 Iron back of sleeve(s)
8 Iron front of sleeve(s)
9 Iron back of blouse
10 Iron front of blouse.

This individual omitted to mention setting the temperature control, and, as in Example A, the over-obvious stage of docking the iron between periods of use.

Remembered analysis has limitations. Familiar task sequences are stored in the brain as scripts and procedures which are expressed accurately as the task is performed, but which may not be accurately recalled. It is therefore much easier to show how a task is done by actually doing it than by attempting to describe how it is done. The more complex, skilled and highly integrated the performance is, the harder it can be to describe.

As shown by the examples, apart from the tendency to forget the obvious, even a well-remembered sequence will only represent the personal method of the analyst. Unless the task has a very rigid sequence, there is no guarantee that others will do it in the same way. The scope for individual variation is apparent in the two examples. In Example B, a steam iron is used, and a different sequence of ironing parts of the garment is employed. A different environment or context may also alter the sequence. It is therefore important to distinguish between a recalled sequence and a sequence which has been observed.

TASK ANALYSIS BY OBSERVATION

The most reliable method of conducting a task analysis is to watch someone doing it and to write down what happens. In ideal circumstances the observation should be repeated for a number of people in a number of different settings in order to understand the 'typical' sequence (or content) and the room for variation.

When observing the task, it is important to identify each separate stage and not to let stages run together even though in practice they occur as one uninterrupted flow of action. Linked stages may form a subset within the task. For example, putting the iron on the ironing board, plugging it in and switching it on form a linked sequence, but each is a separate operation.

If a very long chain of stages seems to be evolving, the analyst needs to look for a point where there is a distinct change in the nature of the performance and subdivide it into two or more tasks.

For example, getting out and setting up the ironing board could be seen as a separate task prior to ironing. Similarly, if the iron is kept at a distance from the ironing station, obtaining it could involve enough separate stages to make it into a preparatory task. Collecting the items to be ironed is yet another preparatory task.

Differentiating tasks can be important when trying to identify the origin of a performance problem. A person who complains of 'difficulty ironing' may be able to iron, but be unable to set up the ironing board or carry piles of laundry.

In analysing the sequence of events, the therapist is also interested in the efficiency of the process. A form of 'time and motion' study may be needed. Are there events which could be omitted, or areas where there are more actions than necessary? Could energy be saved in some way?

PRESENTING A TASK SEQUENCE

Task performance can be represented by written description or, in the case of a set procedure, by a visual representation such as a flow chart or 'tree'.

METHOD ANALYSIS

To some extent, the method is implied by the task sequence; however, the sequence states the order in which things will be done, and not *how* they are to be done. Sequence and method are often confused as anyone who has tried to follow an unfamiliar cooking recipe will have found to their cost.

Here is an example:

Recipe for soda scones (adapted from the *St Michael All Colour Cookery Book*)
Ingredients
225 g plain flour
1x5 ml spoon bicarbonate of soda
1x5 ml spoon cream of tartar
25 g butter
150 ml buttermilk

Instructions (task stages sequence)
1 Sift the flour with the bicarbonate of soda and cream of tartar into a mixing bowl
2 Rub in the butter
3 Make a well in the centre of the flour and pour in buttermilk; mix quickly to soft dough
4 Turn dough onto floured board
5 Knead dough until smooth
6 Roll out until approx. 1.75 cm thick
7 Stamp out into approx. 12 rounds with a 5 cm pastry cutter
8 Leave to stand for 15 minutes before baking
9 Put rounds on heated, greased baking sheet and bake in a hot oven (220°C) for about 10 minutes or until scones are well risen and golden
10 Transfer to wire rack to cool slightly
11 Serve warm with butter and jam and/or cream.

At first sight, this recipe appears explicit. It tells the reader what *materials* are needed. It itemizes *what* is to be done and the *order of doing it*. A therapist will note, however, that it makes several assumptions.

It does not tell the reader to do some essential operations. For example, it is assumed that the cook will understand that it is necessary to switch on (or light) and preheat the oven,

It lists ingredients, but not the *tools or utensils*. The cook is expected to understand from experience that the necessary equipment will have to be assembled before starting to make scones.

More fundamentally, it is assumed that the reader will know *how* the task stages are performed. For example, the instruction 'rub butter into flour' assumes that the cook knows that this means first cutting the butter into the flour with a knife and then using the finger-tips to rub the ingredients together until they resemble coarse breadcrumbs. Hands should be cool and clean, and floured to prevent sticking. Similarly, 'knead dough until smooth' assumes that the cook knows that kneading involves squashing the dough together into a lump, folding it over on itself and repeating this process a number of times until the dough is an even consistency (but not too often so that it becomes overcompacted or sticky).

If one set out to teach a person to make scones, one would not only teach the sequence, but also the method. It is often difficult to describe method in words; it is far easier to demonstrate the actions and explain the judgements and decisions. This is why few cookery books attempt this level of detail.

Description of method and description of order can be combined in a brief summary of task stages. As we have seen, method is often made apparent by the previous level of task analysis, *microanalysis*, where task stages are sub-divided into performance units. This could be added if required.

VARIATION AND VISIBILITY

Once a content analysis and a sequence analysis have been undertaken, two other aspects of task performance can be explored, *variation* and *visibility*. In basic task analysis, it will usually be sufficient to state whether visibility and potential for variation are high, medium or low.

VARIATION

Some tasks have a fixed sequence and set of requirements and there is little room for variation. Others, however, have a more flexible form. *Variation potential* is important to the therapist as an indicator of the potential for the task to be adapted. Low variation potential is likely to mean low adaptability; the task can only be done one way.

Just as the sequence of a task may vary, so may the content. The more visible, routine and rigid the task performance is, the less there is scope for variation. Creative tasks have higher variation potential. These are the tasks which have traditionally been used therapeutically because variation allows scope for adaptation.

For example, a routine self-care task such as cleaning one's teeth permits little variation (one might, perhaps, change one's brand of tooth-paste or buy an electric toothbrush). A variation analysis for a routine ironing task is shown in Table 25.1. A constructive task such as knitting a garment or painting a door, offers a little more scope for variation (colour, type of yarn or paint); a creative task such as painting a portion of a picture or composing a verse of a poem has high variation potential.

Variation may occur in:

- sequence
- practical requirements: tools, materials
- location
- standards.

Visibility analysis

Visibility analysis (Alderton 1998, personal communication) examines the extent to which task performance is observable. Visibility becomes more important at higher occupational levels, but it is an attribute of tasks and therefore requires consideration at this point. The features of high and low visibility performance are contrasted in Box 25.2.

Table 25.1 Variation analysis of the task of ironing a blouse

	Stable elements	Variation
1	Set up ironing board	Use worktop or table with cloth
2	Get iron from store cupboard	May have iron permanently at ironing station
3	Get clean, crumpled blouse	May be kept at a distance from ironing station
4	Plug in iron	Different models have different types of controls. Steam iron will need filling and setting of steam control if used
5	Switch on iron	
6	Set controls	(If steam iron not used, garment may, depending on the material and degree of dampness, require 'damping down' by sprinkling or spraying with water)
7	Iron garment	Parts of garment may be ironed in any order. Garment may be moved frequently or to a limited pattern. Number of times iron is pushed across garment in between docking iron and moving garment is also variable

Box 25.2 High visibility task content versus low visibility task content (adapted from Alderton 1998, personal communication)

Low visibility task content	High visibility task content
• Not easily seen by observer and can easily be overlooked	• Easily seen by observer; hard to ignore
• Does not require use of objects, tools and materials	• Usually requires use of objects tools and materials
• Relates to the cognitive or psychological function of the participant (process skills)	• Relates to the physical function of the individual (sensori-motor skills)
• Involves verbal, symbolic and gestural responses (interactions)	• Is expressed by purposeful actions
• Is performed spontaneously (reactions)	• Tends to become structured and routine
• Difficult to analyse into separate stages	• Can be broken down into stages that are easily identified
• Usually more difficult to teach	• Usually easy to teach
• Intended purpose may be misinterpreted	• Intended purpose is usually apparent to an observer
• Lack of visibility results in others failing to recognize or evaluate the performance	• Performance is readily recognized and evaluated
• Link between causes and effect not apparent	• Clear links between performance and outcome

The effect of visibility on the observer's evaluation of the performance is significant. In the introduction we have seen how judging by appearance has tended to devalue occupational therapy. Much of the practice of occupational therapy is 'invisible' and what is visible appears simple.

The relationship between visibility and the attribution of high status or value is not direct. It is not true to say that high visibility tasks are automatically highly valued – they are valued in proportion to skill, complexity and degree of knowledge.

Most simple tasks are highly visible. For example, when making a cup of tea most of what is being done can be seen. A person who makes the tea, or sweeps the road, is doing something highly visible, but apparently simple and unskilled. The observer will (probably) not value this performance very highly, nor give high status to the performer.

High status and value tend to be attributed to tasks which are highly visible, but which the observer judges to be complex, highly skilled (or in some way incomprehensible). Therefore, the operation of a computer may be viewed as complex by an observer who does not know much about computers, but has a general understanding that they are in some way complex, 'clever' and technical.

In fact, the task of operating the computer may be relatively low in skill. The 'clever' bit is the invisible work which went into the programming to make operation simple.

If, however, the observer understands more about the implications of the observed performance, the 'invisible' aspects may be inferred from observation and valued accordingly. For example, the task of completing a section of an embroidery has both high visibility and low visibility components.

The high visibility elements are the observable performances such as sewing a stitch, or selecting a new thread. Low visibility aspects include choice of suitable stitch to create the desired effect, choice of colour, and ability to follow a design. Anyone with a basic knowledge of embroidery technique will be able to appreciate both 'seen' and 'unseen' aspects of the performance.

It is possible for a task to be mainly 'invisible', for example, doing mental arithmetic is an invisible, cognitive process which only becomes visible at the point when the result is spoken or written down. However, most simple tasks at constructive level are highly visible.

PUTTING THE ELEMENTS OF TASK ANALYSIS TOGETHER

The therapist uses the headings to structure a brief description of the task. This must be concise; a descriptive 'essay' is not what is needed. Once completed, the analysis should enable someone to set up and perform the task with relative ease.

This type of analysis, and the techniques used to undertake it, form the basis of all other forms of activity analysis. An example of basic task analysis is given in Table 25.2.

For further information refer to Watson 1997, Johnson 1996 and Crepeau 1998.

Table 25.2 Example of basic task analysis

Task title	Iron a scarf
Content analysis	
Purpose	To remove creases from a recently washed scarf
Participant	One person. Person specification: an adult (male or female). Knowledge: safe use of iron. Abilities/skills: person must be able to lift and use iron; discriminate between creased and uncreased item; lift, move and fold scarf. Attitudes: values neatness and precision; pays attention to safety
Practical requirements	Equipment: iron; ironing board Materials: creased scarf
Location	Clear space in kitchen; adequate light; adjacent power point. Check no children or animals likely to come into contact with hot iron
Standard	Scarf should be completely smooth with neat edges *and* no wrinkles or creases. No burns or distortions of the material should appear
Sequence analysis	
Sequence and method	1 Switch on iron 2 Get scarf; check type of material; assess required iron temperature 3 Check temperature setting of iron (if necessary reset to required temperature) 4 Feel scarf to check whether degree of dampness is suitable for ironing (if necessary dampen down a little) 5 Place scarf on widest part of ironing board, smooth it out as much as possible by hand 6 Take iron and press down firmly and evenly moving rhythmically across fabric to smooth out portion of scarf; ensure edges do not curl 7 Dock iron safely flat on iron rest, or standing upright 8 Move scarf so that un-ironed portion is on wide part of board 9 Repeat stages 6, 7 and 8 until ironing is completed 10 (optional) Fold scarf into a neat square
Variation potential	Low
Visibility	High

26 Basic activity analysis

An activity takes place at the effective level. It occurs at a particular time and place for a specific purpose. Activity analysis is an organized, structured process in which information is gathered by observation and arranged under headings.

TYPES OF ACTIVITY ANALYSIS

Several systems for analysis have been proposed. It is clear that, while these analytical systems have much in common, there are different intentions in the mind of the analyst. What is wanted may be a *description* of an activity, or an analysis of its *demand* or an analysis of its *potential as therapy*.

Young & Quinn (1992) begin by suggesting that activities can be analysed in a therapeutic setting under three main headings:

1 Permanent and unchanging requirements intrinsic to the activity logical task sequence; sensorimotor requirements; cognitive requirements.
2 Requirements which are always present, but subject to change: space; equipment; materials; cost.
3 Social and cultural perceptions of the activity and its outcome. This might include gender attribution; status; cultural utility.

Apart from sensori-motor and cognitive requirements, the items mentioned all contribute to basic activity analysis, that is, an understanding of the activity itself.

Johnson (1996) gives a detailed analysis model for use when selecting a therapeutic activity. She lists common factors which always need consideration as:

1 Environment: including physical content and arrangement and demand
2 Motivation: facilitation of effective participation; relationship to individual roles and values
3 Appropriateness to developmental and chronological age of intended participant
4 Adaptability of the activity
5 Vocational application: relevance of content to work, leisure or self-care activities which participant might need to engage in
6 Cost implication
7 Safety aspects
8 Time required for completion
9 Potential for individual and/or group work.

This appears to be more like an *applied analysis* since it is done in relation to the needs of a client or clients in the context of a therapeutic situation.

Johnson also describes how to analyse performance components using appropriate frames of reference to identify *demands*. These include: motor/physiological demands; sensory demands; cognitive demands; perceptual demands; emotional demands; social demands; independence and cultural demands.

Crepeau (1998) describes a structure for a descriptive basic analysis of an activity which has six steps:

Step 1 Describe the activity
Step 2 Describe the typical age range of people who engage in this activity
Step 3 Describe the environmental aspects of the performance context
Step 4 List supplies and equipment needed to carry out the activity
Step 5 Describe the safety hazards inherent in the activity
Step 6 List the sequential stages of the activity.

It is useful to to keep clear distinctions between *basic analysis* (which is descriptive), *demand analysis* (which is concerned with skill components and levels of performance) and *applied analysis* (which matches an activity to the therapeutic needs of a client). All are required, but this chapter is concerned with basic analysis as this has to precede the others.

SCOPE AND LIMITATIONS OF BASIC ACTIVITY ANALYSIS

Activity analysis is based on observation. It follows that the performance involved must be something which can readily be observed. This may sound too obvious to be worth stating, but there is an implicit problem which limits the scope of activity analysis.

Some performances are simply too complex for easy observation (Table 26.1). There is too much going on, and the usual approach of dividing performance into tasks cannot be applied. Consider a game of football or tennis played by experts, or a performance by an expert musician or ballerina; how could one easily describe these in terms of tasks or provide a detailed analysis of performance skills? The most one could do is to give a general description as suggested by Crepeau.

Table 26.1 Features of complex activities which are difficult to analyse. A complex activity has two or more of the features listed below. Examples of these activities are also listed.

Features	Examples
Not task-based	Play game of chess
A repertoire of actions, interactions and reactions is used as required on each occasion; no fixed sequence	Play ice hockey Act in a play Drive car in a rally
May involve special methods or techniques	
Explicitly or implicitly rule-governed	
Highly skilled/expert	
Product observable but usually intangible	

In order to analyse these activities in detail, one must possess personal knowledge and expertise, or be a good performer oneself, or a trained coach or critic. One needs to know the rules of the game, or understand the discipline of the dance style. It takes a long time to acquire enough expertise to meet the high performance demand of such activities. If one can gain the requisite knowledge and skill, it might then be possible to provide a reasonable description. Because the participants are deeply engaged in the flow of the activity, it is likely that they too will be unable to analyse and describe what happens.

It may also be possible for an expert observer to do a microanalysis of a small episode of such complex performance, although even that is likely to be difficult. This is the kind of analysis an expert coach might do when seeking to perfect some aspect of performance.

At the opposite end of the spectrum, some performances are hard to analyse because there is too little going on (Table 26.2). A list of tasks would be sparse; the sequence may well be unstructured. The level of physical skill required may be low. The product is intangible. Much of what happens is invisible; it takes place in the mind and experience of the participant. These activities are often creative or recreational. The best person to capture this type of performance is the participant; the outside observer really cannot 'see most of the game' because there is nothing much to see.

Table 26.2 Features of unstructured/low visibility activities which are difficult to analyse. An unstructured/low visibility activity has two or more of the features listed below. Examples of these activities are also listed.

Features	Examples
Low visibility Not task-based	Sit on a beach Read a book Listen to a concert Watch a play
Unstructured No rules, or implicit rules	
Product intangible	
Result may be hard to define or observe	
Moderately variable or highly variable performance	
Variable skill level but physical skill tends to be low	
Variable level of knowledge	

Somewhere between these two extremes come the kind of activities which therapists can and do analyse (Table 26.3). These are typically well structured, highly visible, involve medium levels of skill, and are relatively quick to learn. They are usually appropriate for use as therapy. Both the participant, and an observer will be able to gain a reasonable understanding of what is involved and, with the aid of a well-structured system of analysis, can provide a good description.

Table 26.3 Features of activities which are appropriate for analysis. These activities have two or more of the features listed below. Examples of these activities are also listed.

Features	Examples
High visibility	Simple woodwork project
Well structured and/or sequenced: implicit rules	Plant flowers in a container Get dressed
Task-based: may be specific methods or techniques	Cook a meal
Product tangible or result easily observed	
Moderate level of skill	
Moderate to low variation	

The divisions are not hard and fast; much depends on the circumstances in which the activity is performed and the level of expertise of the practitioner. It is advisble, however, to do a mental checklist of the relevant characteristics before undertaking a detailed analysis (Box 26.1).

DETAILED ACTIVITY ANALYSIS

It should be obvious by now that activities are composed of tasks so, having mastered task analysis, activity analysis becomes easier. Many of the techniques are the same. An activity is a larger, more complex entity than a task, so the description has to be undertaken at a more generalized level of detail.

Box 26.1 Checklist to determine suitability for activity analysis

Activity	Yes	Partly	No
Based on tasks Follows a set performance sequence Uses set methods or techniques Product tangible Result easy to define/observe Requires special knowledge Requires previous experience			
Level of performance	Expert	Competent	Novice/unskilled

Summary
- High visibility/structured activity suitable for detailed analysis by therapist
- Complex activity suitable for general description by therapist
- Complex activity, can be described by expert participant or knowledgeable observer
- Low visibility/unstructured activity can be described by participant

ACTIVITY ANALYSIS: STABLE AND SITUATIONAL ELEMENTS

An activity differs from a task in that there is usually more scope for variation. There are *stable* elements which remain much the same, but in addition there are *situational* elements, which may change each time the activity takes place (Hagedorn 1995a). The degree to which the activity is relatively fixed or capable of change is the degree of *variation*.

STABLE ELEMENTS

The therapist needs to begin with a description of performance. Analysis of stable elements is obtained by *sequence analysis*, listing the tasks which comprise the activity and *content analysis*, summarizing the general purpose and product, and the practical requirements.

The stable elements may be analysed to indicate the *visibility* of the activity; as already explained the activity must have a high proportion of visible elements to be suitable for this type of analysis.

SITUATIONAL ELEMENTS

As noted by Young & Quinn (1992), there are unchanging and changing aspects of an activity.

Situational elements change depending on the context of performance. Context includes the environment, roles and reactions of others, expectations generated by rules, cultural norms, or standards. An activity is given meaning by its context.

Situational elements also include those which give scope for choice in the course of the activity, such as choosing to do *this* but not *that*; changing the sequence in which things are done, or selection of a particular colour or pattern.

These situational elements are important in analysing the type and level of performance demand. Analysis of performance demand requires the combination of the situational and stable elements of activity analysis. Environmental analysis can add depth to this description.

ANALYSIS OF STABLE ELEMENTS

The system is very similar to that used for task analysis. Method is excluded, because that is a more detailed level of description which requires task analysis or microanalysis.

HEADINGS FOR BASIC ACTIVITY ANALYSIS: STABLE ELEMENTS

- Content
  - title purpose/product
  - participant

- resources
    practical requirements
    time
- setting
    location; context; motivating
    factors; stressors
- standards
    intrinsic/extrinsic
- rules
    implicit/explicit
- risks
    Sequence
- procedure
    preparatory tasks
    order of tasks in main activity
    consequent tasks

An example of an analysis of stable elements is given in Table 26.4.

CONTENT ANALYSIS

Title

The title of the activity is often short and relatively uninformative, for example, quiz; art group; baking; woodwork; shopping; go for a walk. The title simply explains the type of activity that is being done.

Purpose

This is a statement of what the aim of the activity is, what will have been achieved when it is finished. This is not, at this point, a statement of *therapeutic purpose*, as that comes later.

Purpose may be stated by a simple sentence, for example, 'Visit supermarket to buy food'; 'Make a garden bench'; 'Participate in a team quiz'; 'Play skittles'.

Product

The product may by now be very obvious and tangible: the product of 'Make a garden bench' is the bench, and there is little scope for variation in this. The product may be expressed as an expected *result* rather than a product: 'Buys food on

list'; or as the overall objective of the activity: 'Win the game'; 'Enjoy the music'.

These three headings – title, purpose and product – plainly overlap; they may be used as required, avoiding unnecessary repetition.

Participant

This involves a brief description of who the participant (or participants) will be. It might include an outline participant specification using a KAVS analysis to identify any prerequisite knowledge, attitudes, values and skills. It may include age or physical characteristics.

Resources

Most activities require resources. These include practical requirements, time, and possible assistance from, or co-operation with, others.

Practical requirements

This is a list of all the tools, machines, objects, furniture and materials needed for the activity. One also needs to list physical resources such as water, light and source of power. This kind of list may be quite extensive: for example, to list all the practical requirements and facilities for making a wooden bench will take some time and thought.

Time

It is useful to state the length of time the activity will take, and the time of day when it will be performed.

Others involved

The activity may be solitary. Otherwise the number of participants is stated, perhaps with a simple indication of the type of interaction involved: co-operative; competitive; leader and group.

Setting

The setting provides the context for performance and, often, the reason for it. The elements of the setting combine to alter the way the participant is likely to perceive engagement in the activity, for example, as pleasant or stressful. Changes to setting are often made for therapeutic reasons so analysis of this is important.

The headings for analysis of setting are:

- location
- context
- motivating factors
- stressors.

The factors identified under these headings are interdependent and combine to describe the setting.

Location

The location is the place, room or type of environment where the activity takes place. This may be relatively fixed; to take a bath one really needs to be in a bathroom. For some activities, there may be options; one normally cooks in a kitchen, but one might cook outdoors on a barbeque or camping stove, or in the galley on a boat.

Context

The context of performance determines its meaning. The therapist might begin with the traditional occupational performance designation of the activity (work; leisure; self-care) as modified by the circumstances.

A more detailed analysis would consider the norms, roles or expectations to which the participant must conform. These are a combination of the location and the situation. The cues to these expectations might be identified.

Motivating factors

These are often implicit and hard to identify, but as the effect of such factors can strongly influence the level and success of participation, it may be worth trying to specify them. For example, in a carpentry workshop the demand of the environment presses for articles to be made; this press will be increased if there are other people engaged in making articles, samples of finished products and a general atmosphere of 'business'. If, on the other hand, the participant is alone in the workshop and there is little visible sign of past or present activity, the participant must rely more heavily on personal motivation to 'get going'.

One might begin by designating the setting as highly motivating, moderately motivating, neutral, or low in motivating factors.

Stressors

Stressors are elements in a situation which are likely to be experienced as negative or over-demanding. Stressors can arise from the context, aspects of task demand, factors in the environment, the location or other people.

A stressor may or may not adversely affect individual performance. At this stage, it may be sufficient to give an approximate value to the expected level of stress as highly stressful, moderately stressful or low in stress factors.

Standards

Explicit or implicit standards of performance influence all our activities. Sometimes, these are very firmly established and give little scope for deviation. More often, there is a range of normal, accepted standards of performance.

Sometimes, the boundaries between acceptable and unacceptable forms of performance are clear, but usually only the extremes of unacceptable or acceptable performance are obvious. There is a large 'grey area' open to interpretation in the middle. In basic analysis of stable elements, the therapist is concerned to describe the generally expected parameters of performance.

The headings for analysis of standards are:

- intrinsic standards – those which are built into the activity and must be met if performance is to be competent.
- external standards – those set by others which may require the participant to perform at a higher or lower level within the range of what is expected. These include cultural standards which a particular group considers important.

Rules

Some activities, such as games, are overtly rule-governed. The rules provide a structure and define the limits of the activity and what may or may not happen in different circumstances. Quite often rules are implicit. These may be rules for culturally acceptable behaviour in a situation or legal rules such as paying for goods in a shop, or procedural rules of the 'if this, do that' variety.

Table 26.4   Example of analysis of stable elements

Activity title	Going to a supermarket to do the shopping
Content analysis	
Purpose	To obtain necessary food and supplies for the home
Product	Shopper obtains items wanted
Participant	The shopper; age 16–90+ male or female
Resources	
Practical requirements	Access to supermarket Means of carrying purchases Means of paying for purchases Sufficient time to complete shopping
Time	Duration: about 1 hour. Shopping can take place between 8 am and 8 pm any weekday
Others	Solitary activity, but other shoppers present and may offer assistance
Setting	
Location	Supermarket
Context	Self-care activity Shopping at supermarket is an accepted way of obtaining items, Participant has role of 'shopper'
Motivating factors	Low: most shoppers regard shopping for routine household items as a chore
Stressors	Moderate
Standards	
Intrinsic	Shopping is completed as required Shopping is done in efficient manner without wasting time or energy Shopper considers budget/economy
Extrinsic	Implicit cultural norms and standards of behaviour while shopping: e.g. being dressed for shopping; not making a noise; being careful with trolley; queuing in turn; not running, dancing; being polite; honesty in paying for goods
Risks	Low; extra attention needed to avoid slipping, tripping and damage to self from accident with trolley
Sequence analysis	
Preparatory activities/tasks	Make shopping list Travel to supermarket
Procedure	Tasks 1 Select trolley (option) 2 Push trolley/select basket (option) 3 Enter supermarket 4 Consult list (option) 5 Navigate to area in which required item is located, pushing trolley 6 Scan shelves to find required item 7 Select required item 8 Pick up item and load into trolley 9 Repeat tasks 4,5,6,7,8 until decide that shopping is completed 10 Push filled trolley to checkout area 11 Find checkout; queue if necessary 12 Unload items onto belt 13 Pack items once scanned and costed 14 Load filled bags onto trolley 15 Pay for items 16 Find exit 17 Leave supermarket, pushing loaded trolley

ANALYSIS OF SITUATIONAL ELEMENTS

These are the elements of performance which are variable. The same headings are used, but instead of listing items which are typical and always present when the activity is performed, the therapist identifies the items which can be varied. At this stage, only items that are normally subject to change or choices are included. Therapeutic analysis and adaptation are carried out at a later stage. An example of a situational analysis is given in Table 26.5.

USE OF ACTIVITY ANALYSIS

This form of analysis expands our understanding of the complexity of an activity. It can promote efficient organization. It forms a basis for *demand analysis* which considers the effect of both situational and stable elements on a potential performer. It may indicate areas of performance which require assessment or provide a basis for adaptation and problem-solving.

The approaches described in Chapter 23 can be used to limit the scope of the analysis or to provide more detail. An episode from the activity may be subjected to task analysis or micro-analysis in order to further isolate problems, teach methods or identify specific performance skills.

The amount of detail required for a comprehensive activity analysis may look daunting, but a basic analysis only has to be done once. It is advisable to build a portfolio of analysed activities which can form the foundation for future therapeutic intervention. This can gradually be expanded to include demand analysis and notes on adaptations.

Table 26.5 Example of situational analysis

Activity	Going to a supermarket to do the shopping	
Content	**Stable elements**	**Situational elements**
Participant	The shopper	May have person to assist. May be taking care of a child/children
Purpose	To obtain necessary food and supplies for the home	May decide to purchase luxury item for special occasion. Budget may be limited
Product	Shopper obtains items wanted	May exercise personal choice. May add or delete items as shopping is done in response to availability of items
Resources		
Practical requirements	Access to supermarket Means of carrying purchases Means of paying for purchases	List is optional Various trolleys available Can use cash, cheque, credit card or store card
Time	Duration: about 1 hour Shopping can take place between 8 am and 8 pm any weekday	Duration varies with length of list and conditions inside store. Some stores open late, or 24 hours, or on Sunday
Setting		
Location	Supermarket	May decide to use local shops Computer shopping and home delivery may be options
Context	Self-care activity Shopping at supermarket is an accepted way of obtaining items Participant has role of 'shopper'	Shopping for luxury items may be regarded as a leisure activity
Motivating factors	Low: most shoppers regard shopping for routine household items as a chore	Motivation may be higher when buying presents, personal items, non-routine items or luxuries

Table 26.5 *(Cont'd)*

Content	Stable elements	Situational elements
Stressors	Moderate	May be high Affected by factors such as noise and crowding, or having to cope with small children. Stress may be reduced when shop is quiet, e.g. late at night
Standards Intrinsic	Shopping is completed as required Shopping is done in efficient manner without wasting time or energy Shopper considers budget/economy	Little variation
Extrinsic	Implicit cultural norms and standards of behaviour while shopping: e.g. being dressed for shopping; not making a noise; being careful with trolley; queuing in turn; not running, dancing; being polite; honesty in paying for goods	Some tolerance, but unacceptable behaviour likely to provoke adverse response from other shoppers or management
Rules	Implicit	Little variation
Risks	Low; slipping, tripping and damage to self from accident with trolley	Risk increases with crowding Wet floors and dropped items increase fall hazard
Sequence analysis		
Preparatory activities	Make shopping list Travel to supermarket	(optional) Various modes of transport If close to home, may walk
Procedure (shortened)	**Tasks** 1 Select trolley (option) 2 Enter supermarket 3 Select basket (option) 4 Consult list (option) 5 Navigate to required item 6 Scan shelves for item 7 Select required item 8 Repeat tasks 4,5,6,7 until shopping is completed 9 Find checkout; queue if necessary 10 Unload items onto belt 11 Pack items once scanned and costed 12 Pay for items 13 Leave supermarket	Various trolleys available Automatic or revolving doors Only if small list Assistance usually available to find or select item Length of queue variable Width of checkout aisle varies Can request help Assistance available Various methods Collect by car and take to car; home delivery services may be available
Consequent activities	Return home; unpack Put items away in cupboard, refrigerator or freezer	Have drink or meal at coffee shop before leaving *Note*: time variation limited, food items must be kept cool and stored as soon as possible

27

Macroanalysis and client-centred analysis

ANALYSIS AT THE ORGANIZATIONAL LEVEL: MACROANALYSIS

Macroanalysis may involve *analysis of an occupation*, or *analysis of an occupational history* which investigates the roles and patterns of participation of an individual across the individual's lifespan to date.

ANALYSIS OF AN OCCUPATION

We have not, so far, developed many detailed descriptions of occupations. Better descriptions would provide information about the overall structure and patterns of occupations, how they link with roles, and how they are affected by culture, gender and other factors.

STRUCTURES FOR ANALYSIS OF OCCUPATIONS

A SYSTEMS APPROACH

In occupational science, occupations are currently viewed as being comprised of inter-related subsystems:

- physical
- biological
- information-processing
- sociocultural
- symbolic–evaluative
- transcendental.

These offer a potential structure for macroanalysis. An example of an analysis of this kind is the article on 'Running as an occupation: multiple meanings and purposes' (Primeau 1996).

'10 P' ANALYSIS

I have suggested a framework for macroanalysis entitled '10 P' analysis (Hagedorn 1995a) to which readers may refer, but this is too cumbersome a process for use in clinical settings so it will not be described in detail here.

This analysis considers occupations under ten headings, indicating attributes which all conveniently begin with the letter p (hence 10 P analysis):

- participant
- principles
- positions
- possessions
- purposes
- processes
- products
- patterns
- practical requirements
- performance demands.

WORK, LEISURE AND SELF-CARE

A more traditional form of macroanalysis is the designation of an occupation as work, leisure or self-care (or similar designations). This is a useful 'shorthand' method of defining the nature of an occupation.

Some occupations have a fixed designation. Occupational therapy, for example, could only be classified as work. In the majority of occupations, designation is situationally determined. Cooking, might be work, leisure or self-care, depending on the context and the intention of the cook.

This form of analysis has limitations. The criteria by which one might allocate an occupation to a category are not well-defined. There are insufficient categories to cover the range of human occupations: for example, is 'worshipping' work, leisure or self-care? None seems appropriate.

In real life, many different occupations interlock, enmesh and enfold which can make classification difficult. Cynkin & Robinson (1990) provide a good review of the problems associated with this classification system.

ANALYSIS OF AN OCCUPATIONAL HISTORY

As a first step, the therapist asks the client to describe past experiences of education, work, leisure and coping with a home. Analysis of this history (with or without the client) can provide insights into roles, interests, abilities and coping skills and potential for development. It may indicate possible causes of maladaptive responses or cycles. Discussion of a personal 'occupational story' can be the basis for development of personal meanings and insights (see Ch. 21).

ANALYSIS OF PATTERNS OF PARTICIPATION

The patterns of performance which occur in an individual's life over shorter or longer timeframes are highly significant. These patterns influence participation at the effective level.

Participation analysis explores the interests and patterns of engagement over varying periods of time. For example, a client might be asked to keep a diary of all activities over a period of 1 or 2 weeks (e.g. idiosyncratic activities configuration, Cynkin & Robinson 1990) or over a year or so (e.g. modified interests checklist, Kielhofner 1995).

An impoverished or unbalanced repertoire of activities, or noticeable changes in the level of engagement can be significant.

Routine or habit analysis can be used to provide a description of integrated patterns of performance in which a number of activities are habitually related over the course of a period of time. One of the important aspects of this analysis is the degree of flexibility or rigidity of such patterns (see Ch. 21).

CLIENT-CENTRED ANALYSIS

Most descriptions of occupational analysis are presented from the therapist's perspective. While there is no doubt that it is an important therapeutic competency, occupational analysis can also be a valuable technique for use in client-centred approaches.

In order to analyse the nature of a performance problem, one has to consider all three points on the occupational performance triangle: the person, the occupation and the environment. The links between different types of performance, the ways in which performance problems interlock and affect each other, and the overall patterns of participation are also important. For this reason, although the analysis may end by focusing on a specific activity, it can be considered as occurring at the organizational level.

As we have seen, the subjective views of a participant are very important. Attitudes and values affect many aspects of performance.

Involving the client in occupational analysis can provide both therapist and client with insight into the causes of performance problems and thus lead into problem-solving or adaptive change.

ANALYSIS OF PERFORMANCE DEMAND AND ABILITY TO RESPOND: SYT ANALYSIS

The method which I have evolved for this client-led, analytical process (Hagedorn 1996) is similar to that described by Holm et al (1998). It can be used with an individual or a group. Because the words 'person, occupation and environment' are not immediately accessible, I have substituted the words 'You, the Task and the Situation', and therefore refer to this form of analysis as 'SYT analysis'.

SYT ANALYSIS

The analysis takes place in stages. It is important to take time to explain the concepts and the rea-sons for doing the analysis before launching into use of the technique.

Stage one: explanation

Before undertaking the SYT analysis, the client should have some grasp of the objectives of the process and the items to be considered under each section.

In order to explain what is involved, the SYT triangle is drawn out using a large sheet of paper (A2 flipchart size is ideal). Draw the SYT triangle (Fig. 27.1) in the centre.

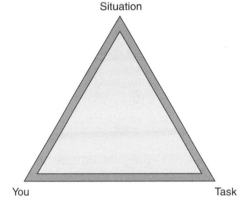

Figure 27.1 SYT analysis triangle

The therapist explains that this is a method of exploring difficulties so that solutions can be considered. Working round the triangle, the therapist explains what is to be considered under each heading (Box 27.1). Where possible, it is helpful to ask the client what the client thinks should be included, attempting to prompt correct responses by leading questions, before adding information of one's own. Cue words are written on the diagram.

Keep the explanations simple and general at this stage and do not get drawn into a discussion of a specific personal problem. Once the client has a general concept of what is required, it is easier to progress to working through an example than to go through a lot of theoretical explanation.

Stage two: problem selection

The client will probably have an initial idea of what the problem is, but the next stage is to get

---

Box 27.1 Items to be considered during SYT analysis

You

Physical abilities	The things you can do
	The things you find difficult
	Limiting factors (e.g. pain; tiredness)
What you know	The level of information you have about the task
	Your experience
	Areas where you are unsure
How you feel	The way you feel about the task
	The way you feel when you have difficulties
Thoughts	The negative thoughts which may come into your head when you experience difficulties

The task

What has to be done	The nature of the task to be done
	The sequence in which the task is done
Tools	The tools or equipment used
Materials	What materials?
Standards	How well has the task got to be done?
	Who says?

The situation

Place	The place where the task is done; characteristics of the place which help or hinder
Access	Ability to obtain items wanted, or to enter areas
Stressor	Anything which makes the task more difficult or frustrating; pressures you experience
Other people	Who else is involved: do they help or hinder?
Expectations	The feeling generated by a situation that certain events or procedures should happen in certain ways

---

the client to identify the problem task or activity with clarity and precision. The title is written at the top of the paper.

Stage three: analysis

Working round the triangle, the client now lists the items which the client feels are part of the problem situation. It does not matter which heading is tackled first; the client may select one, or may jump around the triangle as ideas occur.

The therapist facilitates the process by helping to summarize and capture ideas, prompting deeper thought, and asking leading questions to produce more material.

The area which usually presents most difficulty is identification of negative thoughts. Most clients have no difficulty in saying that they are angry, frustrated, disappointed, guilty; few can spontaneously link these feelings to typical negative thoughts such as 'I'm no good any more'; 'I can't look after my family'; 'I ought to be able to do all the things I used to do.'

The degree to which the therapist needs to 'dig' for this information is governed by the approach. Although making these connections is likely to be helpful to the client, only in cognitive-behavioural approaches is it essential to persevere in making the links.

Negative feelings and thoughts are a normal reaction to loss of function; they are often justified, and this should be acknowledged. Exaggerated or persistent negative thoughts and feelings feed back into negative cycles of behaviour and these may need to be explored and explained. A general awareness that 'bad feelings' tend to make you 'feel bad about yourself' and that this adds to the feeling of having a problem may be all that is needed. It may be possible to encourage the client to see that putting a more positive frame on the situation will help to re-interpret it and reduce the problem. Clients often recognize this spontaneously when they can 'see the whole picture'.

Task analysis: 'traffic light analysis'

When it comes to analysing the task, a simple format which may be called 'traffic light analysis' can be used. The task is broken into stages and these are coded red (stop, difficult), orange (caution) and green (no problem; 'go').

Procedure for traffic light analysis

1. The client lists all the stages in the problem task from start to finish. (Check that no stage has been left out.) The list must replicate individual performance not an imagined or recalled 'ideal'. (The client might actually perform the task and make a list before doing the analysis.)
2. The client is asked to identify the parts of the task which are easy and present no problem. These are marked with green.
3. The client then identifies the task stages which cause the most difficulty, or which cannot be done. These are marked with red.
4. The remaining 'in-between' tasks are marked in orange.

Once the list has been completed, the therapist and the client check it to ensure that it is as accurate as possible, and then discuss the implications.

The first conclusion that often becomes apparent is that only a few of the task stages are actually difficult. There may be several easy parts, and some which are a bit difficult but possible. Really difficult items can then be explored to see what the origin of the difficulty may be.

Stage four: analysis and problem-solving

The final stage of SYT analysis is problem-solving. The client and therapist jointly identify the things which are making the activity or task difficult. Brainstorming for solutions can then be attempted. Again, as far as possible, the client contributes the majority of ideas, and the therapist 'tops up' with missing information. Usually several sorts of action are needed.

Action following SYT analysis

- **the client**
  May need to adapt, e.g.
  – by changing attitudes, recognizing the effects of negative thoughts and feelings and attempting more positive responses, changing priorities, altering standards or expectations, pacing
  May need to learn new skills
  May need more information

- **the task**
  May need to be adapted, e.g.
  – by altering tools and equipment
  – by changing methods

- **the situation**
  May need to be adapted, e.g.
  – environmental adaptations: improving access, changing storage location, altering design
  – reduction of stressors
  – negotiation with others.

Stage five: action plan

Finally, a list of priorities for action, goals and an action plan are produced.

It is important to make goals simple, practical and achievable and to phrase them in a way which enables the client to structure a route to achieving each goal and measuring when it is achieved.

ANALYSIS OF INTERESTS

Clients who have become disabled often cease participation in previously enjoyed leisure activities. This may be because of a limitation which precludes participation, or it may be because assumptions have been made about what is and is not possible.

A client in this situation may be able to participate in the activity in a reduced or tangential way, or alternatively may need to find a replacement interest.

Leisure activities are by definition self-selected and dependent on personal interests and motivations, so any method of exploring them must be client-centred.

A standard approach is to ask the client to list previous interests. A number of questionnaires exploring participation and attitudes to personal leisure are available (see Ch. 13). This may not, however, provide sufficient information about why the client enjoyed these interests and whether the client is going to be able to participate again.

The following technique provides information which helps both client and therapist to gain a better understanding of the motivation to engage in past activities and possible directions for the future.

'WHAT'S IN IT FOR YOU?'

The client selects an activity which the client used to enjoy but has ceased to engage in, or is now finding difficult. This may be a hobby, recreation, sport or special interest. The analysis is done in the form of a 'spidergram' or 'mind map'. It can be compiled by an individual or with contributions from a group.

A large sheet of paper is used on which to draw out the analysis. The starting point is to put the title of the activity in a circle in the centre. The client is then asked to think of all the reasons why the activity was enjoyable. Each reason is put on the sheet with a line connecting it to the central circle. Prompting questions such as 'What did you get out of it?' and 'Why did you enjoy it?' and perhaps a suggestion to get the client started are usually sufficient to produce a comprehensive analysis. Although people cannot usually tell you why they enjoyed an activity if you ask them 'cold' (or they give vague or brief responses), this technique usually facilitates a detailed analysis.

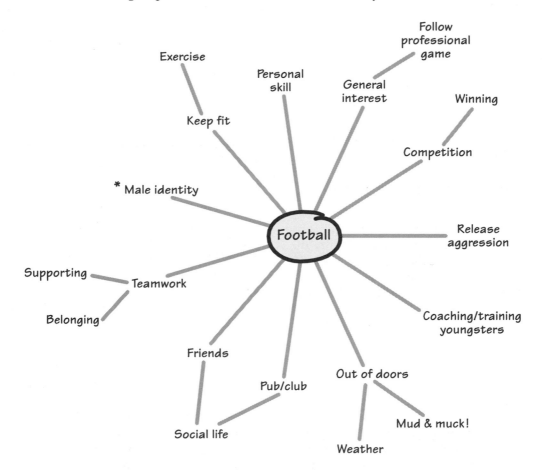

*this figure is based on an actual map produced by a **man** – football may be played by women who may/may not view gender identity as a valued benefit

Figure 27.2 Playing football.

After the analysis has been completed, the picture can be looked at in several ways. Clients may be surprised to find that many of the aspects they enjoyed were actually peripheral to the activity, for example, social contact and friendship. Often there will be some activities that cannot be done, but many others that can. It will be possible to pick out steps that the client can take, do some problem-solving in other areas, and look at ways of starting to participate again.

Alternatively, it may be clear that participation is just not practical, or that the client will not gain satisfaction from partial engagement because it is just 'not like it used to be'. In this case, the therapist suggests to the client that it may be possible to replace the aspects he enjoyed by finding a different activity (or several) which have similar or related features.

The client is often in a similar position to a person who has to change an interest because of advancing age. The difference is that the change may be sudden so there is no time for adaptation. Exploring the differences and similarities between being obliged to give up a favourite activity because of a disability or health problem, and doing so as a natural part of ageing may be helpful.

Figure 27.2 shows an example of a typical analysis. When discussing this diagram with a client, the therapist might prompt the client to identify that he could still watch football, go 'down the pub' with his mates, or take a role in organizing a club or coaching younger players.

Alternatively, the therapist might explore the client's liking for competition, need for release of aggression, need for a social outlet or liking for skilled performance to see if there are other activities which might offer opportunities to provide these experiences.

MAKING A LIFE PATTERN

A similar analytical technique is presented by Baxter et al (1995). This is based on a technique developed by Fanning & Fanning (1990).

The client maps all social and leisure roles as the spokes on a wheel centred on the hub of 'my life'. On each spoke, the client can then add the activities which relate to this role, names of friends associated with it and places the client has been.

Again this technique provides a visual representation which facilitates discussion more readily than a questionnaire.

Demand analysis

FORMS OF DEMAND ANALYSIS

A task places different types of demand on the participant. There is a demand for being *skilled* and able to *do* something, a demand for *knowing* about things, and a demand for *being developmentally ready* to perform. The participant must be able to meet all these demands, either by possessing the required attribute before starting the task, or by being able to learn how to meet demand in the course of participation.

The therapist needs to be able to undertake skill demand analysis, educational demand analysis and developmental demand analysis.

SKILL DEMAND ANALYSIS

SKILL DOMAINS

Knowing *how* to do something is an essential prerequisite for task performance. Even if the task has never been attempted before, the participant needs to have gained a certain level of foundation skills which equip the participant to make a start on mastering new ones.

It is generally accepted that performance can be divided into three skill domains: sensorimotor, cognitive–perceptual and psychosocial. These can be further subdivided into skill components, and, in some cases, these components can be divided still further into highly specific units of skill. Different authors provide somewhat different taxonomies.

These systems are based on the identification of specific skill components: sensori-motor, cognitive–perceptual or psychosocial. The terminology therefore tends to be derived from physiological, neurological or psychological research. Table 28.1 shows the differing approaches taken by recent researchers.

Table 28.1 Proposed taxonomies of skill domains for use in demand analysis

Author	Skill domains
Mosey (1986)	Sensory integration Motor function Cognitive function Psychological function Social interaction
Reed & Sanderson (1992)	Sensori-motor Cognitive Psychosocial
Johnson (1996)	Motor/physiological demands Sensory demands Cognitive demands Perceptual demands Emotional demands Social demands Cultural demands
Crepeau (1998)	Sensori-motor Cognitive integration and cognitive components Psychosocial skills and psychological components

Mosey (1986) provides a very comprehensive list of skills (totalling 99 items, including main and subheadings). She organizes these under the headings sensory integration; motor function; cognitive function; psychological function; and social interaction. She also includes occupational performances, age, cultural implications and other considerations in her analysis. Mosey is admittedly influenced by her interest in the psychosocial components and developmental aspects of occupational therapy, and emphasizes these aspects.

Reed & Sanderson's list (1992) is comprehensive and well balanced. She lists sensori-motor skills (11 items), perceptual skills (10 items), motor skills (11 items), neuromuscular skills (10 items), cognitive skills (20 items), psychosocial skills (12 items) and social skills (7 items). The list is intended to guide assessment rather than

occupational analysis, although the need for analysis is implicit.

Johnson (1996) tends towards the biomechanical approach and gives a structure for detailed activity analysis illustrated by carefully worked out examples. She uses the headings; motor/physiological (3 sections), sensory (5 sections), cognitive (6 sections) and perceptual dysfunctions (4 sections). She also considers emotional, social, independence and cultural demands.

Crepeau (1998) uses a task-focused activity analysis format. Her list of performance components is based on the American Association of Occupational Therapists' Uniform Terminology (1994). It includes: sensory (9 items), perceptual processing (13 items), neuromusculoskeletal (8 items), motor (8 items), cognitive (14 items), psychological (3 items), social (4 items) and self-management (3 items). Crepeau does not give examples, but provides a set of headings for analysis and questions for students.

Although these authors attempt to provide comprehensive lists of skills and skill components, it is clearly difficult for them to avoid being biased by the frame of reference with which they are most familiar.

What these lists share, when viewed as a whole, is a complexity of structure and abundance of descriptive terms which appear quite bewildering to the novice analyst. This is not a criticism of the systems, merely a recognition of the fact that demand analysis is a very complex endeavour.

The reader is advised to refer to as many of these sources as possible before attempting demand analysis because comparison of these systems serves to indicate just how complicated skill analysis can become, and the difficulty of constructing detailed analytical taxonomies.

SOLVING THE PRACTICAL PROBLEMS OF SKILL DEMAND ANALYSIS

It is rapidly apparent when lists of this kind are studied that a comprehensive demand analysis is potentially a huge undertaking which, while valuable as a research tool for understanding human occupation, is not always necessary or practical in a clinical setting.

There are a number of ways of reducing the practical difficulties of demand analysis:

Generalize the analysis	Use the skill domains or select general subheadings only. Summarize the main points.
Use a frame of reference	Select an approach and limit the analysis to the relevant skills.
Restrict the analysis	Select only a small portion of the task for detailed analysis.

GENERAL DEMAND ANALYSIS

General demand analysis is conducted at effective level (chained tasks or activities). This requires a relatively broad approach. The headings: motor demand, sensory demand, cognitive-perceptual demand and social demand can be used to give an indication of the type of skill which is needed.

Physical demand	Is generated by the nature of the movements required during the task.
Sensory demand	Requires identification of, and response to sensory stimulation generated by the task or situation.
Cognitive–perceptual demand	Is generated by aspects of the task or situation which require use of perceptual skill components or cognitive processing.
Social demand	Is generated by the need to interact with or communicate with others.

As additional information, one may give a rating of the level of demand for each item, simply as *high* (requiring a substantial input of the skill and/or high level of effort or skill); *moderate* (a significant amount of use of the skill and/or average requirements for effort or level of skill);

or *low* (minimum contribution from the skill and/or slight effort and low level of skill).

Having previously analysed the content of the activity and sequence of tasks in 'shopping at a supermarket' in some detail in Chapter 26, we can use this as the basis for a demand analysis example.

The tasks are listed in sequence, and then analysed to indicate the type and level of demand. Because of the integrated nature of performance, nearly all skills could be said to be used for nearly every task. It would not, however, be helpful to indicate the use of all four skill domains every time; the skills which are used minimally are therefore discounted and a blank is left.

This analysis demonstrates that shopping requires sensori-motor and cognitive–perceptual skills in approximately equal amounts. There is very little need for social interaction except at

Table 28.2 Summary of general skill demand analysis

Activity Shopping at a supermarket	
Physical demand	Generally moderate, but may be high when loading filled bags into the trolley
Sensory demand	Moderate, but may be high when examining items or selecting produce
Cognitive–perceptual demand	Generally moderate, but may be high when making decisions or if unable to find items
Social demand	Generally low
Potential for variation in task structure or purpose	Low
Context	Self-care activity; culturally well-recognized
Motivational content	Generally perceived as low
Potential stressors	Moderate to high: situationally variable
Risks	Normally low

the cash desk. Physical demand is moderate, but may be high when it comes to handling full shopping bags. Sensory demands are mainly moderate. Cognitive–perceptual demands are low to moderate except when making choices about what to buy. The interactive demands are low, except when relating to the cashier when there is the option to communicate socially. The significant features can be summarized and to complete the picture relevant features from the basic analysis of content and context can also be summarized (Table 28.2).

LIMITATIONS OF GENERAL DEMAND ANALYSIS

This 'broad brush' approach is useful, but it only provides a guide or summary. It is also somewhat subjective; the descriptors are imprecise. It does, however, enable the therapist to decide how appropriate the activity is likely to be before using it therapeutically. It indicates tasks which require more detailed analysis. It may also point to an area where a client might be expected to experience difficulty.

Example of general skill demand analysis: effective level

Activity   Shopping at a supermarket for basic household items

Task		Physical demand	Sensory demand	Cognitive–perceptual demand	Social demand
1 Select trolley	Select		Low	Moderate	
2 Push trolley	Push	Moderate	Moderate	Moderate	
3 Enter supermarket	Enter	Moderate	Low	Low	Low
4 Consult list	Consult		Moderate	Moderate	
5 Navigate to required item, pushing trolley	Navigate		Moderate	Moderate	
	Push	Moderate			Low
6 Scan shelves for required item	Scan		Moderate	Moderate	
7 Select required item	Select		Moderate/high	Moderate/high	
8 Pick up and load into trolley	Pick up	Moderate	Moderate	Low	
	Load	Moderate			
9 Decide when shopping completed	Decide			Low	
10 Push trolley to checkout	Push	Moderate	Moderate	Moderate	
11 Find checkout; queue if necessary	Find		Low	Low	
	Queue	Moderate			Low
12 Unload items onto belt	Unload	Moderate	Moderate	Low	
13 Pack items once scanned and costed	Pack	Moderate/low	Moderate	Low	
14 Load filled bags into trolley	Load	High	Moderate	Low	
15 Pay cashier for items	Pay	Low (hands moderate)	Moderate	Low	Moderate/low
17 Find exit	Find		Low	Low	
18 Leave supermarket with loaded trolley	Leave	Moderate	Moderate	Low	

USING A FRAME OF REFERENCE TO GUIDE DEMAND ANALYSIS

There are several possible approaches to guide a more detailed skill demand analysis. These are based on perspectives on human skills, and the ways in which these may be subdivided. Commonly used approaches have already been summarized in Chapter 23. They include:

Approaches to skill demand analysis	
Approach	**Type of demand**
1. Sensory stimulation	Sensory
2. Biomechanical	Physical
3. Cognitive-perceptual	Cognitive-perceptual
4. Social interactive	Social

The following lists are compiled with reference to the taxonomies produced by Mosey (1986), Reed & Sanderson (1992), Johnson (1996), Crepeau (1998) and the American Association of Occupational Therapists' Uniform Terminology for Occupational Therapy, 3rd edn (1994), with additional material from personal and other sources.

Headings for demand analysis using specific approaches
• Task/activity title
• Occupational designation (work, leisure, spiritual, etc.)
• Brief description of location, purpose, product and participant(s)
• Brief description of content and context of task or activity
• List of tasks having moderate or high demand relevant to the selected approach
• Analysis of the demand relevant skill components in identified tasks (see analysis table)

1. Sensory stimulation approach: Sensory demand analysis

Sensory input during task (indicate source of stimulation)

Vestibular	Olfactory	Tactile	Visual
Proprioceptive	Gustatory	Auditory	Nociceptive

■ *Sensory Skill Demands*

Vestibular	Detect/maintain/change position in space Maintain balance
Proprioceptive	Awareness of/maintenance of position of limbs and joints
Touch	Discrimination: shape, size, form, weight Stereognosis Texture recognition Weight matching, weight judging Gross sensation, fine sensation Temperature discrimination Vibration
Hearing	Pitch, tone, volume; locate source of sound
Smell	Identify/discriminate between smells
Taste	Identify/discriminate between tastes
Vision	Near acuity/far acuity; colour vision, night vision
Nociceptive	Painful or unpleasant stimuli are normally avoided in a therapeutic activity. When the ability to receive sensory input is damaged it may be necessary to identify when normal present sources of potential discomfort.

2. Biomechanical approach: Physical demand analysis

■ *Physical Skill Demands*

Posture

Posture at start of task and any changes to this
Postural alignment (good / bad posture)

Balance requirement for postural control or balance

Movement

Location of movement: list joints involved
Specific movements: list functional movements
(verbs)
Range of movement: specify anatomical
movement and range at each joint
Describe type of movement
- bilateral / unilateral
- active / static / passive
- assisted / resisted
- fast / slow
- repetitive
- jerky / rhythmic

Strength: describe demand for strength as
high / moderate / low

Endurance or stamina: describe demand as
high / moderate / low
Effort intermittent or sustained

Motor skills

Lower limbs
Unilateral use, right / left
Bilateral use
Gross co-ordination
Praxis or motor planning

Upper limbs
Unilateral use, right / left
Bilateral use
Gross motor co-ordination
Fine motor co-ordination
Praxis or motor planning

Hand
Unilateral use, right / left
Bilateral use
Visual / motor (hand / eye) co-ordination
Manipulation and dexterity
Precision
Grip: tip pinch, lateral pinch, tripod pinch,
plate grip, suitcase grip, hanging grip,
cylinder grip, ball grip

3. Cognitive–perceptual approach: Cognitive–perceptual demand analysis

■ *Cognitive Demands*

Initiate and terminate task activity

Interaction with and reaction to surroundings

Orientation: person, place, time, situation, topography

Cognitive processing during task

Attention/concentration: detect, react, select, sustain, shift, track
Association relationships between objects or concepts
Memory
– immediate recall
– delayed recall
– procedural recall,
– rospective recall
Sequencing
Categorizing
Judgement
Selection/choice
Problem-solving
Decision-taking
Planning
Organizing
Abstract/concrete thinking
Logical reasoning
Improvisation
Creativity/imagination
Risk-evaluation and avoidance

Communication

Simple/complex
Verbal/non-verbal

Comprehension

Spoken instructions or information
Written instructions or information

Temporal aspects

Concept of time
Recognizes cues to time
Monitors time
Budgets time

Responsibility

Controls, supervises
Monitors, checks standards

Numerical skills

Calculates
Estimates
Measures, calibrates
Attributes value

■ *Perceptual Demands*

Physical/tactile

Evaluation of size, shape, weight and volume
Stereognosis
Kinesthesia
Body position
Body schema

Spatial

Right/left discrimination
Spatial relations
Evaluation of size, shape weight and volume
Depth perception
Perception of angles/levels

Visual

Recognition of objects
Recognition of faces
Recognition of colour
Recognition of words
Recognition of numbers
Colour discrimination
Colour matching
Figure/ground
Form constancy
Visual closure
Pattern recognition
Pattern matching
Shape recognition
Shape matching

4. Social interactive approach: Social demand analysis

■ *Social Skills Demands*

Type of interaction

Dyadic: structured / unstructured
Group: co-operative group; parallel group,
structured / unstructured, activity based / social
Teamwork: co-operative; competitive

Interactive opportunities/roles of participants

e.g. share, compromise, lead / control, act a part
negotiatedeviate, co-operate, conform / comply,
assert, experiment, follow, explore

Interpersonal skills/communication

Nature/content of communication
 - gives information
 - seeks information
 - instructs
 - socializes / converses

Communication skills
 - physical / non-verbal
 - attention to others
 - gesture / expression
 - direction of gaze
 - touch
 - position in relation to others
 - posture
 - empathy / mirrors

Verbal
 - speaks
 - informs
 - expresses
 - inquires
 - responds
 - prompts / cues
 - times / limits

Listening skills
 - pays attention
 - receives information
 - times:takes turns
 - shares:limits

Expression of emotional reaction to communication by others, e.g.
 - laughs / enjoys
 - surprise / concern
 - empathy / sympathy

Intrapersonal skills

Emotional demands
Expression
Identification
Control

Demands on personal identity
Self-concept
Self-efficacy / control
Self-expression
Insight
Role identity
Responsibility
Attitudes / values

Coping skills
Recognizes stressors
Adapts to stress
Acts to reduce source of stress
Manages personal stress response

Table 28.3 Summary of headings for total demand analysis

Components of physical demand

A. Posture

B. Balance

C. Movement

D. Strength

E. Endurance

F. Motor skills

Components of sensory demand

A. Sensory input during task

B. Sensory skills/discriminations required for task

Components of cognitive and perceptual demand

A. Initiate and terminate task or activity

B. Interaction with and reaction to surroundings: orientation

C. Cognitive processing during task

D. Communication

E. Comprehension

F. Temporal aspects

G. Responsibility

H. Numerical skills

I. Perceptual skills and discriminations

Components of social demand

A. Type and context of interaction

B. Interactive opportunities and roles of participants

C. Interpersonal and communication skills

D. Intrapersonal skills

ANALYSING TOTAL DEMAND

Using an approach has the advantage of focusing the mind on one set of attributes, and dealing with these in considerable detail. Although each list is plainly much shorter than a comprehensive analysis would be, most are quite long. This level of detail is not always relevant or practical.

At the effective level (chained tasks and activities), an analysis of tasks can be done using only the broader headings given in bold type (Table 28.3). Examples of this type of analysis illustrate that a considerable amount of information is provided (Table 28.4).

To obtain a comprehensive picture of an activity one needs to combine all four approaches.

LIMITATIONS OF TOTAL DEMAND ANALYSIS OF TASKS

It will be apparent from the examples of analysis of task demand that it is difficult to set boundaries between task analysis and microanalysis. Inevitably one starts to list specific task stages or components and the relevant skill components.

The boundary is not rigidly fixed; it is a matter of personal analytical style, and the depth of understanding required. It may be worth noting that if one finds oneself getting drawn into detail, it may be advisable to move further down the occupational levels. A task analysis will itemize the task stages, and the skill components of each can then be identified.

DEMAND MICROANALYSIS

It may sometimes be necessary to undertake a microanalysis, for example, in order to analyse specific perceptual or cognitive demands, one needs to look at individual performance units.

Demand analysis of performance units can become highly complicated. At this level, each small movement, each perceptual or cognitive process, each minute recognition of a sensory input has to be accounted for.

Although this is very interesting in the context of research, it is extremely difficult to undertake in a clinical setting, and there is seldom a need for this level of detail.

Without access to the sophisticated equipment now used by neurophysiologists, the therapist can only make informed assumptions about what is going on. A single example should suffice to show how this can be done (Table 28.5).

Table 28.4   Example of total demand analysis of tasks

Activity   Shopping at a supermarket for household items

PHYSICAL DEMAND

General demands	Moderate stamina; lower limbs/trunk: able to walk, manoeuvre trolley, stand, bend; upper limbs/hands: stretch, reach, grasp, lift, place, manipulate

Specific task demands

Push trolley	Walk; upright posture; arms push forward; hand cylinder grip; low/moderate resistance
Enter supermarket	Walk; upright posture; gross movement upper & lower limbs; (may need to open door)
Pick up item	Balance; bend/reach/stretch; grasp; lift (items varied shapes, sizes and weights)
Load trolley	Balance; bend/reach/stretch; grasp; lower/place (items varied shapes, sizes and weights)
Queue	Stand; walk
Unload trolley	Balance; bend/twist trunk; arms reach/stretch; grasp; lift (items varied shapes, sizes and weights)
Pack items into bags	Stand; balance; grasp; manipulate; lift/place
Pay for items	Stand; balance; fine grasp (coins/card); manipulate
Load filled bags into trolley	Arms lift, lower; (filled bags various weights; can be heavy); trunk may bend, twist
Push trolley out of supermarket	Walk; upright posture; arms push forward; hand cylinder grip; moderate resistance

SOCIAL DEMAND

General demands	Shopper must conform with generally accepted social behaviour, and manners. Consideration for others desirable. Casual interaction with staff or other shoppers situational or optional

Specific task demands

Pay cashier	Limited verbal exchanges to ascertain price and pay with money or credit card. Polite acknowledgement/smile. Optional: additional social remarks, comments, humour

COGNITIVE–PERCEPTUAL DEMAND

General demands	Navigation into, around & out of supermarket; reading & following signs or other information; location & selection of products; avoidance of hazards & other people

Specific task demands

Select trolley	Discriminate between types and choose correct size and design
Push trolley	Work out route, and how to avoid obstacles/hazards/people
Consult list	Identify item wanted; recall items already obtained
Navigate to required item	Recall probable location/section; follow signs/cognitive map; visually identify and locate required item
Select required item	Visually locate item; compare similar items (evaluate quality, value, price), decide on item to purchase (or decide not to purchase)
Decide when shopping completed	Check list; compare list with items in trolley; determine completeness
Pay cashier	Evaluate bill; calculate; check correct and affordable; identify best method of payment; find correct money or nearest approximation (or select credit card); check change

SENSORY DEMAND

General demands	High/moderate; supermarket environment designed to provide high sensory stimulation; good vision required in order to navigate, read signs/information, find products, avoid hazards and others; products may be checked and evaluated using touch (weight), visual checks (colour, size, shape), taste and smell; hearing needed to listen to announcements, information, prices

Specific task demands

Push trolley	Maintain grip contact on handle; steer trolley using hand/eye co-ordination
Navigate	Vision: look around and ahead to find clear route; follow signs; read labels
Find item	Vision
Select item	Vision; may also use evaluation by touch, taste, smell.
Handle items	(Pick up; manipulate; lift; pack) vision, touch; appreciation of weight, size
Pay cashier	Vision; touch (handle coins/credit card)

EDUCATIONAL DEMAND

A task or activity which requires considerable prior knowledge or skill has *high educational demand*; it may require special personal attributes which restrict the number of participants. One which can be learnt 'on the job' by most people has *low demand*.

An analysis of educational demand aims to answer questions such as 'What does the participant need to know in order to perform this task? What information should the participant have? What should the participant value? The therapist is interested in the learning *prerequisites* for task performance.

An understanding of educational demand enables one to evaluate whether an individual is *ready* to perform. If there is a mismatch between the state of current learning and the required level, the therapist can decide whether the additional knowledge, attitudes, values or skills need to be taught *before* the task can be attempted, or whether task performance itself will teach the individual what the individual is required to know.

Educational analysis, like other skill demand analysis, can become very complex. As before, if the list becomes too long, it is better to deal with the requirements task by task. Educational demands can be stated as competencies at constructive or effective level, or as behavioural components at acquisitional level (see Ch. 7).

HEADINGS FOR ANALYSIS OF EDUCATIONAL DEMAND

- Title of activity / task
- Overall evaluation of complexity / difficulty of task: simple / basic to highly complex and difficult

---

Table 28.5 Example of microanalysis of demand

Activity Shopping at a supermarket

Task Select required item

Task stages
1 Visually locate item and price information
2 Mentally evaluate price information (option: reject item)
3 Visually examine item (option: handle item)
4 Confirm item matches (or fails to match) requirement
4 Compare item with any similar items; contrast price, quantity and quality (option: handle items)
5 Decide which item to select (reject others)

Example microanalysis: *Task stage* Visually locate item and price information
PERFORMANCE UNITS
1 Scan shelves to locate item
2 Match located item with remembered item
3 Search for applicable price label on shelf; read price information

	Physical	*Sensory*	*Cognitive*	*Perceptual*
Scan shelves to locate item	Turn head L/R up/down	Visual scan	Recall item Name item Read label	Figure ground Colour recognition Object recognition Shape recognition Pattern recognition (e.g. package design)
Match located item with remembered item	Hold head still Fix gaze	Near acuity	Recall item wanted; Confirm match	Object recognition Shape recognition Colour/pattern recognition Size discrimination
Search for applicable price label; read price	Move head Find and focus	Near acuity	Read price Comprehend numbers	Number recognition

Table 28.6 Example of educational demand analysis

Activity   Shopping at a supermarket for food and household items

Level of performance required: Competence

Specific standards or criteria which must be met:
1   All/most items required must be purchased
2   Items must be suitable, of good value and acceptable quality
3   Budget of available money must not be exceeded
4   Shopper must conform to norms of expected social role behaviour

Prerequisite learning

Knowledge
- Understands general concept of 'shopping' and 'buying'
- Understands limits to acceptable behaviour when shopping
- Understands how to judge if item is of good quality and value
- Understands basic principles of achieving a good nutritional balance
- Understands nutritional information printed on food packaging
- Knows metric system weights and measures.
- Understands the significance of 'shelf life' and 'use by' information

Attitudes/values
- Readily conforms to norms of acceptable behaviour
- Values honesty
- Values personal good manners but shows some tolerance of others
- Appreciates the importance of good value
- Appreciates the importance of good quality
- Values economy and keeping within budget

Skills

• Literacy	Able to read directional signs and labels
• Numeracy	Able to use money; can give correct money and correct change (*or* can use cheque, credit card, store card) Can perform simple calculations and comparisons Able to keep within preset budget Able to judge true value of 'bargains' or 'offers'
• Quantifying	Able to judge quantities (number, size, shape, weight, volume) in relation to personal needs
• Navigating Judgement and discrimination	Can recognize and follow signs and cues to location Able to evaluate and compare size, shape, colour, volume, weight and other physical attributes of items Able to discriminate between levels of food freshness and length of time products can be stored after purchase
• Communication	Able to seek information about products
• Exhibits good manners	Able to produce appropriate and polite responses to others; controls personal responses which may be inappropriate, impolite or unhelpful
• Physical skill	Able to handle and steer trolley effectively Able to handle items safely without dropping or spilling Able to handle money

- Level of performance required: novice, competent, expert
- Specific standards or criteria which must be met
- Prerequisite learning
  - KNOWLEDGE (understanding or information)
  - ATTITUDES OR VALUES
  - METHODS, TECHNIQUES, SKILLS.

An educational analysis may often be more appropriate and useful than the more traditional skills analysis because it considers *knowing about (understanding and information)* and *knowing how (skills)*. Skills are described in functional terms, which is also very relevant to occupational therapy. The analysis acts both as the basis for a set of learning objectives and as a basis for evaluation of whether the individual does have the prerequisite learning for the task. An example of educational demand analysis is shown in Table 28.6.

DEVELOPMENTAL DEMAND ANALYSIS

Analysis of developmental demand is chiefly of interest to therapists who work with children, or with adults with congenital or acquired developmental disorders. As this is a somewhat specialized area of practice, only the general scope of this approach will be summarized. Developmental demand considers three areas: physical development, cognitive development and social development.

Physical development

This is usually considered within one of the neurodevelopmental frames of reference. Main considerations include:

Position	How does position relate to the developmental sequence (lie, crawl, sit, stand, step, run, jump)? Will the position inhibit or promote abnormal tone?
Posture and balance	Postural control; balance; righting reflexes and equilibrium responses.
Movement	Proximal or distal; gross or fine; crossing the midline; bilateral integration; laterality.

Sensory development deals with the maturation of the sensory system and the opportunities offered by the task for enhancing sensory input, perception and feedback. In some approaches, vestibular or tactile stimulation are especially important.

Social development deals with stages in the development of personal identity, communication skills, roles and the ability to co-operate with others.

Applied analysis

CONSIDERATIONS IN APPLIED ANALYSIS

The *application* of activities as therapy was one of the first techniques developed by occupational therapists.

In order to apply an activity there has to be a process of matching the selected activity to the needs and interests of the intended participant.

Applied analysis is founded on basic analysis which provides the understanding of the way in which the activity or task is performed, and demand analysis, which describes how this performance may be expected to challenge a participant to respond.

The third element required before an applied analysis can be conducted is an *evaluation of the individual*. This is in two parts, an *occupational profile* which gives a 'pen portrait' of previous occupations and interests and other relevant details, and an *assessment summary and goal plan* which describes the individual's functional abilities and problems or the specific performance consequences of illness or trauma, and specifies an objective for intervention.

Once this information has been assembled, the therapist can evaluate whether the activity is

---

Summary of considerations in applied analysis
• Therapeutic considerations
• Information about:
  – The individual
  – The activity
  – The environment
• Need and scope for adaptation.

---

likely to be suitable and can begin to match the selected activity to the aims and objectives of intervention.

THERAPEUTIC CONSIDERATIONS

These include the aim and objectives of intervention, and awareness of any precautions or contra-indications which may limit the selection of an activity.

Therapy should be based on well-tested assumptions and evidence of effectiveness and the selected activity should make a substantial contribution towards achieving the stated aims.

INITIAL INFORMATION

The therapist must begin by collating all the relevant information about the individual, the aims and objectives of intervention, and the performance demand of a range of potentially useful activities.

The processes used to gather this are described elsewhere in this book; refer to the appropriate chapter if you need to remind yourself about them.

There is a well-worn adage used in information technology 'garbage in, garbage out'. This is highly relevant in applied analysis. If the quality of the initial information is poor, the matching process cannot be effective.

The therapist must not only select an appropriate activity, the therapist must also be able to demonstrate a connection between what has been selected and the needs of the client.

Summary of initial information
- Profile and assessment data for individual
- An indication of the general aim of intervention (e.g. assess, rehabilitate, educate, develop, resettle, maintain)
- Specific objective of intervention
- A summary of the content and context of the task or activity
- A demand analysis of the task or activity and the performance environment.

APPLIED ANALYSIS: SELECTING AN ACTIVITY

Selection of an activity may appear to be a matter of 'applied common sense'. Common sense certainly helps, but it has to be modified by good clinical reasoning. The therapist uses the headings for applied analysis to review the known facts about the individual, and the agreed therapeutic objectives, in relation to the available task options, in order to produce a shortlist of compatible activities.

This process can be structured by asking a set of analytical questions. It is useful for the novice analyst to write the answers in some detail. It is also good practice for a summary of the information to be recorded once the analysis has been completed.

The questions are given in Box 29.1 and a flow chart to guide selection is also presented.

At this point, it may be apparent that only one activity or task is likely to be relevant. The question then becomes how best to present or adapt it and the therapist can move without delay to stage three. On other occasions, there may be several potentially suitable options which require careful comparison and evaluation.

Sometimes, it is not at all clear how best to meet therapeutic objectives. This may suggest that a further period of assessment is required in which the individual is engaged in an activity which is structured to provide more information about skills and abilities, interests, reactions to performance demand and personal attitudes to performance.

IS THE TASK OR ACTIVITY SUITABLE FOR SPECIFIC APPLICATION?

An activity or task has to possess a number of attributes in order to be suited to therapeutic application or adaptation (Box 29.2). Some activities are not suitable because they are too complex, too highly skilled, take too long, require specialized materials and tools, or carry health and safety risks.

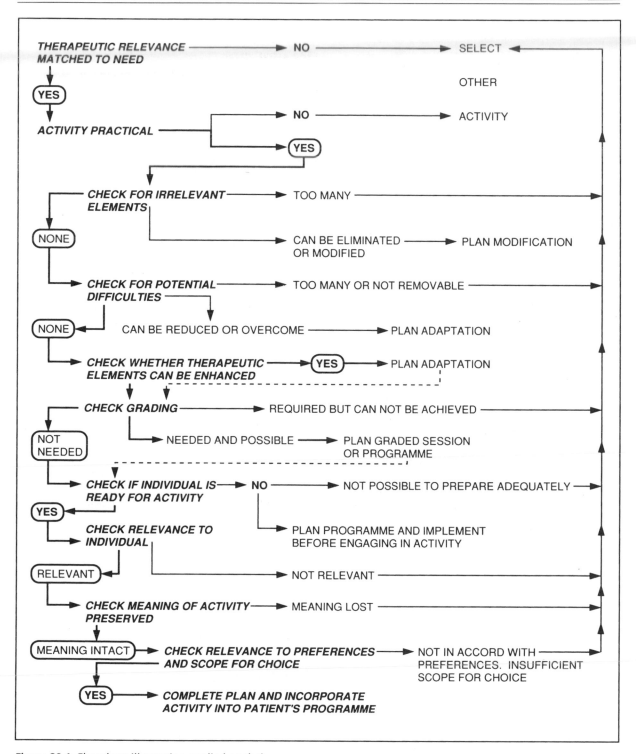

Figure 29.1 Flowchart illustrating applied analysis.

Box 29.1 Checklist for applied analysis

Therapeutic considerations

What is the main aim of using the activity?

What are the objectives?

Are there any precautions or contra-indications?

Is a specific therapeutic approach to be used?

How does this affect activity selection?

Are specific therapeutic adaptations needed?

Will grading be required?

The individual

Occupational performance

Is the dysfunction general or is there specific loss of competence?

If task-related, which task or tasks are involved?

Which skill domain or domains are mainly involved?

At which level of performance is intervention required: acquisitional, constructive, effective, organizational?

Motivational aspects

Has the client expressed any preference for, or concern about, a specific task or activity?

Does the client's occupational history suggest existing skills or interests which may guide selection, or provide motivation?

What type of activity is likely to be perceived as meaningful or relevant?

How may opportunities for personal preference or choice be provided? (Or must choices be limited?)

The activity/task

Which activity or task is likely to be appropriate? List options.

What elements in the performance demand, purposes or product of this activity relate to the roles, needs, abilities and interests of the client?

Is it age appropriate and culturally appropriate?

Are there elements which do not relate to needs/abilities or interests? Are these a major or minor part of the activity?

Are there any undesirable features? If so, can these be eliminated?

Is the activity likely to be practical? (Consider cost, safety, preparation, practical requirements and clearing up.)

Is the activity likely to motivate engagement?

Is the individual ready to meet the performance demand of the activity? If not, is there sufficient time for learning or skill development?

Will adaptations to enable or enhance performance be needed?

Can adaptations be made without losing the meaning and context of performance?

The environment

What environmental requirements does the activity impose?

Will the demand of the environment contribute to therapeutic goals?

Will adaptations to the environment be needed?

Box 29.2 Desirable features of a therapeutic activity

- A degree of familiarity and relevance within a given culture
- Moderately high visibility with an amount of structure
- Moderate to high variability with potential for grading or physical adaptation
- Tasks which individually require low to moderate skill and can readily be taught
- The capacity to be reduced to a series of apparently simple task stages
- Relatively uncomplicated and easily available materials and resources
- The parameters of performance can readily be controlled by the therapist
- Generally non-hazardous or low risk.

OFFERING CHOICES

In therapeutic application, the degree of choice available to the client in the selection of an activity, or the scope for choices about details of process or product, is one of the parameters controlled by the therapist. It is affected by the selected approach; some approaches imply freedom of choice, while others imply that the therapist must be more prescriptive.

Making choices can promote involvement and increase motivation. As a general principle, the therapist will seek to offer options and opportunities for choice whenever possible, but although choice is often described as ethically important, it is not always appropriate. For example, the patient may have a condition which makes choice very difficult or stressful, or the need to treat a specific dysfunction may restrict options. The patient always has one fundamental choice – whether to participate or not.

THERAPEUTIC ADAPTATION OF ACTIVITIES AND TASKS: PRELIMINARY CONSIDERATIONS

A therapeutic activity or task may require adaptation to make it more effective as therapy. Therapeutic adaptation is aimed at producing a specific benefit for the patient. Applied analysis identifies suitable therapeutic tasks or activities, and suggests the nature of the adaptations required. On the basis of an analysis of therapeutic goals, the therapist can identify specific aspects of performance demand which need to be modified to enhance the benefits of participation, or to make performance possible.

TECHNIQUES FOR THERAPEUTIC ADAPTATION

Adaptations can be made by:

- presenting the task in a specific context
- grading the demand of the task
- adapting tools or materials
- altering position of work or participant
- changing elements in the environment.

These techniques are described in Chapter 30.

IS ADAPTATION NECESSARY?

A fundamental principle of adaptation is to do as little as possible to an activity, and to do it unobtrusively. The reason is simple; the meaning and integrity of an activity is closely linked to its context and method of performance. If these things are lost in the course of over-extensive adaptation, the participant is likely to perceive the whole process of therapy as abnormal and much of the benefit is lost.

When changes are obvious, it is important that the patient or client understands why they are necessary and how they may be expected to be beneficial.

However, part of the skill of adaptation is to make subtle changes which enable the therapist to present the activity *as if it is unadapted*.

Although adaptation is often a central feature of application, the therapist needs to remember that the scope of human performance is wide and the demands of tasks and activities are equally wide and varied. It may well be possible to provide the required demand by selecting a different activity, rather than seeking to adapt a marginally suitable one.

There are times when normal participation in a completely normal environment is what is required.

Therapeutic adaptation: approaches and techniques

CHAPTER CONTENTS

THERAPEUTIC ADAPTATION IN RELATION TO OCCUPATIONAL AND ENVIRONMENTAL LEVELS

As a general rule, the amount of adaptation undertaken decreases as one ascends through the occupational levels and expands outwards from the near environment of the individual into the wider world.

At the developmental level and within the near environment, quite extensive adaptation may be required. Grading is especially important, and practical alterations may also be made. Task performance at this level needs to be kept short, simple and highly specific. Performance may be focused on isolated skill domains.

As one progresses upwards into the effective level, the scope for adaptation becomes smaller and the emphasis on 'normal', integrated performance becomes greater. Activities become more demanding, take more time and are more complex.

At the organizational level, therapeutic adaptation is irrelevant, but some functional adaptation may be required.

FEATURES WHICH CAN BE ADAPTED

The features which can be adapted include:

- the environment
  - features in physical environment
  - environmental demand, context and cultural meaning
- the task
  - method
  - sequence
  - temporal aspects
  - standards
  - equipment, tools and materials
- the individual
  - position
  - movement.

ADAPTIVE TECHNIQUES

There is a wide range of adaptive techniques available to the therapist. These are in turn modified by the selected approach.

PRESENTATION OF ACTIVITIES AND TASKS

The way in which a task is presented to patients or clients affects their reactions to it, and can increase or decrease motivation.

The therapist needs to select a context for presentation, which could be one of the following:

- as normal performance (work, leisure or self-care)
- as a simulation of normal performance
- as a way of solving a problem
- as a way of learning or practising a skill
- as a means of developing an ability
- as a way of finding out more about a situation or about personal abilities
- as a means of exercising a limb
- as a route into a new interest or leisure activity.

Once the context is selected, all aspects of the presentation – environment, resources, words used to introduce the task, approach used by therapist, style of therapeutic relationship – need to be coherent, consistent and explicit in reinforcing awareness of what is intended.

GRADING

Grading is an important concept in occupational therapy. It means altering the parameters of performance to increase or decrease the demand.

The therapist must be able to control the parameters with some precision. This means being able to replicate the performance conditions on successive occasions. In order to do this, accurate and detailed records of all adaptations must be kept and updated each time a parameter is altered.

In the traditional form of grading, the therapist challenges the patient to improve performance by continually increasing the demand so that it remains just a little higher than the patient's current abilities. This will be referred to as *progressive grading*.

Regular re-assessment and measurement of abilities are needed to ensure that demand is increased by exactly the right amount and at the right time. Progressive grading must be used with discretion and close attention paid to precautions and contra-indications.

Reverse grading is also possible; in this approach, demand is progressively reduced as abilities deteriorate, but the therapist attempts to keep abilities at their optimum level and to avoid premature loss of ability through disuse.

When working with some patients, especially those who are old, or who have chronic conditions (e.g. arthritis, cardiac conditions, multiple sclerosis, chronic fatigue syndrome or chronic pain syndrome), progressive grading can be counter-productive. This may be because the continual struggle to cope with the 'moving goalposts' is experienced as overly frustrating or stressful, or because it is hard to set a level which stretches abilities without producing adverse effects such as fatigue or pain. In these cases, the therapist can use *proportional grading*.

At the start of proportional grading, a baseline for performance is set based on a thorough assessment of the level of ability of the patient. Having recorded the baseline, the therapist grades the activity to a point somewhat *below* what is currently possible. This may be expressed as a percentage: for example, the patient will work at 80% of maximum capacity.

The assumption is that by working within achievable limits the patient will be less fatigued and likely to sustain effort for longer. This will help the patient to retain motivation, and experience reinforcement from successful participation. Given time, it is likely that performance will improve. At intervals, performance is re-assessed and a new baseline can be set, which means that demand can be increased, although still at a level below maximum. The patient may be taught to monitor aspects of personal performance or physiological responses, and to *pace* the activity to keep within set limits.

Both progressive grading and proportional grading deal with the same general parameters. These include:

- duration or complexity of process
- nature or complexity of product
- aspects of performance demand.

DURATION OR COMPLEXITY OF PROCESS

Crafts and activities traditionally used by therapists were selected principally because they offered extensive scope for grading in both duration and complexity.

Weaving is a good example of this. At its simplest, it can involve weaving a strip of rag or thick wool over and under the large threads of a simple warp strung on a card or frame. At its most complex, it can involve elaborate pattern weaving using several colours on a multi-heddle, traditional craft loom.

As many of these activities are no longer available to the therapist for a multitude of reasons (practical and cultural), finding suitable equivalents demands imagination and ingenuity.

Duration

The length of time for which performance must be sustained has a direct link to the degree of demand and the requirement for expenditure of energy. Tasks which are of short duration, or can be broken into convenient stages, can be structured as performance episodes which are matched to the patient's abilities and therapeutic needs.

Controlling the length of time worked is a simple and effective form of grading, but care must be taken that performance does not become so episodic that process and product become disconnected.

Complexity

Complexity provides cognitive challenges. It is partly a function of duration; in a short time-frame, it is likely that performance will be less complex.

Complexity is also an intrinsic feature of tasks and activities. Complexity may come from having to integrate many different processes and skills, or from the need for high level judgement or decision-taking.

NATURE OR COMPLEXITY OF PURPOSE OR PRODUCT

Activities used as therapy typically have high visibility products, either in terms of something which is made or a familiar purpose with a well-structured, cultural context such as playing a game or participating in a quiz.

Cooking and gardening provide good examples of activities which have numerous possible purposes and products from the very simple to the highly sophisticated.

SPECIFIC PERFORMANCE DEMAND

Demand analysis indicates the intrinsic nature of tasks or environments. The therapist is faced with the task of making these demands relatively more or less difficult. This involves modification of components or parameters which create demand.

INTRINSIC GRADING

Some activities have an inbuilt grading of effort or complexity. This may mean that the most difficult or resistive tasks come first. For example, most woodwork projects require resistive tasks such as sawing, planing and chiselling at the earlier stages, whereas relatively less resistive tasks such as sandpapering or varnishing come last. This can create a problem if the therapist is looking for a task which can be progressively graded. It may mean that patients finish a product made by someone else rather than starting their own and this may reduce motivation.

On the other hand, an activity such as stool seating can begin with an unresistive task such as sanding and varnishing the stool frame. It progresses through the first stage of seating which is moderately resistive but at the final stage when the last few sections of weaving are completed, it can become highly resistive.

GRADING OF PERFORMANCE DEMAND

Box 30.1 Examples of specific parameters which may be graded

Physical demands
- effort or strength required
- resistance to or assistance to a movement
- range of movement
- duration of movement episode
- number of movements or repetitions of a movement
- postural requirements
- speed of movement
- need for balance
- degree of co-ordination or dexterity
- degree of accuracy

Sensory demands
- degree to which each sense is brought into use
- level of sensory discrimination required

Social interactive demands
- requirement for communication skills
- information content of communication
- requirement for co-operative working
- requirement for self-control
- role demands

Perceptual demands
- level of perceptual discrimination
- speed of discrimination

Cognitive demands
- number of routine versus non-routine operations
- information content
- requirement for abstract processing
- requirement for judgement or decision-taking
- complexity or simplicity of performance structure at each stage
- number of stages in task activity
- requirement for speedy reactions
- level of responsibility
- stressors

GRADING ADAPTATIONS TO METHODS AND SEQUENCES

Grading adaptation to methods and sequences include:

- breaking the task into small stages
- leaving out task stages
- introducing rests
- changing the usual method
- changing the usual tools or equipment
- changing the usual materials.

Adaptations to temporal aspects

These include:

- limiting the duration of the task
- extending the duration of the task
- doing a task at an 'unusual' time of day
- emphasizing temporal aspects (time, seasonal connections, relationship to past, present, future)
- setting goals of performance in relation to a set length of time (e.g. make y in x minutes; try to 'beat the clock')
- emphasizing the monitoring of time (do this for 5 minutes; check this in 10 minutes).

Adaptations to standards

Standards may be lowered:

- reduce requirement for quality
- reduce need for accuracy or judgement
- reduce normal parameters of speed; quantity
- have wide spectrum of acceptable performance.

Standards may be increased or emphasized:

- have a narrow band of acceptable performance
- show good examples of finished products
- set explicit targets
- ensure work is overtly checked and evaluated.

ADAPTATIONS TO DESIGN OF TOOLS AND EQUIPMENT

ADAPTATIONS TO EXISTING DESIGN

Therapists have spent decades inventing and making innovative (sometimes bizarre) adaptations to standard tools, workshop equipment or games. These are usually provided in the context of physical rehabilitation.

REMEDIAL APPARATUS

In the 1960s and 1970s, in the attempt to provide more specific and more readily controlled demands, workshop machinery designed for physical rehabilitation was created. These included lathes, bicycle fretsaws, and upper limb rehabilitation devices such as the wire-twisting machine and the FEPS (a device for promoting flexion/extension/pronation/supination at the wrist). Many of these have now passed into history.

The effect of this was, however, to replace *creation of product* with *non-productive movement*. The workshop machine which also provided exercise became simply an exercise machine.

The legacy of this remedial workshop equipment is a new generation of adaptive devices for computers, and other special equipment. The challenge for the profession is to create equipment which is not only therapeutic but also purposeful and productive, in keeping with contemporary culture and the fundamental assumptions of occupational therapy.

Adaptations to the design or structure of tools or equipment are sometimes referred to as physical adaptations.

EXAMPLE OF PHYSICAL ADAPTATION: REMEDIAL GAMES

Remedial games are widely used. Unfortunately, use is often stereotypical and loses the purpose and fun derived from playing the game. This may be due to lack of choice of game (there are numerous possibilities) or lack of competition.

Apart from solitaire, all games require a partner who will genuinely try to win.

Games using pieces or men which are (or were) commonly played in the UK include chess; draughts and its variations (e.g. fox and geese); Chinese chequers; nine men's morris; noughts and crosses; dominoes; solitaire. In addition, there are several games originating in Africa and Asia which use pieces (originally pebbles or shells), often with boards having carved-out holes.

Examples of the adaptations that can be made include:

- adaptations to pieces:
  - wooden dowel pegs of different diameters
  - pins or nails moved by hand or with tweezers
  - nuts and bolts to screw and unscrew
  - bottle or jar tops to screw and unscrew
  - wooden discs of various diameters
  - shaped pieces: blocks, crosses, octagonal
  - marbles or pebbles
  - pieces with holes to fit over pegs
  - weighted pieces: tins, jars filled with sand; old weights
  - very light pieces; polystyrene, foam, balsa
  - velcro loops or hooks
  - pieces to move (hook or push) with feet or stick
  - finger loops or hand loops for lifting
  - added textures for visual or tactile discrimination
  - colours
- adaptations to boards:
  - extra large size for table
  - very large for use on floor
  - with holes for pegs, or dowel for pieces with holes
  - brighter colours
- adaptation of position:
  - on a sloping support on a table
  - on a vertical frame
  - on a wall
  - on the floor.

For further examples of how to adapt gardening and computer operation, refer to Johnson (1996) and Turner & McCaul (1996).

ADAPTATIONS TO TOOLS AND EQUIPMENT: TECHNIQUES OF THERAPEUTIC ADAPTATION USING SELECTED APPROACHES

From the starting point of the existing equipment and methods, the therapist must plan how to make demand precisely match treatment objectives.

These alterations may change physical demand, cognitive-perceptual demand, social demand, or a combination of these.

BIOMECHANICAL APPROACH: CHANGING PHYSICAL DEMAND

This means planning how to alter shapes, sizes, lengths or weights. This process implies some understanding of leverage and mechanical forces coupled with a good knowledge of human anatomy and movement.

It also involves evaluation of position of the patient, the movement the patient makes and the position of objects which the patient will use.

Type of movement

Can the nature of the movement be adapted? For example:

- one hand used instead of two (or both instead of one)
- a leg used instead of an arm
- a movement eliminated (or promoted) by positioning the patient or the work in a different way or restricting movement at one joint
- one movement converted into another, for example, pull to push; twist to push; crossing the mid-line from side to side instead of moving backwards and forwards.

Position of patient

Consider whether there should be any change from the normal working position.

- Should the patient:
  - sit (decide height; support; design of seat; mobile or fixed)
  - stand (with or without support)
  - lie down (prone or supine)
  - move (turn, bend, stretch, reach, walk)?

Adapting the task, tools, materials, equipment

Providing assistance to movement

Movement is assisted by anything which counteracts gravity or promotes free movement with minimum effort or frictional resistance.

Examples of adaptations to provide assistance to upper limb or lower limb movement:

- support the forearm in a buoyancy sling (a sling suspended from a spring attached to an overhead support or gantry)
- support the forearm on a 'skate' (a board or gutter support on wheels or ball-bearings which slides freely across the table surface)
- work with gravity assistance, either in horizontal plane or where effort occurs mainly when moving from high to low
- provide mechanical or electrical assistance (e.g. powered tools gearing; pulleys, springs)
- select materials which are intrinsically less resistive
- reduce weights of materials or tools
- emphasize movements which swing, slide, glide; avoid tasks which need static grip or holding of position, or which demand pulling, pushing or lifting.

Increasing resistance to movement

Resistance demands increased effort or strength. Working against resistance promotes stamina.

Examples of adaptations to increase resistance:

- select materials which are intrinsically more resistive
- increase the weight of materials or tools
- emphasize movements which require static holding or gripping, pushing, pulling, or lifting

- work against gravity, that is, when effort occurs mainly when working from low to high
- add mechanical resistance from springs, gears, brakes.

Altering the position of tools and materials:

- Should these be:
  - close to patient (visible; in easy reach)
  - positioned so as to demand a specific movement or to obtain materials or tools (high; low; to the side; on the floor)
  - at a distance from patient (to promote walking, lifting, carrying)?

Changing size and shape

- Can size be increased? For example: padded handle, oversized game piece (is this to assist grip or to provoke a specific movement?)
- Can size be decreased?
- Will a different shape promote a specific grip or movement?

Altering length:

- A longer handle or tool may increase range of movement but the effects of leverage also need to be considered. If the fulcrum is near, the user effort will be decreased, but if it is further away, effort will be increased.

COGNITIVE–PERCEPTUAL APPROACHES

In adapting activities within cognitive – perceptual approaches, the main consideration is the amount and quality of information provided. Information is inherent in all aspects of the situation. For example, tools and materials, sensory input, instructions and symbols, spatial relationships, environmental distractors, all have cognitive – perceptual implications.

Adaptations are required in order to:

- simplify the task
- reduce the amount of information

- increase the amount of information
- enhance a specific kind of information
- increase the complexity of the task
- improve learning or transfer of learning.

Reducing or increasing the amount of information

Reducing or increasing information can, paradoxically, serve two purposes. It can enhance understanding and cue behaviour, or it can reduce cues and increase the need for cognitive processing. It all depends on what you choose to leave out or put in. These techniques are often combined.

This is best explained by an example. Consider the difference between a crossword puzzle in which one is given difficult clues and minimal cues to how the crossword grid has been designed, and a small crossword puzzle where the starting letters for short words are provided with a simple definition, and one just has to complete the answers.

In both examples, information has been removed. In the first example, the helpful parts of the information are left out, and the information provided is given in an obscure form, so that extensive information-processing and problem-solving are needed. In the second example, anything extraneous is removed, only helpful information is given, cues are provided by giving the first letter of each word and the task is reduced to one of simple recall or word-finding.

Enhancing information content

Reduction can *enhance* information content and *simplify* the task by:

- removing all objects not immediately associated with the task
- reducing the number of objects needed for the task
- ensuring objects are familiar and clearly recognizable
- providing a readily identified context for use
- putting objects in a logical relationship to each other and to the user

- removing options and choices
- removing distractors in the near environment
- reducing the amount of information presented at a time
- reducing the need for judgements and discriminations.

Addition can enhance information content and improve task performance by:

- providing clear instructions
- providing feedback which shows the user that each stage has been performed correctly
- providing extra cues such as a distinguishing colour or shape
- enhancing cues to the context of performance.

Obscuring information content or increasing complexity

It may be necessary to obscure or reduce information content in the context of assessment. Cognitive – perceptual information content in real-life situations is very variable and people often need to be able to discriminate between relevant and irrelevant information, or need to solve problems using restricted information.

When learning to transfer a new skill into an unfamiliar situation, it is necessary to gradually increase complexity, introduce novelty and withdraw assistive information.

Reduction can *obscure* information content by:

- removing helpful cues to use such as position, relationship of objects or indications of context
- removing instructions
- providing information in small but unrelated 'packages'
- not reinforcing correct decisions or correcting wrong ones.

Addition can obscure information content by:

- providing several options or choices
- increasing novelty
- adding content which is not directly relevant to the task
- adding to peripheral distractors

- providing too much information at once
- providing several different kinds of information simultaneously
- extending the chain of tasks which must be undertaken.

EXAMPLE OF ADAPTING INFORMATION CONTENT

Making a cup of tea

Enhancing information

The therapist prepares a space on the kitchen worktop and removes all other items nearby. The therapist provides essential items for tea-making: a mug, a tea bag, a spoon, some milk in a marked carton and a kettle which is already filled and plugged in. These items are arranged in close association. The patient has agreed to make a cup of tea. The patient is presented with the layout and given the cue 'Here is what you need to make your cup of tea.' As the tea is being made, the therapist occasionally intervenes with a prompting comment such as 'The kettle has boiled now'; 'Do you want milk in your tea?'

Obscuring information

The therapist prepares the kitchen ensuring that items required are located in various drawers and cupboards. Tea is in a high cupboard with other items. Milk is in a jug in the fridge. The kitchen worktop has the usual clutter. The patient has agreed to make a cup of tea and is told 'Here is the kitchen. The tea is in the cupboard over there and the cups are down here. I'll come back in about a quarter of an hour. Enjoy your tea.'

SOCIAL INTERACTIVE APPROACHES

Interaction is promoted by situations which demand communication between people and some degree of co-operative endeavour.

Adaptations to promote interaction may include:

- changing a task normally performed by one person into a shared or group endeavour
- introducing shared or group decision-taking
- reducing the amount of tools or materials so that users must share
- sharing task stages between participants so that a 'production line' is set up
- making some items unavailable so that users must ask for them
- structuring seating, table layout, and other aspects of environment to promote interaction
- making small table games into large versions (floor or vertical) for use with groups
- adapting equipment for active games (e.g. making it lighter, larger, safer, suitable for use when seated).

Functional adaptation

CHAPTER CONTENTS

Therapists provide adaptations to enable people to perform functional activities (work, leisure or self-care) or to enhance performance abilities. Adaptations may be short-term or long-term.

SHORT-TERM ADAPTATIONS

Short-term adaptations are required to overcome a problem which is the result of an illness or injury which has temporarily affected functional performance. The expectation is that adaptations can be progressively removed until normal performance is restored.

These adaptations frequently focus on the basic self-care or instrumental activities of daily living which are essential for personal well-being. Alterations are usually straightforward and can include: changes to task content, structure, demand, the way people move or position themselves, modification of normal tools and equipment, or provision of special equipment.

These adaptations are normally suggested and provided by the therapist, and there is an overlap between this type of adaptation and therapeutic adaptation. Because the problem is not expected to last, the client is usually ready to accept temporary changes, and the dynamics of the situation are different. This chapter will deal with long-term or permanent adaptations which present far more challenges to both therapist and client.

LONG-TERM ADAPTATIONS

Long-term adaptations are required when a person has a chronic disability. These adaptations are frequently provided in the client's own home or workplace, and may relate to activities of daily living or to work or leisure activities. Adaptations can include changes to methods, pacing techniques, risk-reduction techniques, modification of tools and equipment and environmental changes.

Emphasis is often placed on making changes to the task or the environment. It is, how-ever, important to check first whether the individual's function may be improved by specific treatment.

Providing adaptations instead of therapy may sometimes appear to offer a rapid and practical solution. However, this is like a doctor treating the symptoms of a disorder rather than the cause. If the underlying problem can be treated, the need for other action may be removed or reduced, which may in the longer term be more cost effective.

Second, if there is no scope for therapy, it is important to consider whether the client can become more adaptive because by doing so the need for adaptations to tasks or environments may become unnecessary.

HELPING THE INDIVIDUAL TO ADAPT

Functional performance is a combination of knowledge, attitudes, values and skills which the individual learns and then assembles and uses to meet the demand of each task or situation. Individuals can adapt to a disability by making changes to what they know, to how they perceive situations or value aspects of their lives, by learning new skills, and by changing the ways in which these elements are organized and used. The need for adaptation varies with the nature and severity of the disability and the personal circumstances of the client.

It is a fundamental assumption of occupational therapy that all individuals have the potential to learn and develop, and therefore to change in an adaptive manner, and that it is the role of the therapist to assist in this process.

The degree to which individuals are capable of adapting is, however, variable. It is as if there is a kind of adaptive continuum, from being highly adaptive through to having miminal capacity for adaptation.

A person who is highly adaptive will take action to make the necessary changes (often without need for intervention from a therapist), and is open to suggestions about how to do so. A person who is not adaptive is unlikely to initiate change, and may well resist it.

This adaptive capacity is a complex entity. It is difficult to be sure how much it is innate, stemming from predispositions of the mind and personality, and how much it is a learned response.

Learning is certainly important. The input derived from the results of previous participation shapes future reactions. If participation is successful and satisfactory, it promotes further engagement; similarly, successful attempts at being adaptive promote further attempts. Conversely, unsuccessful attempts reduce motivation to try again.

It is possible for people to become fixed in maladaptive cycles which limit their capacity for change. If the therapist can intervene to change the cycle into a positive one, it may be a first step towards a more adaptive approach to life.

The capacity for adaptive change is adversely affected by depression and other affective disorders, and by cognitive dysfunction. It is also influenced by age, and by cultural and religious beliefs and values. Learning difficulties also reduce the ability to adapt.

It can be difficult to assess the extent of an individual's capacity for adaptive change, yet the degree to which this capacity is present affects the outcome of intervention.

Some indicators of adaptive and non-adaptive attitudes and behaviours are summarized in Box 31.1. While these may give a useful guide to the client's current adaptive state, the therapist must beware of making assumptions about how they may predict the future.

The therapist must also beware of adopting negative attitudes to people who appear to be 'hard to help'. Because therapists are usually highly adaptive themselves, and because they value adaptation, it is easy to fall into the trap of thinking 'adaptive change = good; failure to change = bad'.

People have the right to choose what to change and how to change it. They also have the right to choose not to change anything. Given the complex nature of change itself and of human reactions to it, we should not automatically assume that adaptive change is always the best solution. There are times when doing nothing is preferable.

What all clients require is sufficient information about their personal situation or condition and the available options and strategies so that they have a rational basis for their decisions. It is principally the way in which this material is presented that is affected by presence or absence of obvious adaptive potential.

Box 31.1 Indicators of adaptive potential	
Adaptive individual	*Unadaptive individual*
Has a pattern of lifelong learning and personal development	Does not show a pattern of personal development or learning
Has adapted to previous stressful changes	Has not adapted well to previous stressful changes
Has already taken some positive action in the current situation	Has taken no action in the current situation
Shows positive attitudes to suggestions or information	Shows generally negative attitudes to suggestions or information
Shows realistic appraisal of situation	Does not show realistic appraisal of the situation
Is moderately optimistic	Is either pessimistic or over-optimistic
Has previously had flexible routines and patterns of performance which have changed and evolved over time	Previous routines and patterns are rigid and inflexible and show little change over time
Has a moderate to good perception of self-efficacy	Has a poor perception of self-efficacy
Has an internal locus of control	Has an external locus of control
Shows problem-solving skills	Does not show problem-solving skills
Has no cognitive dysfunction or learning difficulty	Does have cognitive dysfunction or a learning difficulty

FACILITATING ADAPTIVE CHANGE

Because of the inextricable link between thoughts, feelings, attitudes, values and behaviours, a cognitive–behavioural approach is often effective in prompting adaptive change. If the client can accurately identify the features of a problem situation and their effects on thoughts, feelings and behaviours, then helpful attitudinal shifts may be made which promote problem-solving and positive action.

This approach is only possible with clients who do not have cognitive dysfunctions which impede learning or analytical thinking.

The therapist provides information and teaches techniques by which problems can be explored and solved. The therapist acts as a 'sounding board', enabling the client to explore all aspects of the situation in an impartial manner. The therapist should not seek to influence the client during this process because, apart from any ethical considerations, attitudinal changes require insight and a degree of cognitive restructuring which only the individual concerned can achieve.

LEARNING HOW TO NAME AND FRAME PROBLEM SITUATIONS

Although the symptoms of a functional problem may be apparent ('I can't go shopping'), the causes of the problem may be obscured by assumptions, attitudes and the way the problem is mentally defined and framed. Some of these assumptions may be based on lack of information, misconceptions, strong personal perceptions, ideas or emotions, reaction to past experiences, or habitual modes of thinking about the world.

If these strands can be identified and untangled, it may be possible to define the problem more accurately. One method of doing this is to get the client to do a SYT analysis (situation; you; task: see p. 213) which analyses the effects of task demand, environmental factors, other people, and personal abilities, thoughts and feelings on the problem situation.

LEARNING HOW TO RECOGNIZE NEGATIVE CYCLES

There are several common negative or maladaptive cycles which prevent adaptive change.

SELF-FULFILLING PROPHECY OF FAILURE

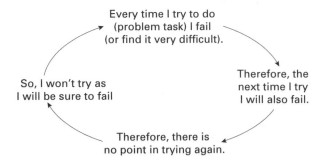

In this cycle, the individual begins to limit activities to within strict, self-imposed boundaries. The expectation of failure closes off the possibility of trying to find alternative ways of doing the task. If this attitude begins to extend across a range of activities, a spiral of decreasing participation is set up.

A similar construct is 'there's no way out':

There is no way out of this situation, and no-one can help.

So I'm not going to look for a way out or go to anyone for help.

These cognitive patterns are quite normal, in that most people experience them in a minor form at some point in their lives. Because of this they can be hard to detect, either by an observer or the person concerned. The associated thought-patterns become habitual and not fully articulated. In exaggerated form, they become very obvious to others, if not to the person involved.

ACTIVITY CYCLING

This term describes a pattern of performance in which the amount of activity varies widely over longer or shorter timeframes.

It typically occurs when a person has a chronic condition which restricts the energy available for task performance, or where symptoms are produced in response to activity which limit performance (e.g. chronic pain syndrome, chronic fatigue syndrome, multiple sclerosis, rheumatoid arthritis).

The individual allows task performance to be governed by how the individual feels; when the individual feels good, the individual pushes ahead to work hard to catch up with tasks, often getting tired or experiencing pain in the process. Once the work is completed, the individual 'collapses' for a period in order to recover. On recovery, the whole cycle starts again so that the pattern of performance is one of continually alternating peaks and troughs. The pattern can extend across a day, or a week, or over longer periods.

This 'push–push–push, now rest' pattern of performance is quite normal for some people. It works well if there is sufficient energy available to recover rapidly. It ceases to be so effective when capacity to recover is limited by a chronic condition or disability.

The problem is that, while in the short-term work does 'get done', in the longer term more time may be spent in recovering than in working. Another disadvantage is that priority is typically given to chores which are perceived as essential, and no energy is left for social or recreational activities. Consequently, life becomes a continual struggle to cope with relatively mundane tasks without experiencing any compensatory enjoyment.

In some conditions, the need to monitor physical sensations such as pain in order to know whether to start or stop work operates a neurophysiological mechanism which actually exacerbates the unpleasant sensations.

'I OUGHT TO BE ABLE TO… I MUST…'

People who engage in activity cycling may describe many of their tasks as 'things I must do' (or 'ought to do').

Most people have some 'musts and oughts' in their lives. These are things which they strongly feel they should do, usually for others, and often to a high standard. Typically, again, these are household chores and duties, the processes of which are not actually enjoyed although the end result may be valued.

If not done, or not done to the desired standard, the individual feels guilty, anxious or frustrated. These feelings and the negative thoughts which may accompany them set up a cycle of physical stress.

The problem with 'musts and oughts' is that they may induce the individual to place emphasis on things which have the superficial appearance of importance but actually are not that essential when compared to other aspects of life. The negative emotions aroused by failure may impede problem-solving and can also interfere with enjoyment of other aspects.

Clearly, some tasks really are 'musts' but it is worth challenging the validity of the designation, and attempting to balance these tasks with others which have a wider personal meaning.

HELPING THE INDIVIDUAL TO LEARN ADAPTIVE TECHNIQUES AND COPING STRATEGIES

The antidote to most of these patterns is first to recognize that they exist, to attempt to challenge any habitual negative thoughts, feelings or behaviours and to replace them with more positive and adaptive ones. A combination of planning, prioritizing and pacing and other coping strategies can be used to ensure that a balanced repertoire of activities is carried out in an effective manner which suits the individual.

LEARNING HOW TO PLAN AND PRIORITIZE
Setting priorities

It can be difficult to identify what is truly important in a person's life. It is important that the identification is done by the client, and not by the therapist who may impose personal preferences and standards on the individual.

For example, a disabled mother wants to cook, wash, shop, clean the house and look after the children. However, she also wants to play with her children, find time for her husband, meet her friends, and perhaps have a job or a personal interest. Which of these items is most important? This is an impossible question. Each of those involved in this situation is likely to have a different perspective. The client is likely to feel that she wants to (or should) do all these things. Plainly self-care is essential, and children do have to be looked after.

A better question may be 'Which of these things could someone else do for you?'. It is likely that someone could do some of the household chores, even take over some aspects of child care. But no-one else can experience playing with her children or being with her husband on her behalf.

Working through a simple flowchart (Box 31.2) can help to set priorities and leads into planning and problem-solving.

LEARNING HOW TO IDENTIFY AND SOLVE PROBLEMS

Some clients are already good problem-solvers, but sometimes an individual has not mastered the analytical thinking required or 'can't see the wood for the trees' and needs assistance to work through this. The following seven-point plan enables therapist and client to jointly work through the problem and arrive at a solution.

Setting priorities can be difficult. If there are many problems, it can be more effective to whittle them down by starting with the easy ones first, even if these are not the most important. By removing small problems, the client gains positive experience of problem-solving and being adaptive, and the remaining 'big problems' may then appear less daunting.

This approach to problem-solving fits well with client-based assessments of need such as the Canadian Occupational Performance Measure.

Box 31.2 Setting priorities

Does the task **have** to be done? → No → Forget it

↓

Yes

↓

Do I enjoy doing it? ——————→ No

↓ ↓

Yes ←———————— Does it have to be done by me?

↓ ↓

↓ No

How often? How well? ↓

↓ ↓

Can it be made easier? How? Delegate it

A SEVEN-POINT PLAN FOR PROBLEM-SOLVING

Stage one – What is the problem?
- What are the client's priorities? What does the client most want or need to do?
- List the top few goals (not more than five) in priority order.
- If appropriate, spend some time exploring priorities and challenging 'musts and oughts'.

Stage two – Where is the problem?
- Select one or two problems to work on. Decide whether the problem originates in the abilities or reactions of the client, or in the task demand, or the physical or social environment (or a combination of these).
- If in the task, is this due to method, tools or intrinsic demand? Can particular difficulties be located? (Use 'traffic light analysis' p. 214) Could changing these avoid the need for a physical adaptation?
- If in the environment, what aspects contribute to the problem? Consider physical environment, social or cultural aspects and other people. Could small changes remove the need for a larger one?
- If with the client, does the difficulty stem from lack of physical ability, attitudinal problems, or the way the client has thought about (named and framed) the problem? Is it likely that therapy or education might remove any of these problems, thus removing or reducing the need for adaptation?

Stage three – Brainstorming
- Select one problem and get the client to brainstorm all possible solutions. Include all ideas, even 'silly' or impractical ones, as these can make the exercise less sober and sometimes lead to other good ideas. The therapist can add ideas which the client may not think of or be aware of.

- Consider all the ideas and make a shortlist of those which seem acceptable or practical.

Stage four – Is the solution practical and acceptable?

- How does the client view potential solutions? What are the views of others affected by the proposals?
- What are the implications of any options, e.g. in terms of cost, permissions, disruption to lifestyle, disruption to home environment, effects on other users?
- Is the gain worth the effort and/or cost?

Stage five – Negotiate an agreed solution

- Discuss all aspects with the client. Agree what can (and cannot) be done.
- Record all agreements.

Stage six – Action plan

- The client makes a personal action plan, or therapist and client jointly work out a plan.

Stage seven – Monitor progress and review results

- It may be necessary to set some criteria by which the success of the outcome can be measured.

RETRAINING IN COMPENSATORY TECHNIQUES

Learning new methods

If an individual has lost previous abilities, a period of readjustment is needed, together with training and practice in new methods and compensatory techniques. For example, the physically disabled client may need to learn to use a prosthesis, to become independently mobile in a wheelchair, to cope with tasks one-handed, or to walk with a guide dog.

Learning to adapt to a disability takes time. It may be necessary to provide more assistance or extra adaptations while this process is continuing.

Learning joint protection techniques

Joint protection techniques are taught to clients with rheumatoid diseases with a view to reduc-ing strain on affected joints. These techniques can be combined with pacing and energy conservation and provision of small items of equipment (see Hammond 1996).

Learning how to recognize and reduce risks

Disabilities can increase risk of accidents. Risk-reduction techniques focus on teaching the individual, or a carer, to recognize potential hazards and take action to remove or reduce them, or to reduce risky behaviours. Specific medical conditions may bring specific risks.

For example, an elderly person with osteoporosis who is prone to fall may be taught to recognize slip and trip hazards (avoiding or removing them), and to avoid certain risky activities such as climbing on a chair to change a light bulb. A diabetic needs to recognize the warning signs of impending hypoglycaemia.

Learning how to plan and pace

Pacing is a technique which involves spreading the amount of effort expended evenly over a period of time. Pacing is designed to avoid fatigue and adverse effects of meeting task demand while still achieving a steady flow of work.

In its simplest form, it involves the client in making a programme or plan of what has to be done and breaking the activities up into manageable 'packets' which are well within the capacity of the individual. These packets are interspersed with planned rests or with different types of tasks. At the same time, care is taken to ensure that a variety of activities, self-care, work, social or recreational, are included so that some meaningful personal balance is maintained.

In a more complex form, pacing becomes a way of life. The principle is similar to that of proportional grading. The client decides how much of a particular task or type of movement can usually be managed, and then plans to do an amount which is somewhat less than this.

This may require the client to formulate *baselines* for certain aspects of performance.

For example, the client may decide that 10 minutes is usually long enough for standing, and then sets a limit for standing at 8 minutes. Then, whatever the client is doing, the client will always rest or change position after 8 minutes of standing. (In some situations the client may also need to avoid sitting down *before* the set time is up.)

Activity is governed by predetermined criteria such as time, a task stage or a distance walked.

By working well within capacity and including rests and changes of task and position, effort can be sustained over a longer period. Specific techniques such as relaxation or simple exercises or stretches can be included in the plan. By sticking to the plan, attention is focused away from unpleasant symptoms which inhibits the physiological mechanisms that promote awareness of them. The problems caused by the peaks and troughs of activity cycling are removed.

This technique takes time to acquire and requires a degree of self-discipline and organization which some clients cannot master, but it can be very effective. It may be combined with adaptations to tools or the environment to further enhance performance.

ADAPTATIONS TO TASK CONTENT AND DEMAND

As already noted, it is useful to identify with precision the point or points at which problems arise before doing anything else. If the problem does seem to lie with the nature of the task demand, a secondary analysis can help to pin this down further (see 'traffic light analysis' p. 214).

The problem-solving sequence can then be followed to identify an adaptive solution. This might involve delegating parts of the task, learning a new method, changing the tools or equipment or some aspect of the environment, using pacing or some other coping strategy, or any combination of these.

ADAPTATIONS TO TOOLS, EQUIPMENT OR FURNITURE

Adaptations to tools and environments are of two kinds. Minor adaptations include provision of small items of special equipment, adaptations to existing items, or small alterations to the home such as grab rails.

Major adaptations involve building work to alter a home or provision of large and expensive items of equipment. Major adaptations are primarily environmental, so they will be described in Section 5.

TO ADAPT OR NOT TO ADAPT?

There is a temptation on the part of both novice therapists and some clients to view home adaptation as the 'easy answer' to most problems.

Although adaptations can transform lives when correctly used, they are not always appropriate and the therapist needs to take time to work with the client to evaluate whether or not adaptation is the best solution, and if so, what should be adapted.

The problem-based checklist given earlier may assist in this decision-taking process.

It is essential to spend time going round the home with the client to listen to the client's descriptions of problems and to watch the client performing problem tasks.

SOURCES OF ADAPTIVE EQUIPMENT

The manufacture and design of adaptive equipment is now a large and profitable industry. The continual production of new items and 'gadgets' challenges the therapist to keep up to date. It can be difficult to find time to evaluate all the available equipment. In the UK, there are many sources of information such as regularly updated information lists or databases, demonstration centres, charities, trade fairs, catalogues and publications.

There is still scope for the innovative and adaptive 'do it yourself' approach, or for design and production of 'one-off' items, with the assistance of professional designers or an organization such as REMAP.

MINOR ADAPTATIONS

Typical adaptations are summarized in this section. More detailed information about home adaptations is given in Section 5.

Altering the position of objects and furniture

A good starting point is to look at where things are kept or placed and to decide if these positions are optimum. Equipment and furniture need to be positioned where there is good access and where they promote and enhance use. Some individuals do take a practical view of such considerations and spend time working out the best position for items to be kept or used. In many homes, however, items get positioned almost by chance and once a position is established, the user does not think to question it. At other times, position may be dictated by aesthetic considerations rather than function, or by poor architectural design.

The therapist has the advantage of seeing a room with fresh eyes, and may quickly identify problems such as clutter, hazards, lack of space, unhelpful relationships between objects, poor access and awkward storage.

Modification of existing tools or equipment

Small changes can make a great deal of difference, for example, changing the shape of a handle, adding extra grips or handles, extending the length of a handle or fixing tools down to enable use (see Ch. 30).

Advising on new tools, equipment or furniture

A list of recommendations might include, for example, acquiring items which are powered instead of manually operated, lighter versions of tools or appliances or furniture of more suitable height or shape.

Provision of small aids to daily living

To help the activities of daily living, aids to mobility, reaching, carrying, dressing, washing, toileting, bathing, eating, cooking and housework could be provided.

Provision of minor home adaptations

These include fitting items such as grab rails, providing small ramps, alterations to thresholds, installing alarm systems, making minor changes to controls on appliances or electric switches, rehanging doors, and many other small changes to existing fittings or structures.

Environmental analysis and adaptation

32

Introduction to environmental analysis and adaptation

ENVIRONMENTAL ANALYSIS AND ADAPTATION

Occupations can be analysed and adapted to provide therapy or enhance function; so can environments. A combination of occupational and environmental analysis provides an understanding of performance demand.

It will have become apparent after reading Sections 3 and 4 that it is impossible to disentangle consideration of the environment from analysis or adaptation of task performance or the abilities and patterns of performance of the user. In practice, the participant, the task and the environment must be considered at the same time. These interactions have been described in this book, and are also explained in other recent occupational therapy texts. Dunn et al (1998) provide a useful summary under the heading of 'the ecology of human performance'. The processes are only presented separately in this text as an aid to understanding the different techniques and emphasis required for each.

COMPONENTS OF THE ENVIRONMENT

Occupational therapy theorists during the 1980s such as Reed (1984) and Mosey (1986) have described the environment as being composed of physical (natural and human constructs) and sociocultural elements (people and social and cultural rules, expectations and symbols). These are sometimes referred to as non-human and human environments; however, the physical, 'non-human' environment contains much that is due to human intervention. The different forms of environment may be referred to as 'environmental contexts' defined by Spencer (1998) as 'the location of occupational performance in space'.

In the American Association of Occupational Therapists' Uniform Terminology (1994), the following definitions are used:

Physical environment: non-human aspects of contexts: includes the accessibility to and performance within environments having natural terrain, plants, animals, buildings, furniture, objects tools or devices.

Social environment: availability and expectations of significant individuals such as spouse, friends, and caregivers. Also includes larger social groups which are influential in establishing norms, role expectations and social routines.

Cultural environment: customs, beliefs, activity patterns, behaviour standards and expectations accepted by the society of which the individual is a member. Includes political aspects such as laws that affect access to resources and affirm personal rights. Also includes opportunities for education, employment and economic support.

PHYSICAL ENVIRONMENT

The physical environment contains tangible, observable objects. Objects may be either inanimate (physical; non-human) such as natural features or man-made constructs or organic (non-human), including living things such as plants or animals. Inanimate and organic objects have physical properties and characteristics which may be fixed or subject to change.

Physical properties include shape, size, colour, texture and temperature. The object may make noises or emit scents. It may have kinetic properties – it may move or vibrate.

Inanimate objects

Inanimate objects include:

Tools and equipment	These are used to perform tasks. Most tools are powered by human effort but some small electric machines are called 'power tools'.
Machines	A machine has a power source which is other than human. Machines include electrical household appliances, office machines, modes of transport and factory machinery.
Artifacts	Anything which is man-made. An artifact may be utilitarian, decorative or symbolic.
Furniture	Items made for human use in and around the home or other building.
Furnishings	These are the soft, decorative items such as cushions, curtains and hangings used in the home or other indoor areas.
Decorations	Items which have only an ornamental purpose.
Signs	Signs convey information of some kind.
Constructs	These are built or assembled; for example, houses, roads, bridges and dams.

Inanimate objects may be classified as functional, non-functional or hazardous; ornamental or symbolic.

Functional objects are useful, practical items. The object has a utilitarian purpose, it is used *for* something. For example, a cup, a book, a knob, a hook, a knife and a vegetable are all useful.

Non-functional objects have neither practical use nor ornamental or symbolic value. They include discarded materials and rubbish; clutter; objects which are in the wrong place; objects which have ceased to work.

Hazardous objects present risks to the user or people near them. The risk may be intrinsic, such as toxicity, heavy weight or sharp edges, or circumstantial owing to injudicious positioning, proximity or careless use.

Ornamental objects: some objects are purely ornamental, such as sculpture, paintings, interior decorations, garden flowers or personal jewellery. *Ornamental* features are those which enhance the appearance of an object without having utilitarian value. Ornament may include colour, pattern, textures, form, and use of precious or costly materials.

Symbolic objects are those which have a meaning other than that derived from its appearance or use. Some symbols are widely understood but others come from personal experience or memory. The rose may be, according to context, a commodity to be sold, an aesthetic object in a garden or room, a token of love, a wedding buttonhole or the logo of a political party.

Religious and cultural aspects of objects can change them from being mundane to being significant to the individual. They may form a group which means more than when the objects are separated.

Organic objects

Organisms are other living creatures, both plants and animals.

SOCIAL ENVIRONMENT

The social environment contains:

People who contribute to the environment by means of behaviours. Other people and the things which they do or say have a profound impact on our perceptions of the environment.

Social cues which originate in learned understandings of what kind of social behaviour is expected in a specific physical environment and the implicit or explicit *roles* and *rules* which govern behaviour within it.

CULTURAL ENVIRONMENT

The cultural environment is often complex and hard to define because it originates from a combination of concepts, expected behaviours and valued symbols which influence the actions of a group of people.

It may be possible to observe externalized aspects of culture in the physical environment such as clothing, decorative features, art, religious objects or food.

Behaviours such as rituals, customs and performances may be typical of the culture.

It is, however, much less easy to understand the importance of beliefs, taboos, attitudes and values, or the way in which a particular culture views its members in relation to the rest of the world. Culture also encompasses political structures and beliefs.

Unless one is a member of a culture, one is by definition excluded from it as an outsider. Therapists are more aware than they used to be of the necessity to understand the culture of the client, especially when the client belongs to a minority group. However, there is also a need to be sensitive to less obvious subcultures such as regional groups, particular socio-economic groups or age-related cultures.

ENVIRONMENTAL DEMAND

In the 1990s, influenced by open systems and ecological theories, descriptions of the contents of the environment and the effects of these on occupational performance have been elaborated. These theories stress the interactive or 'transactional' (Law et al 1995) nature of environmental components with the behaviours of organisms which live within it. The emphasis has moved from description of the *content* to analysis of the *effects* of the content and the information it provides for the user. These effects are referred to as environmental press or demand.

Social models of disability have also served to stress the effects of the environment in reducing or increasing the effects of dysfunction.

Kielhofner and Barris were among the first theorists to work on the ecological systems model in relation to human occupation, showing how behaviour affects and alters the environment, and how these changes are perceived by the individual, which in turn changes behaviour in a continual cycle of input, throughput and output.

My personal model of the mirror-image, external and internal environments shows how occupations act as the bridge between the wants and needs of our 'inner selves' and the external world. If we change what is done and aspects of the environment in which it is done, we cannot help but change something within ourselves to a greater or lesser extent.

Kielhofner (1995) gives a very clear account of the content of the environment and its influence on occupation. He argues that 'the characteristics of the environment *afford* a range of opportunities for occupational behaviour because they represent specific potentials for action'. He also states that the content of the environment *presses*: 'strongly recruits or requires particular behaviours'.

Nelson (1988) has described *occupational form*: 'an objective set of circumstances independent of and external to the person'. Form is a complex concept, including the materials, physical context and content of task performance and the subjective elements such as social or cultural context and expectations and personal values and standards.

Recent discussions of the environment in relation to occupational therapy explore and summarize these ideas (see Corcoran & Gitlin 1997, Fougerollas 1997, Spencer 1998).

All these theories combine to emphasize the crucial importance of the environment in the person–environment–occupation transaction. Competent performance decreases in a hostile, stressful, deprived or inappropriate environment.

OBJECTIVE AND SUBJECTIVE COMPONENTS OF DEMAND

In order to understand the nature of environmental demand on the individual, the therapist must take account of both *objective components* (directly observable physical, social or cultural content) and *subjective components* (how the individual perceives, understands and reacts to the content of the environment, and the social cultural or symbolic aspects of it). Together these combine to afford opportunities and affect the nature of performance.

Although the objective physical and social components can be described with relative ease, given practice, it is much harder to take account of the subjective components. These must be inferred from observation of reactions and behaviours, or elicited from the individual by careful and patient questioning.

ENVIRONMENTAL LEVELS

In Chapter 6, a description of *environmental levels* arranged in relation to the proximity to the user is given.

Of particular interest to the therapist using the COPE taxonomy is the *resource area*, which comprises the *immediate environment, near environment and used environment*.

NESTING OF LEVELS

Environmental levels nest inside each other like a Russian doll, so that the largest level contains all the rest. A comprehensive environmental analysis would have to consider so many components that it would quickly amass far too much material. When analysing the content or demand of an environment, the therapist has to place an artificial boundary on the area to be examined, considering only the factors which are relevant to the user within the defined limit. An example of considerations at each level is given in Table 32.1.

TECHNIQUES OF ENVIRONMENTAL ANALYSIS

ANALYSIS OF THE IMMEDIATE ENVIRONMENT: MICROANALYSIS

This is concerned with things which are within arms' reach of the user. Typically, in the context of task performance, this will include items arranged on a table or working surface, including tools, utensils and materials.

These items provide resources for task performance and information about what is to be done and the effects of action. Items need to be visible and accessible if they are to be used.

At the developmental level, small adjustments to layout and content of the immediate environment can have a disproportionate effect on demand and therefore on the success or failure of the user.

As one is working in such small spaces in the immediate environment, content, demand and adaptation can be considered at the same time.

ANALYSIS OF THE NEAR ENVIRONMENT

The near environment is a portion of the working space currently occupied by the user. It includes both the items which are within reach

Table 32.1 Objective components of the environment: examples of content at different environmental levels

Level of environment	Constructs	Objects and artifacts	Organisms and natural features	Physical resources
Immediate	Floor/ground Wall Door Window Surface	Tool Furniture Material Small machine Utilitarian object Small aesthetic object Small ornament Book Disc or CD Clothing	Small animal Small plant Human	Power point Switch Tap
Near	Room Storage cupboards Shelving	Large tool, equipment or machine Decorations Furnishings Lights Large ornaments	Large animal Large plant Human	Source of heat Source of light Source of water Drain
Used	House Garden Street Shop Library Park Road Bridge Field	Means of transport Signs Sculpture Recreational objects/ equipment	Landscape Trees Natural features People	Public utilities

and the items which are easily accessible, by changing position or walking a few paces.

The near environment has physical content, the objects, organisms and people which are within it, and also symbolic and situational content which is produced by the totality of content and its meanings to the individual. *Content analysis* explores both the physical and situational content. The combined effect of these produces environmental demand. The nature of this is summarized using *demand analysis*.

If the environment is in a therapeutic setting, it may be necessary to change it in some way and this requires *adaptive analysis*; in order to relate the need for adaptation to individual needs *applied analysis* is used.

ANALYSIS OF THE USED ENVIRONMENT

The used environment contains all the resources routinely available to the client. This might include a dwelling, its surroundings and access to local goods and services.

Content analysis needs to be undertaken at the effective level, considering the user's overall pattern of daily or weekly activities. This may be described as *mesoanalysis* to distinguish it from other forms of environmental analysis.

The way in which the user performs in and interacts with an environment is evaluated by means of a *functional assessment* (see Chs. 20 and 21).

MACROANALYSIS

This is a research tool for therapists, sociologists, environmental psychologists, human ecologists and others. It involves an analysis of the ways in which the totality of the environment – physical, geographical, organic, social and political – interacts to affect human life and occupations. Methods for undertaking this kind of complex review are influenced by philosophical theories about the nature of reality and our perceptions of it and techniques of analysis are still being evolved.

ADAPTATIONS TO THE ENVIRONMENT

The environment can be adapted to enhance performance by five basic techniques:

- by *removing* something
- by *adding* something
- by *altering* something
- by *positioning* something
- by *enhancing* something.

Although the actual techniques used to adapt demand may be relatively simple, judging what, or how much to adapt, and what the effect may be on the user is a different matter. This requires good clinical reasoning and judgement.

Environments may be adapted in order to provide therapy or to improve function.

APPROACHES TO ANALYSIS AND ADAPTATION

As with other processes, a frame of reference may be selected in order to focus or limit analysis. The relevant approaches have already been described in Chapter 23.

FOUNDATION SKILLS

The foundation skills for environmental analysis and adaptation are:

- observation
- measurement
- recording
- drawing simple plans.

33

Analysis of the environment

ANALYSIS OF THE IMMEDIATE ENVIRONMENT

MICROANALYSIS

Microanalysis, as the name implies, is concerned with minute examination of the environmental components within arms' reach of the user which contribute to or detract from task performance.

Once the environment has been analysed, modifications can be made, if required, in order to improve task performance or to enhance awareness of surroundings.

COMPONENTS OF MICROANALYSIS

Microanalysis involves analysis of the '5 Cs':

- content
- convenience
- comfort
- cues
- communication.

Content

The immediate physical surroundings of an individual consist of two- or three-dimensional objects and supporting surfaces or constructs – table, worktop, seat, bed, wall, ceiling and ground. It also includes materials and other resources required for task performance.

Convenience

Objects occupy space and usually have physical relationships to each other as arranged on a surface, and to the individual.

They are nearer or further away from each other. They have functional relationships. The physical arrangement of objects required for a task and the ease of access to them are important.

One of the key areas of the work of an ergonomist is design of workstations and the layout of tools and materials in a manner which facilitates use.

Lack of convenience increases fatigue, makes a task take longer and may promote stress.

Comfort

Physical comfort

Physical comfort is an attribute of the immediate environment in relation to the tasks and positions of the user. Objects need to contribute to comfort to promote competent performance. Lack of comfort makes the task stressful, fatiguing and limits the optimum length of engagement.

The human body operates best when homeostasis is readily maintained, so extremes of heat, cold, noise, wetness or any unpleasant sensation affects performance and may pose a threat. If the source of some highly unpleasant sensation is in the immediate vicinity, the person is likely to want to move away fast.

Psychological comfort

Personal perceptions of safety vary widely but a feeling of safety and security normally contributes to a sense of well-being and effective performance. Within the immediate environment, psychological comfort is closely linked to physical comfort. Familiarity also tends to contribute towards psychological comfort; surroundings, tasks and contexts which are unfamiliar may be experienced as threats. There are, of course, exceptions where a sense of risk is experienced as pleasurable, but this is usually a somewhat artificial, well-managed and limited form of risk, for example, a seat on a 'white knuckle ride' at a theme park.

Cues

Cues to expected behaviour within the immediate environment come from the combined effects of the information content of objects, surfaces and people.

The objects and surfaces in the immediate environment give the person cues about the nature of the environment and what the person is expected to do in it. Sitting at a table in front of a place-setting and a plate of food cue eating. Standing by a set of brushes, paints and paper suggests engagement in art. A till and a moving belt containing items of shopping cue pricing and exchanging money. Sitting on grass suggests gardening or a picnic.

Adults are usually adept at sorting out the correct cues to performance; they have learned how to do this. But cues may be ambiguous, or give too little or too much information.

If there is damage to perception or information-processing, the objects may fail to cue behaviour, cue inappropriate behaviour or result in unproductive 'fiddling'.

A person with a sensory deficit such as blindness needs special cues in the person's immediate environment to compensate for the deficit. Patients suffering from dementia or brain damage may need an environment in which a limited number of objects are carefully placed to give precise cues to behaviour (see Corcoran & Gitlin 1997).

Social cues are especially important for the reasons described above. Humans need to communicate clearly. This depends on both verbal and non-verbal communication. If the individual cannot properly see or hear the person who is trying to communicate, the individual cannot sort out the cues to the expected social behaviours. Consequently the individual may misunderstand, feel threatened or produce an inappropriate response.

Environmental cues also provide information about potential hazards which may be outside the immediate area, for example, smells, sounds, sense of heat, warning signals.

Communication

Other people in the immediate environment of an individual – within arms' reach – are within a highly sensitive zone of proximity.

Touch is one of the first means of communication which humans experience, and it remains deeply significant throughout life. Only a person who is well-known to the individual and liked by the individual is likely to be welcomed readily within this close personal space or be permitted to touch without asking.

A stranger who invades personal space without invitation is usually perceived as a threat. Anyone who has been unwillingly jammed into close proximity with strangers in a crowd will know the uncomfortable feeling this engenders.

Most cultures have a strict code of expected behaviours to make close approaches to another person safe and comfortable. There are explicit or unstated rules about 'safe' distances and 'safe'

forms of touching or communicating. Certain people – medical practitioners, priests – may have 'cultural exemption' to cross the permitted boundaries in special contexts. Westerners will readily remove their clothes for a medical examination by a doctor in a hospital or surgery, but not at a formal, social occasion.

TECHNIQUES OF MICROANALYSIS
Content analysis

Using the '5 C' headings as a structure for observation and description, the therapist can give an account of a circumscribed environment (Box 33.1. Analysis should be strictly limited to what is within reach. This may be with or without the user. If the user is present, it is possible to gain more information about comfort and convenience. The therapist may be involved personally as a participant to gain direct experience of the environment.

Box 33.1   Example of microanalysis: word-processor workstation

Content
Physical objects – utilitarian
Furniture
- computer desk
- movable support shelf
- typist's swivel chair
- wooden footrest

Fittings
- small shelf on wall

Tools
- word-processor screen
- keyboard and printer
- pens, various

Artifacts
- clock
- toast rack (used to store disks)
- pen holder
- book on worktop
- books in shelves behind user (in reach if chair is swivelled)
- journal

Materials
- used disks
- paper
- computer disks in box
- boxes of printer ink cartridges (packaging decorated)

Resources
Light
- from window and spot bar (not in reach)
- angle lamp

Heat
- adequate: radiator (not in reach)

Power
- two double power sockets above worktop

Convenience
- generally good

Comfort
- adequate
- potential hazard from overuse of word-processor and VDU

Cues
- work environment

Communication
- phone out of reach

Note Listing content without a visual representation of it does not provide sufficient information for therapeutic analysis.

It may help to make a diagram showing the position of objects, or to take a photograph or video recording.

As with all analysis, the key is accurate observation and clear description. This takes practice. Ideally, your description should be so clear that, given the objects you have described, someone else could use your description to reconstruct the environment.

Demand analysis

When a user is working within the confines of an immediate environment, most of the demand comes from the intrinsic task requirements and this needs to be analysed.

The immediate environment may contain some cues to the nature of the setting and the expectations for behaviour within it. For example, objects may suggest work, a self-care task or a leisure activity. People in close proximity may suggest intimacy or risk.

Environmental demand is usually more apparent in the near or used environments because the cues provided are more abundant.

ANALYSIS OF THE NEAR ENVIRONMENT

OBJECTIVE ANALYSIS

Analysis of the near environment is similar in general structure and approach to content analysis of the immediate environment but the area of observation is extended. This may include the whole of a small room, or a defined area within which the user is moving.

The '5 C' headings can be used, but the content of each section is expanded (Box 33.2).

SUBJECTIVE ANALYSIS

Subjective analysis is concerned with the way in which content influences how an individual perceives and understands an environment and how the individual feels about it. The purpose of this analysis is to attempt to link reactions to the content of the environment. It is not, therefore, sufficient to discover how a person feels, but to try to track back to *what* it is in the environment which prompts this reaction.

Box 33.2   Headings for objective analysis of the near environment

Content
Inanimate objects
Functional objects
e.g. tools, utensils and equipment, machines and appliances, receptacles and containers, furniture, utilitarian furnishings, clothing, signs, means of transport materials

Non-functional objects
e.g. discards and rubbish, misplaced objects, items not needed for task, broken items

Hazardous objects
e.g. toxic materials, fire or source of extreme heat, source of extreme cold, slip or trip hazards, sharps, objects of extreme weight, unstable objects

Decorative objects
e.g. pictures or photos, ornaments, artworks or sculptures, flowers or flowering plants, hangings, soft furnishings, decorative finishes, non-utiltarian clothing, jewellery

Symbolic objects
e.g. religious objects, cultural artifacts, memorabilia

Constructs
e.g. parts of a building, shelving or storage, fitted worktop, curtilage of building, amenity landscape, roads, pavements

Organic objects
e.g. plants, pets, domesticated animals, pests, humans

Convenience and comfort
e.g. layout or position, access to objects or resources, need to move to obtain objects or resources, suitability of furniture, risks or hazards

Cues
e.g. relationships between object, information, social or cultural meaning

Communication
e.g. proximity of others, communication technology, information content

Areas to be explored may include:

- feelings about features of the environment: positive/negative/neutral
- perceptions of safety/risk
- personal meanings associated with content
- perceptions of role within the environment
- desire to interact with or withdraw from the environment
- symbolic material.

DEMAND ANALYSIS

The content of the environment demands a response. The response may be a simple action, reaction or interaction. It may be in the form of task performance or it may be a cognitive or emotional recognition of meaning.

Physical demand

A demand for a physical response comes mainly from physical content. Steps need to be climbed; uneven surfaces have to be negotiated with care; a shelf must be reached by stretching or using a step ladder. The presence of tools may demand that they are used in some way.

Cognitive demand

Information content

The amount of cognitive processing required by an environment is directly related to the richness and degree of organization of its content and the speed with which this changes. A bland, static environment with little content requires little cognitive evaluation. An environment which is full of changing information needs constant and rapid appraisal and appropriate reactions.

If this content is well-presented, for example, in displays on an instrument panel, the user can react to it with relative ease. If it is disorganized, the user may feel overwhelmed and be unable to process the amount of information.

The therapist needs to identify the sources and types of information being presented in order to decide if this should be changed in any way.

Stressors and distractors

Items in the environment which distract attention or increase stress levels tend to decrease competence. These may be an integral part of some environments, for example, in some factories or offices. The cause may be temporary – a pneumatic drill being used on the road outside; although the drill is not within the near environment, the noise of it is.

Quite often, however, the distractors are unintentional and stem from faults in design or placement of objects. Users often become habituated to permanent distractors and learn to filter these out of their awareness; someone new to the same environment, however, may notice these things and find them intrusive or disturbing. Occupational therapy departments are often full of equipment and objects which the therapist is familiar with and no longer perceives as strange, but these objects may be perceived by the new user as unfamiliar, distracting or even threatening.

Signals of risk

These are items in the environment which act as signals to the user to take care or avoiding action.

Occupational demand

Humans tend to construct their environments for a purpose. The purpose is conveyed by a combination of design, content and learned meanings. At home, specific environments are constructed for sleeping, eating, cooking, toiletting and relaxing. Entering part of a church or temple suggests prayer and worship; sitting down in a theatre suggests watching a play. The user learns to respond with the appropriate occupational behaviour in each area.

It is therefore important for the therapist to understand how this type of demand is generated so that it can be re-created or simulated when engaging the client in therapeutic activities.

Social or cultural demand

This type of demand presses the user to conform to a set of social or cultural behaviours. We should be quiet in church or in a library but we may shout and jump up and down when watching a football match. The information may come from the occupational demand of the environment but it also stems from observation of the appearance and actions of other users.

AMBIENCE

Creation of 'ambience' or 'atmosphere' is the task of interior designers and architects. The very smart hotel foyer is deliberately designed to impress and to suggest exclusivity, opulence and luxury. The fast food restaurant is designed to make people move faster and eat more quickly; it emphasizes the recreational aspects of food consumption and low cost in a way that attracts young people. It is instructive to the therapist to observe how the designer achieves these effects by use of colour, materials, cultural images and social cues, and to analyse how people adapt their behaviour in response to these cues.

This form of demand is a combination of factors in the immediate, near and used environments and is also considered at a higher level where the total impact of surroundings can be appreciated.

HEADINGS FOR DEMAND ANALYSIS

Physical demand   List all features which require the user to produce an action.

Cognitive demand   Information content.
Stressors and distractors.
Signals of risk.

Social or cultural demand   Features which have social or cultural meaning.
Design features, décor and ambience.
Appearance and behaviour of other users.

ANALYSIS OF THE USED ENVIRONMENT

The used environment includes the whole of a home and its curtilage (the adjacent outside areas) together with the area outside of the home which an individual uses to obtain resources, to work, or to engage in social, cultural, spiritual or leisure occupations.

MAPPING THE USED ENVIRONMENT

Understanding the constituents of the used environment may help therapist and client to appreciate patterns of engagement. A restricted resource area may indicate dysfunction, social isolation or poverty. This type of analysis can also serve to indicate the barriers to use.

Various techniques can be used to make a 'map'. A list of shops, services, friends' homes or recreational resources could be made. It can be difficult for clients to remember these, and it may be better to draw out a simple map of the area or to use a real map and ask the client to point out the places the client uses.

The 'spidergram' can also be used. Taking a large sheet of paper, the client's home is represented by a circle in the middle, and the client then draws out lines to various places used. The mode of transport can be indicated. It may be necessary to ask about places which used to be visited and to explore reasons why they are not used any more.

BARRIERS TO USE: ACCESS AND ATTITUDES

PROBLEMS WITH ACCESS

There can be little doubt that environmental barriers to access by disabled people create a major part of the handicapping effect of a disability.

The barrier may be in the form of inaccessible transport, architectural barriers, poor design features, or lack of provision of information in a form which the disabled person can access.

Recent UK legislation places a duty on the owners of all buildings used by the public to make them accessible to disabled people.

However, more subtle barriers exist in the form of attitudes of the disabled person or others, expectations about the needs and wishes of disabled people, cost, political priorities, and a host of other factors which may require consideration.

The therapist works with disabled clients to identify and overcome barriers. Having identified aspects which are causing a problem, it is usually necessary to follow this up by a visit to the area, preferably with the client, so that specific problems can be noted and potential solutions explored.

Solutions may involve adaptation of the environment, remembering that in this context adaptations to the knowledge, values, attitudes and skills of others comprise part of the environment which have just as much impact on performance as physical content. The solution may equally lie in an adaptation to the task or to the user's behaviour.

34

Therapeutic adaptation and management of the environment

ADAPTING THE ENVIRONMENT IN THE CONTEXT OF THERAPY

The therapeutic environment consists of locations, objects and people. It includes tools and materials. It operates at several levels, from the layout and content of the immediate or near environment, to the demand created by the general therapeutic milieu.

Therapeutic adaptation is related to the needs of an individual or, sometimes, a group. The aim is to provide treatment or enhance performance. Environmental adaptations often involve changes to the physical environment which are obvious and practical. More subtle changes to social and cultural aspects of the situation may also be made. The therapist may also need to exploit existing aspects of an environment in order to maximize therapeutic opportunities, without making actual alterations.

Management of the environment includes deliberate use of the totality of its content and resources in a therapeutic context.

As therapists use many different enviroments and situations, this makes it difficult to describe environmental adaptations in detail. In this chapter, some examples will be used to demonstrate basic principles which can be generally applied.

TECHNIQUES OF ENVIRONMENTAL ADAPTATION

The techniques of environmental adaptation are based on:

Removing	Taking away distracting or unwanted content.
Adding	Bringing additional material, objects or information into the environment.
Altering	Changing the shape or design of objects or structures.
Positioning	Looking at objects in relation to each other or the user.
Enhancing	Improving aspects of the environment and focusing the attention of the user on them.

In the immediate and near environments, these techniques will usually be employed in relation to an approach which emphasizes a specific aspect, for example:

Approach	Aspect which is emphasized
Biomechanical	Movement; posture
Neurodevelopmental	Position; posture
Cognitive	Information content; relationships between objects; links between objects and actions; exploration
Perceptual	Material which requires use of perceptual discrimination
Sensory	Material which stimulates senses
Social	Communication between people
Educational	Opportunities for learning

PRESENTATION

Once the task or activity is selected, the modifications to the environment will be selected to enhance the presentation of materials and tools as required by the approach. Presentation also includes the occupational context of performance as work, leisure or self-care.

ADAPTING THE IMMEDIATE ENVIRONMENT

These adaptations affect the area nearest to a user. The immediate environment might be a table top or the operating controls of a machine. The near environment is the surrounding area containing the resources for task performance. Some alteration in this area may be required to support what is done in the immediate vicinity of the user.

This type of adaptation is useful in a variety of situations:

- to improve the design of a workstation, the layout of tools and materials or the information content of the area
- to improve performance of simple daily living tasks by promoting access to tools or materials and providing cues to use

- to promote awareness of the environment or stimulation from it
- to simplify and reduce available information
- to enhance information to compensate for sensory deficits
- to promote learning
- to enhance therapeutic attributes of a task.

EXAMPLES OF ADAPTATION OF THE IMMEDIATE ENVIRONMENT

1. Adaptations to enhance dyadic interaction

Remove   Objects which act as a barrier between therapist and the client. Sources of distraction in near environment – noises, other people, busy activity; or in immediate environment – unnecessary objects.

Add: Good lighting; avoid glare. Make sure therapist's face is well-lit, not silhouetted against the light. Comfortable seating; (if standing, avoid fatigue). Ensure person has aids to communication to hand, e.g. spectacles (clean); hearing aid (working); pen and notepad. If demonstrating, ensure all tools and materials are available.

Alter   Size of print if written material is used. Use pictures if required.

Position   If seated, have face level with that of patient. If standing, ensure patient can see you without having to adopt an uncomfortable posture. Select position of self and furniture and choose location to emphasize the nature of the communication: friendly, authoritarian, teaching, counselling. Avoid mismatching

environment with nature and purpose of communication.

Enhance   Comprehension – provide a little information at a time. Ensure explanation or information is understood before passing to next topic. Ensure language and manner of communication are appropriate to age and culture.
Non-verbal communication – use appropriate expressions and body language to reinforce meaning. Use gestures sparingly and with purpose.

2. Adaptations to promote movement

Remove   Any obstacle to the desired movement.

Upper limbs

Add   Examples:
Arm supports, e.g. fixed sling, buoyancy sling; skate; ball-bearing arm rest
Handles, e.g. padded, flat, round, shaped
Levers, extended handles; lever tools increase movement and decrease effort (or may increase effort, depending on position of fulcrum).

Alter   Shape or size of used objects.

Position   Place objects or tools further from user to promote stretching and reaching. Use shelves, racks and boxes. Place objects nearer to reduce movement to smaller range.

Lower limbs

Add   Examples:
Mobility aids, e.g. frame, stick, crutch, rollator
Wheelchair; powered chair, glide-about; chair with castors to 'scoot'.

Position   Place object at a distance from user to promote walking/mobility.

3. Adaptations to enhance information content of environment

Remove	All objects unconnected with task. Distractions in the near environment.
Add	Objects which provide clear cues to use. Prompts from therapist if required.
Alter	Size, colour, texture.
Position	Ensure all required objects are within visual field of user. Place objects in logical and functional relationship to each other.
Enhance	Ensure tools and materials are easily seen. Improve visual contrast by placing dark objects against a lighter ground (or the reverse).

4. Adaptations to challenge process skills

Remove	Place some necessary items out of sight in container or cupboard. Remove sample giving cues to task product.
Add	Some items within view which are not required for the task so that selection is required.
Position	Items out of sequence or with no logical organization.

These examples should be sufficient to indicate the way in which a small part of the environment can be manipulated to make performance easier or more challenging.

Further examples can be found in Allen (1985), Turner & McCaul (1996) and Corcoran & Gitlin (1997).

THERAPEUTIC ADAPTATION OF THE USED ENVIRONMENT

SIMULATED AND PROTECTED ENVIRONMENTS

In the traditional, occupational therapy department, environments which simulate those found in the home or workplace are often provided. These environments provide opportunities for safe exploration and learning, and for assessment of function in an analogue of real-life situations.

A typical example is the 'daily living suite' which comprises a kitchen, bedroom, bathroom and lavatory. These rooms may be designed and furnished to look like a typical home, or may contain a mixture of normal and adapted equipment.

Work environments may also be simulated, for example, a clerical work area, woodwork shop or garden.

A leisure area might be a lounge, a patio with a barbeque, or a games room.

In any simulated environment, it is important to maintain a consistent and appropriate approach to design, furnishings or equipment. A certain amount of theatrical 'set dressing' may be needed in some situations, but items which are obviously fake or cannot be used (e.g. a dummy fireplace with a painted fire) are best avoided as they can appear to patronize users.

Advantages of simulated environments

As recovery takes place, the individual is likely to pass through stages in which the individual needs to practise activities in order to gain confidence, consolidate gains in function and take 'safe risks'.

The occupational therapy area enables this process to take place in an environment which is, to some degree, controlled and protected. This environment can readily be adapted without inconvenience.

In the case of an activity area, the environment provides realistic opportunities and challenges to engage performance.

Limitations of simulated environments

The most obvious limitation is that the environment, however carefully designed to be user friendly and homely, is *not* home (or *not* the workplace or *not* the busy street) and can only be an inadequate substitute for the real, risky and unpredictable world.

Skills which have been learned in protected settings, where a lot of cues to performance are available, may not be transferred to novel situations where the cues are less helpful and the distractions or stressors much higher.

A person may perform better in a protected environment, thus giving a false impression of independence; equally, the person may perform less well than in a familiar setting. Assessment conducted in a simulated environment can only provide *a guide* to probable performance in the real world.

In institutional settings, especially those which are modern and purpose-built, it is hard to avoid bland, 'hotel style' furnishings in therapy areas. Features which are required for health and safety reasons inevitably have to be included which would not be present in the ordinary home; over-zealous adaptations of this kind (e.g. an industrial style ventilator in a kitchen) may need to be resisted.

Despite these limitations, simulated environments do provide useful opportunities which 'bridge the gap' between care settings and more challenging environments.

OUTDOOR AREAS

People normally spend much of their time out of doors, even if it is only in transit from one building to another. Work may be based outside, especially heavier jobs. Many leisure and recreational activities take place in the open air. Despite this, therapeutic use of external environments is often overlooked, or considered only in terms of therapeutic horticulture.

Use of an outdoor area can be divided into active use and reactive use. In active use, the participant engages with objects and features of the outdoor environment and performs tasks or activities connected with them. In reactive use, the participant passively enjoys features of the outdoor world and the experience of being out of doors, or uses the area for activities which are unconnected with the outdoor location.

Active use

- Use for assessment, e.g. work assessment; mobility assessment; activities of daily living
- Therapeutic activity, e.g. horticulture; outdoor games; outdoor social activities
- Provision of sensory stimulation, e.g. plants for colour, smell, texture; swing for vestibular stimulation
- Use as an educational resource
- Use to promote fitness, e.g. running, jogging, sport.

Reactive use

- Rest area
- Leisure area, e.g. eating outside; unstructured activity enjoying plants, birds, insects
- Social area
- Relaxation/meditation area.

THERAPEUTIC HORTICULTURE

Since the mid-1980s, horticulture has been used as therapy, both in rehabilitation, and in education and training of people with learning difficulties. There is specialist literature on this, and in England, some courses in horticultural therapy are now available. Gardening tasks can be performed in the context of work, leisure and self-care and are readily broken into stages and graded. Horticulture also has considerable potential as an educational medium.

Therapeutic horticulture spans a wide range of activities from modest 'patio gardening' in containers during fine weather, to allotments, glasshouses, and full-scale, year-round, commercial production.

Whether designing an active or reactive outdoor area, therapists who do not have personal expertise in horticulture are advised to seek help from a trained horticulturalist or horticultural therapist.

A therapeutic garden is unique in that there are two sets of needs to be met, those of the user and those of the plants. The design of hard landscape, selection of appropriate plants, consideration of continuing maintenance, and organization of activities require considerable skill and knowledge and there are many pitfalls for the inexperienced. However, horticulture is an immensely rich and rewarding activity and the effort to extend therapy into external areas is well worth while.

MANAGEMENT OF THE NEAR AND USED ENVIRONMENT

Environmental management includes management of all the resources within it, human and non-human, in order to create an appropriate demand for a specified activity.

The following will be used as examples:

- organizing a room for a social group activity
- room management technique
- arranging a room for an interview
- organizing a visit to a community location.

ORGANIZING A ROOM FOR SOCIAL OR GROUP USE: PRACTICAL CONSIDERATIONS

When organizing any group activity, there is a 'checklist' of environmental practicalities (physical and human) which need to be considered in advance. Usually, the organizing therapist decides what is needed, and then either takes appropriate action or delegates this to others. Practical considerations include:

- preparation and clearing up
- setting up the room
- staffing
- equipment and materials
- precautions, health and safety aspects and emergency procedures
- refreshments and access to lavatories
- getting clients to and from the group.

Preparation and clearing up

Group activities may take place in an occupational therapy area, in which case, although preparation and clearing up take time which must be allowed for, the necessary resources are usually to hand. However, preparation time is easy to underestimate, particularly for a 'special event' or if there are unusual requirements.

When using an area which is 'borrowed', especially if it has other uses and users, preparation and clearing up become more of a problem. As well as the practicalities of gaining access, the (sometimes sensitive) views and needs of other users have to be considered. Sometimes, advance negotiations are necessary to smooth the way and ensure that others are not inadvertently upset or inconvenienced.

Leaving things as one found them (or perhaps as one wished one had found them!) is important if one wants to use the area again.

Frequently-used items can be organized into boxes and stored in cupboards or on trolleys for convenience. Wise therapists pay attention to security and check that nothing has 'walked' before the group begins.

Setting up the room

This means creating an environment which is suited to the activity, both in its functional arrangement and its demand. Specific therapeutic objectives must also be considered.

People will interact better if they have visual contact with each other and a degree of propinquity. Layout of furniture is important, but changing layout alone is not sufficient, the environment should also contain cues to the expected social or cultural behaviour. While good management of the environment will do much to promote interaction, this is unlikely to happen without additional facilitation from the therapist either through use of self, or by selection of a suitable activity, or both.

The arrangements in Figure 34.1 show the ways in which the same room could be rearranged to provide for different activities with a group of clients. Selection of chairs and tables which suit the majority of users and the type of use is also important.

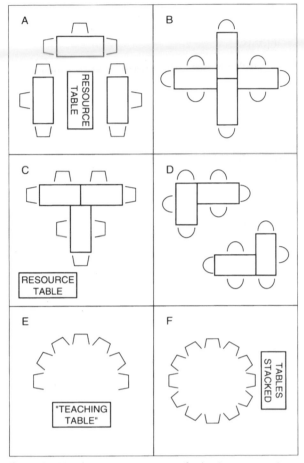

Figure 34.1 Various arrangements of a basic room setting.

Staffing

Humans are an important resource in the environment. The number of staff, their experience and grade, and the roles they will have during the activity should be decided in advance. Unless clients are very independent and capable or other staff are readily available nearby, most group activities require two members of staff in order to cope with any unexpected event. A group should not normally be left alone once an activity starts (unless this is a planned part of therapy).

Staff to assist with personal care may be required as well as staff to assist with the activity. Volunteers can often provide useful input in group activities, but should not be used as 'replacement staff'.

Equipment and materials

A simple checklist will help to ensure that nothing is forgotten. It is wise to have 'spares' of essential items. It may also be necessary to have additional items to use in case the group gets through material faster than expected, or the activity is obviously failing to generate participation.

Adapted equipment for social activities (especially for older people) needs to be designed with care. The result of enlarging equipment such as games' boards, or painting items in bright colours to make them more visible may be to make these items look 'childish'.

Precautions, health and safety aspects and emergency procedures

Precautions arising from the special needs of clients should have been considered before arranging the activity. The usual precautions concerning accidents, spillage, rubbish or clutter, trip, slip or fall hazards, and lifting apply.

In addition, any precautions required when handling, storing or using materials or tools need to be considered. All staff involved should understand these and special instructions should be explained to clients.

All staff involved should be aware of emergency procedures, fire alarms, emergency exists, evacuation procedures, how to obtain first-aid or medical assistance, how to cope with a cardiac arrest, and any other necessary procedure for the safety and security of clients.

Refreshments and lavatories

Arrangements for making or obtaining refreshments usually need to be made in advance.

In an unfamiliar area, it is important to find out what facilities are available and to find and inspect the nearest lavatories, checking that access is suitable for clients.

Getting clients to and from the group

This can be a logistical nightmare if the clients have to be transported over any distance; travel often takes far longer than it should.

Clients may be expected to come to the group on their own, but if they need assistance, such as portering, or if transport has to be booked, arrangements must be made in advance, and may need to be checked on the day. (Despite the temptation to do so, therapists should resist being expected to act as porters except in exceptional circumstances; this is not an effective use of qualified staff time.)

ROOM MANAGEMENT TECHNIQUE

A further example of this comprehensive resource management approach is provided by *room management*. This technique has its origins in behavioural learning, but I have been unable to trace the originator of it.

The technique arose from the observation that in a large group staff time was often dissipated by dealing with incidents or client needs or the general running of the activity to the exclusion of specific therapy. Human resources need to be used effectively within the therapeutic environment, especially when dealing with clients with special needs.

The technique is designed to ensure that clients in a large group each receive at least one period of individual attention focused on a specific therapeutic or learning objective.

To achieve this, each member of staff (often from several disciplines) is given a specific role in managing the group.

The way in which this works is best illustrated by an example:

A group of 12 elderly people with early dementia is involved in an art group with four members of staff. The clients have differing abilities; some are physically disabled, others inclined to wander. Once set up, the art group activity is planned to last for 30 minutes.

The elderly participants are seated in groups of four at three tables. The most dependent clients in wheelchairs are nearest the exit door. The most mobile 'wanderers' are furthest from it.

One member of staff has the role of seeing to toileting needs, general comfort and posture, and making sure clients are safe. This person is not involved in the activity.

All the clients are supplied with paints and paper and for the first 5 minutes three staff take one table each and help the clients to start painting.

Once the general activity has got under way, one member of staff takes on the role of 'activity manager' and circulates round the tables giving general advice, help and encouragement, providing fresh materials and 'keeping things going'.

The third and fourth members of staff each have a list of four clients who have specific therapeutic goals. They spend 5 minutes with each person working for the specified goal.

In this way, eight members of the group get focused individual attention which they might otherwise have missed.

ENVIRONMENTS FOR INTERVIEWS

The environment should reflect the style and purpose of the interview. A formal interview requires a formal setting with traditional, hard-edged furniture (Fig. 34.2). The interviewer will sit at a distance from the interviewee, perhaps by sitting behind a desk.

An informal interview needs a setting and furniture arrangement which promotes a relaxed atmosphere (Fig. 34.2). The participants need to sit adjacent to each other with good visual contact, but avoiding intrusive proximity.

In any interview setting, privacy is essential, and this usually means finding a separate room and closing the door. It is difficult to discuss intimate details when there is only the polite fiction of privacy provided by a screen or drawn curtain; however, many medical interviews are conducted in this environment. The demand of the hospital or clinic environment acts to remove usual barriers to disclosure, but this should not be taken as a licence to make lack of privacy acceptable.

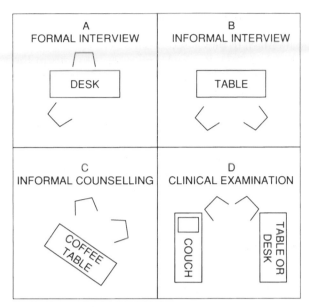

Figure 34.2 Arrangement of desk and chairs for an interview.

ORGANIZING A GROUP COMMUNITY VISIT

Visits to locations or events in the community are valuable and enjoyable therapeutic group activities. It may be felt that a visit offers little scope for therapeutic adaptation of the environment. This may be true, but management of human and practical resources and aspects of the environment are still required. Where potentially vulnerable clients (or those who may themselves cause problems to others) are to be taken on a visit, careful planning is essential.

Pleasant though it may be to have a spontaneous 'trip out', any visit to a location away from base needs planning with all the meticulous attention to detail of a military operation (see Box 34.1).

For the clients (and perhaps for the staff), a visit is often a trip into the exploratory area, away from the usual and familiar surroundings. This sense of adventure can be strong, even when the destination is not particularly unusual or exciting. The therapist needs to use the excitement and stimulation of exploration for therapeutic advantage, while maintaining the essen-

tial sense of safety which enables exploration to occur.

Box 34.1 Checklist for organizing a visit
• Have stated therapeutic aims for the visit • Have a documented local policy and procedure, including what to do in an emergency: check this if unsure • Plan use of human resources • Check the location before the visit • Consider health and safety issues • Plan a detailed itinerary.

Therapeutic aim

The visit, like any group activity, should have a clear therapeutic purpose and be structured to achieve this. Although there may be limited scope for overt therapy while out, there is usually considerable scope to use the visit as a basis for a variety of therapeutic or educational activities both before and after it happens; indeed, this may be the most important aspect of going on the visit.

A policy on visits

Management issues

If visits are undertaken, it is sensible to have a policy document covering all the local procedures. Like all such policy documents, this requires review at intervals.

It may be necessary to specify management aspects such as methods of paying for visits, whether staff are expected to pay for themselves, staff insurance, eligibility to drive vehicles, ratios of staff to clients, and need for medical or other permission to go out.

Notification of the visit

Someone needs to know, in advance, that the visit is to take place. Permission may need to be given, not only for the nature of the visit, but also for the inclusion of individual clients. A written record of the place to be visited, names of clients and staff going out, time of departure and expected time of return, and any other relevant details should be left with a responsible person.

Emergency procedures

There should be clearly understood, simple procedures for dealing with any emergency which might occur in the course of the visit. It is wise for the organizer to have a mobile phone to keep in touch with base or obtain emergency help.

Medication policy

If clients need to take medication while on the visit, this can cause problems; occupational therapists should not normally administer medication. This means that, unless the client is self-medicating (or accompanied by a relative who normally deals with medication), a nurse must accompany the client on the visit to take responsibility for this.

Client care

Clients need to be appropriately dressed and may need to have protective clothing, hats, sunscreen or sunglasses. Some clients with special needs may have personal supplies or equipment which must be taken with them.

Staffing

Staffing ratios for visits usually need to be higher than for an indoor activity and must be geared to meeting any special needs of clients. Staff must have an appropriate mix of qualifications and experience.

Checking the location

The place to be visited must be checked out well ahead of time. It may be necessary to inform the proprietor that a visit is planned. In general, venues are happy to accept small parties of disabled visitors and often go out of their way to help, but some may, for justifiable reasons, be unable to accept large groups.

Facilities such as tea-rooms or lavatories need checking; general access, parking and hire of wheelchairs need to be reviewed. Health and safety aspects need to be checked.

Plan the itinerary

A detailed, timed schedule for travelling to and from the visit and programme while on the visit help to ensure that the trip keeps on schedule and that sufficient time for each stage, not forgetting rests and refreshments, is included. A long time spent travelling may counteract the benefits of the visit. It is preferable to have a short, successful and enjoyable visit than an overambitious and overextended one.

If it is an outdoor event, it is wise to have a plan to cope with wet weather.

SUMMARY

Adaptation and management of the environment require clear aims, close observation and attention to detail, and good organizing ability. Like other aspects of occupational therapy, the effort which has contributed to production of the desired effect should ultimately become 'invisible' to the user.

35 Analysis and adaptation of the home environment

As care has shifted from institutions into the community, the role of the occupational therapist in enabling and enhancing occupational performance in the home environment has become well established as an essential service.

THE PURPOSE OF A HOME ASSESSMENT VISIT

There are several reasons why a home visit may be made:

- to check if the home is suited to the needs of the client, and to advise on and provide adaptations or services
- to observe the client performing activities of daily living in the client's own home and to assess, in conjunction with the client, whether such performance is adequate to meet the client's needs
- to check on safety and advise on accident prevention. This may include a review of the contents and state of repair of the home, or of the practical or social resources available to the client
- to gain an insight into the client's lifestyle, relationships, and sources of personal stress or support
- to advise a carer on management of a frail or disabled individual
- to provide therapy in the home environment.

The amount of environmental analysis required will depend on the purpose of the visit. In some cases, a general impression is sufficient, whereas in others a detailed evaluation of one area, or even the whole home, may be needed.

USING A CLIENT-CENTRED APPROACH

When undertaking a home visit for any reason, a client-centred approach is essential for both ethical and practical reasons. The purpose of a visit must always be to facilitate the attempts of the client to identify and solve the problems which are relevant and meaningful to the client. It is both unethical and ineffective to attempt to impose actions or solutions which are not actively accepted by the client.

Clients are understandably more willing to comply with advice and adopt solutions when they have been closely involved in the process of problem-solving.

A person's home is personal territory. The therapist may not enter uninvited or without consent. There are implicit rules concerning the behaviour of the therapist in the role of guest and the occupier in the role of host. These rules and roles vary with age and culture.

The therapist crossing the threshold for the first time must instantly acquire sufficient cues from the appearance and behaviour of the client and the nature of the environment to respond with an appropriate set of social behaviours, and to gear the timing of any actions with great care, respecting the attitudes and values of the client.

First impressions govern much of any subsequent transaction. Only after a therapeutic relationship has been established for some time can participants discard first impressions to build up a more accurate picture of each other. If the initial assumptions are incorrect, the intervention may start off on the wrong track. When in doubt an age-appropriate, culturally acceptable, polite social manner is the best starting point.

When visiting a client in the community, the therapist steps into the unknown, and is often alone. The client may be task orientated and greet you with 'So, you have come about my shower?'; you then have a convenient opening for your exploration of the environment. Far more often, however, the client has little idea of why you are there, or of how you could help the client. The client may be more comfortable with 'tea and chat' (or an equivalent) as a starting point, and would find a swift analysis of the bathroom facilities odd and intrusive.

The home visit is likely to engender a range of expectations, positive and negative, for the occupier. Before any examination of the environment can take place, the therapist must therefore spend some time in explanation.

The need for the visit must be clear. Expectations must be realistic from the outset. The goals of the occupier need to be discussed and clarified and the needs of any other resident considered. Above all, it is essential to avoid making promises unless you are certain they can be kept.

WANTS VERSUS NEEDS

A dilemma which may confront the community occupational therapist is that what the client wants may not be what the therapist perceives that the client needs, or, more fundamentally, what resources are geared to provide. Working in a client-centred approach does not mean that every 'want' can be met.

The contest between wants and needs affects us all. I might 'want' a large house with a swimming pool; what I need is a sound roof over my head. Somewhere between these two extremes, and closely connected to the amount of money I have available, is a compromise.

It is necessary to be very explicit, from an early stage, about what is, and is not, likely to be possible, and to steer the client towards a realistic appraisal of what can be done.

However, a dogmatic refusal to consider anything more than basic needs will plainly not value or respect personal preferences and meanings which may have a disproportionate significance for the client.

For example, to keep clean one really only 'needs' some warm water in a basin, soap, a flannel and a towel. But if the client strongly values the experience of a 'a good hot bath' which will make a significant difference to perceptions of well-being in an otherwise restricted and unre-warding life, and if this is achievable, perhaps this wish should not simply be dismissed as an unrealistic 'want'. If washing is also required for a religious purpose, it becomes much more important. The therapist may at times need to act as an advocate for the client in communicating the background to the client's needs.

It seems that for the foreseeable future, resources are constrained. Yet, at the same time, the expectations and aspirations of clients are legitimately increasing. The therapist can be placed in a difficult position when trying to steer a course between conflicting priorities and demands.

ANALYSIS OF THE HOME ENVIRONMENT

CONTENT ANALYSIS

Gaining an overview of the used environment

An overview is useful to set the home in context. The size, layout, location and outdoor areas are likely to be significant, both practically and socially.

The setting and access to resources such as shops, public transport, leisure facilities or other people are also important. In practical terms, it is a very different matter to live in an isolated cottage in the countryside or a flat high in a tower block. In social terms, however, either may be isolating, or sociable, depending on the support network of the resident. The degree of availability of resources can enhance or impede performance.

The interior of the home may give an indica-tion of affluence or poverty, but the therapist should again beware of assumptions. Affluence may be due to past, rather than present, circum-stances, or an illusion created by credit purchas-es. Apparent poverty or lack of repair may mask an eccentric millionaire.

The contents of a home give some evidence of personal taste, culture and lifestyle. Personal standards of tidiness, cleanliness and décor can

be assessed. This may give an indication of whether the client is coping as well as the client always did, or whether there is a dissonance between observations of the client, the client's history and the client's environment.

Personal objects may suggest interests or events in a life history. The degree to which clients have taken control of their environment and personalized it for their own use may also be indicative. Very controlling people who like everything 'just so' with each ornament arranged in the exact spot and not a speck of dust in sight may find it hard to adapt. Creative people who have already designed or adapted areas for their own use may be more receptive.

People who have made no effort to personal-ize their living areas or who accept poor décor or repair although it could be improved may be alienated or dysfunctional in other ways, but equally may simply have adopted a value sys-tem which is different from that of the therapist or the local culture.

These cues should not be accepted at face value but can be used by the therapist to test out hypotheses about the client and the client's needs, to spark discussion or to build rapport.

Objective content analysis of a room

Content analysis of a room is usually utiltarian; the therapist needs to know the layout of the room, what is there, its position, and what it is used for.

It is best to make a written description and room plan. A checklist can be helpful. Memory is unlikely to be accurate about details. It may be necessary to make measurements, not only of the size of the room, but also of the space available for moving around, or the precise dimensions of furniture or doors.

Contents to record include:

General layout	Size, shape, space, height of ceiling; type of walls and flooring; windows, doors, built-in fitments, changes of level, steps.

Services	Heating, lighting, power points, plumbing, drainage, ventilation.
Furniture	What it is, what it looks like; state of repair; dimensions.
Personal possessions	Clothes, toiletries, personal items.
Domestic equipment	Tools, utensils, machines, electrical equipment.
Decorations	Décor, significant pictures, ornaments, rugs, soft furnishings.
Leisure equipment	TV, music, books, games, sports.

In addition, the following areas are usually considered:

Resources	Does the client have the resources needed for activities of daily living. This may include consideration of practical necessities, money, social support networks, and social services already provided.
Access	Can the client get to items and places the client needs inside and outside the home?
Safety	Are there risks or hazards in the environment? Is there safety equipment available?
Utility	Are items to be used of the most practical, and functional design for the client?
Layout	Are items in the best relationship to each other to promote effective and efficient use, reduce fatigue and enhance performance?

Checklists for home assessment

There are a number of published checklists to guide and record observations of the home environment. These are often designed with accident prevention in mind. One of the most comprehensive is the Home Safety Checklist (Clemson 1996). This is not readily available in the UK, but an address is given in the reference section. However, assessment of the home without taking account of the behaviour and needs of the client is insufficient.

Subjective content analysis of a room

A room can provide insights into a client's personality, interests, occupations, roles and past life.

It is sometimes illuminating to ask the client to talk about a 'favourite' room, or an area or objects within a room. Prompts such as questions about how things were chosen, or where they came from, or whether there are any special personal meanings or memories attached to them usually elicit very interesting material.

This environmentally-linked storytelling can facilitate the development of a therapeutic alliance, because it enables the client to understand that the therapist values the client as a person with a unique past and special experiences and interests. The therapist needs to keep a focus on occupational aspects, or the session may become simple reminiscence which, while interesting, is of little therapeutic value.

ADAPTIVE ANALYSIS

This is complementary to content analysis. The therapist needs to relate the observations of content to the needs of the client and to make judgements about whether or not these are compatible.

Although it is useful for the therapist to observe the environment to ascertain this information, it is far more helpful to involve the client in demonstrating how the environment is used and how it meets, or fails to meet, the client's needs.

Once environmental deficits have been identified, the therapist can work with the *client and any other* resident to identify solutions, adaptations and improvements.

THE ASSESSMENT HOME VISIT

An assessment home visit is made in order to assess the ability of the client to cope at home following admission to hospital or care facility, to evaluate the suitability of the accommodation and to identify any home modifications, equipment resources or services which will be needed to support the client in the community.

The client is taken home, by the therapist or by ambulance, the assessment takes place *and the client is then returned to care*. This type of visit is sometimes called a 'discharge home visit' since it precedes discharge from care. This is misleading. It is important to avoid being placed in the position of taking a decision to discharge the client 'on the spot' and leaving the client behind to cope. This is an inappropriate decision for a therapist, and in simply practical terms it allows no time for essential resources and services to be provided.

When taking a patient home from hospital, the therapist has the advantage of having already established a therapeutic alliance with the individual. The reasons for the visit, what it may achieve, and what is likely to happen as a result can all be explored before the event.

The client may well view the visit with anxiety as some kind of 'test' or 'examination' which must be passed if the client is to return home. Anxiety rises in proportion to the desire to be 'back home'. The therapist may need to spend some time in reassurance, emphasizing the practical, problem-solving value of the visit, while acknowledging the possibility of a negative outcome, and alternative options, if that seems likely.

It is usual for the therapist to be accompanied by a colleague or assistant as a safeguard in case of an emergency and as a protective measure, especially if the visit is to an otherwise unoccupied home. If necessary, arrangements can be made for others to be there, either to support the client, or to assist in explaining about what is available.

It is good practice to have a written procedure for a home visit that deals with practical arrangements and also explains what will happen in the case of an emergency.

PROCEDURE FOR AN ASSESSMENT HOME VISIT

The procedure will need to be tailored to local circumstances but in general it should include:

- a statement of general objectives for the visit
- note of any circumstances under which a visit is not appropriate
- transport system and policy on therapist drivers using own cars
- list of persons to be notified and method of notifying all concerned
- health and safety issues
- policy on coping with untoward incidents during visit:
  - illness or accident
  - death of client
  - refusal of client to return to care
  - assault on staff
- Reporting procedure.

It is also helpful to have a checklist (Box 35.1) to ensure that everything necessary is taken on the visit and all arrangements have been made. The

---

Box 35.1 Checklist for discharge home visit

- List of people to be notified about the visit.
- List of people participating in visit with confirmation of notification of appointment time and place and telephone number for contact if visit is cancelled.
- List of items to be taken on the visit:
  - keys to home or location of these
  - personal possessions of client
  - essential medication (check if client is self-medicating, otherwise a nurse will be needed)
  - assistive equipment used by client
  - supplies for snack and hot drink (either to be prepared by client or in case of transport delay)
  - rug; hot water bottle if home is unheated in winter
  - mobile phone for use in emergency: emergency phone numbers, including client's GP
  - assessment checklists or case record forms
  - equipment needed by therapist, e.g. tape measure.

list can be a long one, and it is easy to forget essential items. This is particularly important when the client (often an elderly person) lives alone.

HOME ADAPTATIONS

Alterations to a person's home may be made in order to enhance performance, increase safety or improve resources.

Adaptations can be subdivided into *minor* adaptations – those which have relatively low cost and do not require substantial alterations to the design or structure of the home – and *major* adaptations – those which are costly and usually involve substantial work on the building.

In the UK, the provision of major and minor adaptations is governed by complex legislation. Local authorities have specific duties to provide some help and services, but for others the level of provision is discretionary. This means that local provision is influenced by the available resources and the way in which the local authority chooses to interpret the legislation. Because of this variation, and because legislation is subject to alteration, no attempt will be made to explain the detail of it here.

In general terms, assistance is available to clients who are 'substantially and permanently handicapped', and to their carers. The client's financial circumstances dictate whether or not a contribution is made to the cost of major adaptations. Minor adaptations are normally free, although some authorities charge for items up to a specified amount.

Therapists who are employed by social services departments need to understand both the primary legislation and any local interpretations in detail in order to provide an effective service to clients. It is not surprising, in view of the amount of detail and the fact that services may be provided by different agencies, that clients often find it difficult to understand their entitlements or the range of services available. Therapists may find themselves in a difficult position when trying simultaneously to act as the advocate for the client, and the agent of local policy.

MINOR ADAPTATIONS

Minor adaptations to the physical environment are provided to promote mobility and safe functional use of the environment. The usual principles of adding, removing, altering or repositioning content apply. Minor adaptations include:

Type of adaptation	Examples
Improvements to access	Alterations to doors, small ramps, grab rails, stair rails, changes to steps, paths, access to garden
Safety measures	Fire precautions, fall prevention, accident prevention, personal call alarm, telephone, security
Improved mobility	Use of wheelchair; transfers – bed, chair, toilet, bath or shower; use of stairs, steps; chair or bed raise
Personal activities of daily living	Assistive devices to enable washing, personal hygiene, dressing, eating
Instrumental activities of daily living	Assistive devices to enable cooking, cleaning, laundry, home maintenance reorganization of furniture or fitments

MAJOR ADAPTATIONS

Major adaptations include installation of large equipment such as a lift or a special shower, major alterations such as provision of an adapted bathroom and toilet, or extension to the home, for example, a ground-floor bedroom.

This is a very demanding area of work because it covers a wide area of knowledge and requires co-ordination of resources from many different fields.

When working with the client on a major adaptation, the therapist has a number of important functions to perform:

- explore solutions and options with the client, ensuring that the most practical, efficient and cost-effective solution is adopted
- act as a consultant on adaptations and equipment
- draw up outline plans or a design brief

- assist the client to obtain the services of experts to implement the plans, such as architect, structural engineer and builder
- promote access to grant aid and available resources
- co-ordinate and facilitate progress on the project.

This implies an accurate assessment of the current and future needs of the client, up-to-date knowledge of adaptive equipment, a basic understanding of the practicalities of adapting and extending buildings, and a knowledge of the planning process, relevant legislation and any local limitations.

It can be difficult to reconcile the aspirations of the client with the constraints of available resources. Major adaptations should normally be undertaken only when other solutions have been explored and found unsatisfactory. A great deal can be achieved by rearrangement of existing content and provision of simple equipment. A change of home may be a better long-term solution than an unsatisfactory compromise adaptation.

Clients who have deteriorating or terminal conditions present particular challenges and need very sensitive management, especially when the realistic timescale for undertaking a major adaptation can extend over a year or 18 months or even longer.

INFORMATION ON HOME ADAPTATIONS

For information on designing rooms for disabled people, the standard text is still Goldsmith (1984), although there is now renewed interest on access and design. Organizations which deal with specific disabilities can usually provide advice. Books on ergonomics can also be helpful.

Assistive equipment is continually being developed and improved. The therapist needs to keep up to date by reading the trade press, attending exhibitions, obtaining catalogues and referring to databases which are regularly reviewed.

ADAPTATIONS FOR SPECIFIC DISABILITIES

Most texts on physical occupational therapy include explicit information about adaptations which are appropriate to particular conditions or types of problem (see Turner 1996, Neistadt & Crepeau 1998: Treatment of occupational performance areas). In addition, some texts give more general information about environmental adaptation (Christiansen & Baum 1997).

When considering home adaptations, the emphasis has, until recently, been on promoting mobility and movement-related function. In the past 5 years, there has been more interest in changing the information content of the environment in order to influence behaviour (see Corcoran & Gitlin 1997). Accident prevention and risk-reduction have also been studied, particularly in relation to fall prevention, and here too the links between environment and behaviour need to be considered.

36

Health and safety and accident prevention

ENSURING SAFETY IS A LEGAL REQUIREMENT

Although it is accepted that living is intrinsically a risky business, therapists, like other workers, have a duty to act to eliminate or minimize risk.

Any environment used by the public is subject to regulations concerning hygiene, safety, accident prevention, fire prevention and dealing with emergencies. The environment must be constructed to minimize hazards, promote safety and permit escape.

In a work environment, all users of an environment are responsible for keeping it safe. Hazards must be noted, removed and reported. The need for repairs must be notified. Principles of health and safety must be followed at all times.

SAFETY IN INSTITUTIONAL SETTINGS

Therapists should conduct regular risk assessments of their areas, and should also remain vigilant when using an area controlled by someone else. The Health and Safety Executive produces many useful free leaflets giving advice on identifying hazards and managing risks. Most larger institutions have a Health and Safety Officer to whom one can go for advice. In some areas official inspectors have the right to examine and report and to require improvements.

THE DEPARTMENTAL SAFETY AUDIT

The principles of a departmental safety audit are:

Risk assessment — Inspection and observation are required to identify potential risks and hazards. Risks should be related to the users: some users are more vulnerable and require extra precautions. Risks can be caused by objects that are present, and also by objects that are absent, and by the behaviour of users.

Reporting — Any risks identified should be recorded and reported.

Action — As far as is practical, risks should be removed or reduced. Training should be given to promote safe behaviours.

Review — At intervals, the area should be reviewed to see that accident-prevention measures are in place and no further risks or hazards have been identified.

The following notes give basic guidance on the main areas which concern a therapist.

FIRE PRECAUTIONS

Fire is caused by a combination of a source of heat, an inflammable substance and oxygen. Fire prevention is based on the principle of keeping these three elements separated.

Occupational therapy departments may contain readily inflammable substances such as paint, glue, solvents and thinners and potentially inflammable materials such as paper. Readily inflammable substances should be kept in a locked, fire-retardant, metal cabinet in a cool place; a few substances have low flash points and may ignite in strong sunlight. Craft activities may produce inflammable waste such as wood shavings, dust or used rags soaked in solvent. These need to be removed promptly. Metal waste bins are much safer than plastic ones.

Fire exits must be clearly marked, kept unobstructed and easy to use. There should be a conveniently located fire alarm and everyone should know how to raise the alarm and how to recognize alarm signals. Fire extinguishers should be suitable and accessible, and everyone should understand how to use them. Most institutions have regular fire-prevention training sessions, and advice from a fire officer can be obtained if required.

MEDICAL EMERGENCIES AND FIRST-AID

There should be a clear procedure for dealing with any medical emergency such as a cardiac arrest. Patients taken ill may also need care. The environment must contain the instructions and, if necessary, basic equipment to deal with these events.

First-aid items such as dressings for cuts may be needed by both patients and staff. Protective plastic gloves should be worn when dealing with an open injury. There should be a designated first-aider in each area. It is worth noting that a nurse or a therapist is not regarded as qualified to give first-aid without additional training. First-aid material should be kept in an easily accessible place in the correctly marked box.

HYGIENE

Kitchen hygiene is especially important because an occupational therapy kitchen may be used by many people whose standards and abilities vary. Some of the requirements are drawn from commercial catering regulations and may make the kitchen less 'user friendly' and domestic in character, such as the need for a separate basin for washing hands instead of using the sink.

Correct food storage is important, and high standards of cleanliness for equipment, worktops and utensils need to be maintained. Dishcloths, cleaning cloths and drying cloths should be separated, changed frequently and kept clean. It may be helpful to have one person with responsibility for checking on these items and procedures.

Disinfectants and cleaning substances should be used correctly and stored safely away from food.

Personal hygiene is equally important. Staff need to have facilities for hand-washing, and protective clothing if dealing with a transmittable infection. A disinfectant policy may be in force.

STORAGE

Storage should be designed to ensure that items can be reached easily, and that users can conform with manual handling regulations or fire precautions. Hazards from badly stacked items which might fall and hurt someone need to be avoided. Stable steps should be available to reach high shelves.

Storage of tools and materials in areas used by patients who are unable to evaluate risk or who may attempt self-harm requires great care, close supervision and a very detailed system of checking.

There are separate regulations for handling, storing and disposing of hazardous substances (COSHH) and although the therapist may use few of these substances, any which are in use must be treated correctly.

An alarmingly large number of commonly used domestic or garden products is potentially toxic. The therapist needs to read all the 'small print' and must ensure instructions for use and storage are followed.

USE OF TOOLS AND EQUIPMENT

Risks are caused by incorrect use, so it is necessary for the therapist to observe use by patients, and also by others in the environment.

Sharp or heavy tools present particular problems. Most occupational therapy workshops have tool cupboards with well-designed holders, or shadow boards to display tools. It is necessary, however, to check that tools are in place and to carry out regular maintenance. A blunt tool can be more dangerous in use than a sharp one.

It may be necessary to restrict the use of some items by isolating switches, or locking away parts. Guards must be used when fitted. Instructions and warnings need to be prominently displayed in the best position to alert users to

precautions, and training in correct use must be provided.

Office regulations cover the use of equipment such as computers and word processors, and draw attention to hazards such as unstable filing cabinets and fumes from photocopiers.

The therapist must be well-versed in the use of all equipment present in an occupational therapy area.

SLIPS, TRIPS AND FALLS

These are caused by factors such as obstacles, trailing electrical cables, clutter, slippery or uneven surfaces, poor storage and bad lighting and lack of repair. Since many of these hazards originate from human activity, the therapist needs to exercise continual vigilance, and any hazard should be dealt with at once.

DISPOSAL OF WASTE

Hospitals have clear systems for waste disposal and usually code different types of waste. Ordinary refuse, kitchen waste and clinical waste may be handled differently. Infected waste may need special treatment. Correct disposal of sharps – especially used needles or blades – is vital, particularly because of the risk of hepatitis or HIV. Any accidental injury must be instantly reported and dealt with.

In non-hospital settings, disposal systems may be more lax, and potential hazards consequently greater.

ITEMS IN NEED OF REPAIR

There should be a system of planned inspection and maintenance for any items which require it. This extends from maintenance of plumbing and electric systems to maintenance of tools or special equipment such as hoists and wheelchairs.

Any item in need of repair should be immediately withdrawn from use, marked as unfit for use, and a repair carried out as soon as possible.

Repairs to the fabric of a building or to larger items of furniture or floor coverings should also be promptly requested.

No unsafe or unhealthy item or area should be used by either staff or patients.

PHYSICAL ELEMENTS

Sources of heat or extreme cold need special care. The general levels of noise, temperature and light should be within acceptable limits. These are defined by regulations. If protective equipment is needed (e.g. ear protectors; goggles), these must be readily to hand.

For some environments, there are also regulations about the amount of space required by each worker.

MANUAL HANDLING

The fact that numerous working days are lost each year because of back injuries and strains caused by incorrect lifting has prompted strict manual handling regulations to be brought into force. Regulations governing lifting and handling impose limitations on load and emphasize the need to use lifting and handling equipment wherever possible. All staff who need to handle heavy objects have to be trained to do so correctly.

Lifting a person or helping someone to move is also now governed by regulations, which may be subject to local interpretation. In hospitals and care homes, 'no lift' or 'minimal lift' policies may be used. It is important to understand how to use lifting equipment such as hoists and sliding boards.

There can be a mismatch between rehabilitation procedures – where a therapist gives physical assistance in order to enable a person to recover independence – and care policies which prohibit manual help. Overly rigid interpretation of 'no lift' rules can impede rehabilitation.

SAFETY WHEN WORKING IN THE COMMUNITY

The principles of health and safety apply when visiting a person's home. If the environment is for some reason unsafe (perhaps a floor is about to collapse with dry rot or an aggressive dog guards the door), the therapist may reasonably refuse to enter it: such extreme circumstances are fortunately uncommon.

THE HOME SAFETY AUDIT

It may be necessary to assess a home or other environment for risks, including slip, trip and fall hazards, fire, electrical safety and toxic emissions (e.g. carbon monoxide). Although a therapist can reasonably be expected to evaluate many of these risks, expert technical help has to be obtained when judging electric safety, gas emissions and structural defects.

Checklists for home safety assessment and guidance for clients are available from the Royal Society for the Prevention of Accidents.

There are implicit assumptions in risk-reduction: first that accidents are largely preventable, and second that an unsafe environment contributes substantially to increased risk. While largely true, both statements represent oversimplified views of a complex problem.

It is not difficult to recognize when a home is dangerous. Poor repair, clutter, uneven or slippery flooring, dangerous wiring, lack of fire precautions or blocked exits are immediately apparent. There is no doubt that reducing hazards in this situation will directly improve safety.

However, the environment is only one point on the occupational performance triangle. The person using the environment and the tasks the person is performing in it also need to be considered. Each of these three elements can be placed somewhere on a continuum between safe and unsafe. It is the interaction between the user, the task and the environment which increases or decreases risk.

In traditional functional assessment, the three elements – user, task and environment – are often considered in isolation. The user is assessed to see if the user is able to perform tasks. Tasks are evaluated for risk content. The home environment is examined to detect hazards. This approach can be misleading because the outcome is only predictable at the opposite extremes and because the dynamic interactions between environment, task and user may be overlooked.

It is a reasonable assumption that a safe user in a safe environment doing a safe task is at low risk. It is equally obvious that an unsafe user, doing a risky task in a hazardous environment is at very high risk. However, there is a large 'grey area' between these extremes.

Probability may suggest that if two out of the three elements are unsafe, there will be a higher level of risk. This would be true if all the elements were equally weighted, but this is not the case.

The contribution of the user is particularly important; a 'safe' user may be able to compensate for somewhat risky elements in a task or an environment, whereas an 'unsafe' user may well be at risk even when both task and environment are safe. The task or the environment may be extremely unsafe, thus outweighing the safety of the other two.

When conducting a home assessment which is aimed at judging whether the client will be at risk, it is therefore essential to observe the client undertaking tasks within the home and interacting with the environment.

These observations can help the therapist to avoid making arbitrary recommendations which, while based on sound theories, may not be appropriate, as shown in the following example.

A woman who has had a minor fall is assessed to see whether there are risk factors in the home environment which may increase the probability of another fall. The therapist notices a rug with a curled edge which might be a trip hazard, and an unmarked, small step on the landing which could cause a fall. However, as the therapist goes round the home with the client, she observes that the client takes care to step over the rug, and also automatically remembers the step.

In discussion, the client explains that she has lived with these features for many years and is accustomed to avoiding them. The therapist points out that these are hazards which could increase risk of falling but the client does not want to take any action to change the situation. The therapist accepts that the client is not put at unacceptable risk by these features because she shows good coping and avoidance strategies. Adults have the right to take reasonable risks in their daily lives. However, the therapist points out that visitors may not be so aware of these hazards, and suggests that the client alerts them to the need to step over the rug and avoid missing the step. The client has not thought of this, and agrees to warn her guests, and also suggests putting a brighter light on the landing to show up the step.

PRINCIPLES OF DEALING WITH RISK

The occupational performance triangle is a sound guide to risk assessment in all environments. It follows that it is also a useful guide to risk management. These principles are the same in any environment: therapeutic, work, recreational or home.

ENVIRONMENTAL HAZARDS

Techniques of dealing with these are based on the principles of environmental adaptation already noted:

Remove	Features or objects which are unsafe.
Add	Features or objects which contribute to safety.
Alter	Aspects of design to reduce risk and promote safety.
Position	Items to reduce risk and promote safe use.

OCCUPATIONAL HAZARDS

The risks which are inherent in human activities are now much better documented and understood.

As well as dealing with the safety of places, tools and materials, it is necessary to look at the task.

Task analysis can indicate potential problems such as repetitive strain, fatigue or poor posture. Adapting the method used to perform the task (as in manual handling) or the duration and sequence of performance, increases safety.

THE USER

The user is a key component; as already illustrated, if the user is 'unsafe', other safety measures have reduced efficacy.

The quality of being 'unsafe' can stem from many causes, physical, psychological, cultural and social. It can be difficult to identify precisely why risk-taking behaviour is present or persistent.

The main approach to user safety is education and training. This needs to be simple, appropriate and repeated as experience unfortunately shows that habitual patterns of behaviour are hard to break. It is far better to educate people to be safe *before* they commence a task than to try to change unsafe behaviour afterwards.

References

Allen C K 1985 Occupational therapy for psychiatric disorders: measurement and management of cognitive disabilities. Little Brown, Boston

American Association of Occupational Therapists 1994 Uniform terminology for occupational therapy. American Journal of Occupational Therapy 48:1047–1054

American Association of Occupational Therapists 1995 Position paper: occupation. American Journal of Occupational Therapy 49(10):1015–1018

Arndottir G 1990 The brain and behaviour: assessing cortical dysfunction through activities of daily living. Mosby, St Louis

Ashworth P D, Saxton J 1990 On competence. Journal of Further and Higher Education 14(2):1–25

Atkinson R L, Atkinson R G, Smith E, Benn D 1993 Introduction to psychology, 11th edn. Harcourt Brace, Florida

Austin C, Clark C R 1993 Measures of outcome: for whom? British Journal of Occupational Therapy 56(1):21–24

Barnett R 1994 The limits of competence: knowledge, higher education and society. SRHE and Open University Press, England

Bateson M C 1996 Enfolded activity and the concept of occupation. In: Zemke R, Clarke F (eds) Occupational science the evolving discipline. F A Davis, Philadelphia

Baum C, Edwards D E 1993 Cognitive performance in senile dementia of the Alzheimer's type: the kitchen task assessment. American Journal of Occupational Therapy 47:431–436

Baxter R, Friel K, McAtamney A, White B, Wilkinson S 1995 Leisure enhancement through occupational therapy. College of Occupational Therapist, London, p 51

Berg K, Wood–Dauphinee S, Williams J I 1995 The balance scale: reliability assessment for elderly residents and patients with acute stroke. Scandinavian Journal of Rehabilitation Medicine 27(1):27–36

Bronfenbrenner U 1979 Towards an experimental ecology of human development. American Psychologist 22:513–531

Bucks R S, Ashworth D L, Wilcock G K, Siegfried K 1996 The Bristol activities of daily living scale. Age and Ageing 25:113–120

Bullock M 1990 Ergonomics: the physiotherapist in the workplace. Churchill Livingstone, Edinburgh

Burnard P 1996 Acquiring interpersonal skills: a handbook of experiential learning for health professionals, 2nd edn. Chapman & Hall, London

Canadian Association of Occupational Therapists (CAOT) Townsend E et al (eds) 1997 Enabling occupation: an occupational therapy perspective. CAOT, Ottawa

Carkhuff R 1969 Helping and human relations, vol II. Rinehart & Winston, New York

Carkhuff R, Berensen B 1977 Beyond counselling and therapy, 2nd edn. Holt, Rinehart & Winston, New York

Chaparro C, Ranka J (eds) 1997 Occupational performance model (Australia). Monograph 1. Co–ordinates Publications, PO Box 59, West Brunswick, Victoria, Australia

Christiansen C, Baum C (eds) 1997 Occupational therapy enabling function and wellbeing, 2nd edn. Slack, New Jersey

Clarke F A 1993 Occupation embedded in a real life; interweaving occupational science and occupational therapy. American Journal of Occupational Therapy 47:1069

Clark F 1997 What can occupational science do for occupational therapy? (Material from workshop handout) OT Australia, Australian Association of Occupational Therapists 19th National Conference 'Making a difference', Perth

Clark F, Ennevor B L, Richardson P L 1996 A grounded theory of techniques for occupational story telling and occupational story making. In: Zemke R, Clarke F (eds) Occupational science the evolving discipline. F A Davis, Philadelphia

Clemson L 1996 Home fall hazards. Co–ordinates Publications, PO Box 59, West Brunswick, Victoria, Australia

Cole M B 1998 Group dynamics in occupational therapy: the theoretical basis and practical application of group treatment, 2nd edn. Slack, New Jersey

College of Occupational Therapists (COT) 1992 Employment assessment and preparation in occupations. COT, London

College of Occupational Therapists 1994 Core skills and a conceptual foundation for practice. COT, London

College of Occupational Therapists (COT) 1995 Code of ethics and professional conduct for occupational therapists. COT, London

Corcoran M, Gitlin L 1997 The role of the physical environment in occupation performance. In: Christiansen C, Baum C (eds) Occupational therapy enabling function and wellbeing. Slack, New Jersey

COSHH. Care of Substances Hazardous to Health 1990 regulations

Creek J (ed) 1997 Occupational therapy in mental health, 2nd edn. Churchill Livingstone, Edinburgh

Crepeau E B 1998 Activity analysis: a way of thinking about occupational performance. In: Neistadt M E, Crepeau E B (eds) Willard and Spackman's occupational therapy, 9th edn. Lippincott, Philadelphia

Csikzentmihali M 1993 Activity and happiness: towards a science of occupation. Occupational Science 1(1):38–42

Cynkin S, Robinson A M 1990 Occupational therapy and activities health: toward health through activities. Little Brown, Boston

Darnell J L, Heater S L 1994 Occupational therapist or activity therapist – which do you choose to be? American Journal of Occupational Therapy 48(5):467–468

Delbeq A L, Van de Ven A H 1971 A group process model for problem identification and program planning. Journal of Behavioural Science 7(4):465–492

Dombrowki L B, Kane M A 1997 Functional needs assessment treatment guide. The Psychological Corporation, London

Doyle P 1994 Marketing, management and strategy. Prentice Hall, London

Dunn W, McClain L H, Brown C, Yougstrom M J 1998 The ecology of human performance, In: Neistadt M E, Crepeau E B (eds) Willard and Spackman's Occupational therapy, 9th edn. Slack, New Jersey

Eakin P 1989a Assessments of activities of daily living: a critical review. British Journal of Occupational Therapy 52(1):11–15

Eakin P 1989b Problems with assessments of activities of daily living. British Journal of Occupational Therapy 52(2):50–54

Eakin P, Baird H 1995 The Community Dependency Index (CDI). British Journal of Occupational Therapy 58(1):17–22

Fanning T, Fanning R 1990 Get it all done and still be human: a personal time management workshop. Open Chain Publications

Farrar-Edwards D 1997 The effect of occupational therapy on function and well-being. In: Christiansen C, Baum C (eds) Occupational therapy, enabling function and well-being. Slack, New Jersey

Fenton S, Gagnon P 1998 Treatment of work and productive activities: an industrial rehabilitation approach. In: Neistadt M E, Crepeau E B (eds) Willard and Spackman's Occupational therapy, 9th edn. Slack, New Jersey

Fisher A G 1994 Assessment of motor and process skills (AMPS) Research edn. 7.00. Department of Occupational Therapy, Colorado State University, Fort Collins

Fisher A, Kielhofner G 1995 Skill in occupational performance in Kielhofner G (ed) 1995 A model of human occupation: theory and application, 2nd edn. Williams & Wilkins, Baltimore

Fleming M H 1994 The therapist with the three-track mind. In: Mattingly C, Fleming M H (eds) Clinical reasoning. Forms of inquiry in a therapeutic practice. F A Davis, Philadelphia

Fleming A, McAughtrie M, Mitchell R, McNaughton L 1997 Learning disabilities. In: Creek J (ed) Occupational therapy and mental health, 2nd edn. Churchill Livingstone, Edinburgh

Folstein M F, Folstein S E, McHugh P R 1975 Mini mental state: a practical method for grading the cognitive state of patients for the clinician. Journal of Psychiatric Research 12:189–198

Forsyth K, Sulamy M, Simon S, Kielhofner G 1998 A user's guide to the assessment of communication and interaction skills. University of Chicago, Illinois

Foster M 1996 Assessment. In: Turner A, Foster M, Johnson S (eds). Occupational therapy and physical dysfunction: principles, skills and practice. Churchill Livingstone, Edinburgh

Fougerollas P, The influence of social environment on the social participation of people with disabilities. In: Christiansen C, Baum C (eds) Occupational therapy enabling function and wellbeing, 2nd edn. Slack, New Jersey

Fricke J 1993 Measuring outcomes in rehabilitation: a review. British Journal of Occupational Therapy 56(6):217–221

Gage M, Noh S, Polatajko H J, Kaspar V 1994 Measuring perceived self–efficacy in Occupational Therapy, American Journal of Occupational Therapy 48:783–790

Gerrard B A, Boniface W J, Love B H 1980 Interpersonal skills for health professionals. Reston Inc (Prentice Hall), Reston, Virginia

Goldberg D P, Williams P 1988 A user's guide to the General Health Questionnaire. NFER–Nelson, Windsor, Berkshire

Golding E 1989 The Middlesex Elderly Assessment of Mental State (MEAMS). Thames Valley Testing Co, England

Goldsmith S 1984 Designing for the disabled, 4th edn. Royal Society for British Architects, London

Golledge J 1998a Distinguishing between occupation, purposeful activity and activity, part 1. British Journal of Occupational Therapy 61(3):100–105

Golledge J 1998b Distinguishing between purposeful activity and occupation, part 2: why is the distinction important? British Journal of Occupational Therapy 61(4):157–160

Grandjean E 1988 Fitting the task to the man: a textbook of occupational ergonomics, 4th edn. Taylor & Francis, London

Hagedorn R 1995a Occupational therapy: perspectives and processes. Churchill Livingstone, Edinburgh

Hagedorn R 1995b The Casson memorial lecture 1995: An emergent professional – a personal perspective. British Journal of Occupational Therapy 58(8):324–331

Hagedorn R 1996 Use of occupational analysis with clients on a pain management programme. College of Occupational Therapists Annual Conference unpublished paper

Hagedorn R 1997 Foundations for practice in occupational therapy, 2nd edn. Churchill Livingstone, Edinburgh

Haglund L, Henriksson C 1995 Activity – from action to activity. Scandinavian Journal of Caring Sciences 9(4): 227–234

Hammond A 1996 Rheumatoid Arthritis. In: Turner A, Foster M, Johnson S (eds) Occupational therapy and physical dysfunction. Churchill Livingstone, Edinburgh

Hansen R A 1993 Ethics in occupational therapy. In: Hopkins H, Smith H (eds) Willards and Spackman's occupational therapy, 8th edn. Lippincott, Philadelphia

Hargie O, Saunders C, Dickson D 1994 Social skills in interpersonal communication, 3rd edn. Routledge, London

Hasselkus B, Rosa S A 1997 Meaning and occupation. In: Christiansen C, Baum C (eds) Occupational therapy enabling function and wellbeing, 2nd edn. Slack, New Jersey

Helfrich C, Kielhofner G 1994 Volitional narratives and the meaning of occupational therapy. American Journal of Occupational Therapy 48:319–326

Helfrich C, Kielhofner G, Mattingly C 1994 Volition as narrative: an understanding of motivation in chronic illness. American Journal of Occupational Therapy 48:311–317

Henderson A 1996 The scope of occupational science. In: Zemke R, Clarke F (eds) Occupational science the evolving discipline. F A Davis, Philadelphia

Holm M B, Rogers J C, Stone R G 1998 Person–task–environment interventions: a decision making guide In: Neistadt M E, Crepeau E B (eds) Willard and Spackman's occupational therapy, 9th edn. Slack, New Jersey

Hopkins H L, Smith H D (eds) 1993 Willard and Spackman's Occupational therapy, 8th edn. Lippincott, Philadelphia

Horvath A O, Symonds B D 1990 The relationship between working alliance and outcome in psychotherapy: a synthesis. Paper presentation, Society for Psychotherapy Research, Wintergreen, VA

Ilott I 1995 Let's have a moratorium on activities (the word not the deed). British Journal of Occupational Therapy 58(7):297–298

Jacobs K (ed) 1991 Occupational therapy: work related programs and assessments, 2nd edn. Little Brown, Boston

Jacobs K 1993 Work assessment and programming. In: Hopkins H, Smith H (eds) Willard and Spackman's occupational therapy, 8th edn. Lippincott, Philadelphia

Jacobs K, Bettencourt C M 1995 Ergonomics for therapists. Butterworth–Heinmann, London

Jeffrey L I H 1993 Aspects of selecting outcome measures to demonstrate the effectiveness of comprehensive rehabilitation. British Journal of Occupational Therapy 56(11):394–400

Jenkinson C, Coulter A, Wright L 1993 Short form – 36 (SF36) Health survey questionnaire: normative data for adults of working age. British Medical Journal 306:1437–1440

Johnson S E 1996 Activity analysis. In: Turner A, Foster M, Johnson S E (eds) Occupational therapy and physical dysfunction, 4th edn. Churchill Livingstone, Edinburgh

Kanny E 1993 Core values and attitudes of occupational therapy practice. American Journal of Occupational Therapy 47:1085–1086

Kaplan K, Kielhofner G, 1989 Occupational case analysis interview and rating scale. Slack, New Jersey

Karhu O, Kansi P, Kourinka I 1977 Correcting working posture in industry: a practical method of analysis. Applied Ergonomics 8:4

Kielhofner G 1995 A model of human occupation theory and application, 2nd edn. Williams & Wilkins, Baltimore

Kohlmeyer K 1998 Evaluation of performance components. In: Neistadt M E, Crepeau E B (eds) Willard and Spackman's occupational therapy, 9th edn. Slack, New Jersey

Krupnik J L, Sotsky S M, Simmens S, Moyer J, Elkin I, Pilkonis P A, Watkins J 1996 The role of the therapeutic alliance in psychotherapy and pharmacology outcome: findings in the National Institute of Mental Health treatment of depression collaborative research program. Journal of Consulting and Clinical Psychology 64(3):532–539

Lamport N K, Coffey M S, Hersh G I 1989 Activities analysis handbook. Slack, New Jersey

Laver A, Powell G 1995 The structured observation test of function (SOTOF). NFER–Nelson, Windsor, Berkshire

Laver–Ingram A J 1997 Occupational therapy assessment and evaluation. Conference proceedings VAOT

Law M 1998 Client centred occupational therapy. Slack, New Jersey

Law M, Letts L 1993 A critical review of scales of activities of daily living. American Journal of Occupational Therapy 43(8):522–528

Law M, Baptiste S, Carswell A, McColl M A, Polatajko H, Pollock N 1994 Canadian Occupational Performance Measure (COPM). Canadian Association of Occupational Therapists, Toronto

Law M, Cooper B, Strong S, Stewart D, Rigby P, Letts L 1997 In: Christiansen C, Baum C (eds) Occupational therapy, enabling function and wellbeing. Slack, New Jersey

Letts L, Scott S, Burtney J, Marshall L, McKean M 1998 The reliability and validity of the safety assessment of function and the environment for rehabilitation. (SAFER tool). British Journal of Occupational Therapy 61(3):127–133

Lewin J E, Reed C A 1998 Creative problem solving in occupational therapy. Lippincott, Philadelphia

Levine R E, Brayley C R 1991 Occupation as a therapeutic medium. In: Christiansen C, Baum C (eds) Occupational therapy: overcoming human performance deficits. Slack, New Jersey

Lewis J M 1998 For better or worse: interpersonal relationships and individual outcome. American Journal of Psychiatry 155(5):582–589

Lloyd C, Maas F 1992 Interpersonal skills and occupational therapy. British Journal of Occupational Therapy 55(10):379–382

Loupajarvi T 1990 Ergonomics analysis of workplace and postural load In: Bullock M I (ed) Ergonomics: the physiotherapist in the workplace. Churchill Livingstone, Edinburgh

Mahoney F I, Barthel D W 1965 Functional evaluation: the Barthel Index. Maryland State Medical Journal 14:61–65

Maslow A H 1970 Motivation and personality. Harper & Row, New York

Matheson L N, Bohr P C 1997 Occupational competence across the life span. In: Christiansen C, Baum C, (eds) Occupational therapy enabling function and wellbeing, 2nd edn. Slack, New Jersey

Mattingly C, Fleming M H 1994 Clinical reasoning: forms of inquiry in a therapeutic practice. FA Davis, Philadelphia

McColl M A 1997 Meeting the challenges of disability: models of service for people with disabilities. Australian Association of Occupational Therapists 19th conference proceedings, Perth

McFadyen A K, Pratt J 1997 Understanding the statistical concepts of measures of work performance. British Journal of Occupational Therapy 60(6):279–284

Miller R J, Walker K F (eds) 1993 Perspectives on theory for the practice of occupational therapy. Aspen, Gaithersburg

Mosey A C 1986 Psychosocial components of occupational therapy. Raven Press, New York

Mullins L J 1993 Management and organisational behaviour, 3rd edn. Pitman, London

Munroe H A 1992 Clinical reasoning in community occupational therapy: patterns and processes. PhD thesis, University of Aberdeen

Murdock C 1992 A critical evaluation of the Barthel Index Part 1 British Journal of Occupational Therapy 55(3):109–111

National Centre for Medical Rehabilitation Research (NCMRR) 1993 Research plan for the NMCRR. (NIH publication no. 93–3509) NCMRR, Bethesda

Neistadt M E 1998 Overview of evaluation. In: Neistadt M E, Crepeau E B (eds) Willard and Spackman's occupational therapy, 9th edn. Lippincott, Philadelphia

Neistadt M E, Crepeau E B (eds) 1998 Willard and Spackman's occupational therapy, 9th edn. Lippincott, Philadelphia

Nelson D L 1988 Occupational form and performance. American Journal of Occupational Therapy 42:633–641

Nelson D L 1996 Why the profession of occupational therapy will flourish in the 21st century. American Journal of Occupational Therapy 51(1):11–24

Oakley F, Kielhofner G, Barris R, Reicher R K 1986 The role checklist: development and empirical assessment of reliability. Occupational Therapy Journal of Research 6:157–170

Oborne D J 1987 Ergonomics at work, 2nd edn. Wiley, Chichester

O'Donnell M 1992 A new introduction to sociology, 3rd edn. Thomas Nelson, Walton–on–Thames

O'Neil H 1995a The assessment and treatment of problematic anger, Part 1 British Journal of Occupational Therapy 58(10):427–431

O'Neil H 1995b Anger: the assessment and treatment of problematic anger, Part 2, British Journal of Occupational Therapy 58(11):469–472

Ottenbacher K J, Christiansen C 1997 Occupational performance assessment. In: Christiansen C, Baum C (eds) Occupational therapy enabling function and wellbeing, 2nd edn. Slack, New Jersey

Pattie A H, Gilleard C J 1979 Manual of the Clifton Assessment Procedures for the Elderly (CAPE). Hodder and Stoughton Educational, Sevenoaks

Pelonquin S 1998 The therapeutic relationship. In: Neistadt M E, Crepeau E B (eds) Willard and Spackman's occupational therapy, 9th edn. Lippincott, Philadelphia

Pheasant S 1986 Bodyspace anthropometry, ergonomics and design. Taylor & Francis, London

Polatajko H J 1992 Naming and framing occupational therapy: a lecture dedicated to the memory of Nancy B. Canadian Journal of Occupational Therapy 59(4): 189–200

Polgar J M 1998 Critiquing assessments. In: Neistadt M E, Crepeau E B (eds) Willard and Spackman's occupational therapy, 9th edn. Lippincott, Philadelphia

Primeau L A 1996 Running as occupation: multiple meanings and purposes. In: Zemke R, Clark F (eds) Occupational science the evolving discipline. F A Davis, Philadelphia

Reed K L 1984 Models of practice in occupational therapy. Williams & S Wilkins, Baltimore

Reed K L, Sanderson S N 1992 Concepts of occupational therapy, 3rd edn. Williams & Wilkins, Baltimore

Reilly M 1962 Occupational therapy can be one of the great ideas of 20th century medicine. American Journal of Occupational Therapy 20:61–67

Rogers J C 1982 Order and disorder in medicine and occupational therapy. American Journal of Occupational Therapy 36:29–35.

Rogers J C, Holm M B 1989 The therapist's thinking behind functional assessment. In: Royen C B (ed) American Occupational Therapy Association (AOTA) self-study series – Assessing function. AOTA, Rockville

Rogers J C, Holm M B 1998 Evaluation of activities of daily living (ADL) and home management. In: Neistadt M E, Crepeau E B (eds) Willard and Spackman's occupational therapy, 9th edn. Slack, New Jersey

Rohmert W, Landau K 1983 A new technique for job analysis (English edition). Taylor & Francis, London

Rosa S A, Hasselkus B R 1996 Connecting with patients: the personal experience of professional helping. Occupational Therapy Journal of Research 16(4):245–260

Ryan S E 1992 Clinical reasoning: a descriptive study comparing novice and experienced occupational therapists. MSc dissertation, University of Columbia

Schkade J, Schultz S 1997 Occupational adaptation model. In: Christiansen C, Baum C (eds) Occupational therapy enabling function and wellbeing, 2nd edn. Slack, New Jersey

Seedhouse D 1988 Ethics: the heart of health care. Wiley, Chichester

Shah S, Cooper B 1993 Commentary on 'a critical evaluation of the Barthel Index'. British Journal of Occupational Therapy 56(2):70–72

Singleton W T 1972 Introduction to ergonomics. World Health Organization, Geneva

Smith N, Kielhofner G, Watts J 1986 The relationship between volition, activity pattern and life satisfaction in the elderly. American Journal of Occupational therapy 40: 278-283

Spencer J C 1998 Evaluation of performance contexts. In: Neistadt M E, Crepeau E B (eds) Willard and Spackman's occupational therapy, 9th edn. Lippincott, Philadelphia

Stewart A M 1992 The Casson memorial lecture: Always a little further. British Journal of Occupational Therapy 54(8):297–300

Tinetti M 1995 Tinetti balance and gait evaluation. Journal of Gerontological Nursing: June 15–16

Training Agency 1988 Development of assessable standards for national certification – Guidance notes 1–6. Training Agency, UK

Trombley C A (ed) 1989 Occupational therapy for physical dysfunction, 3rd edn. Williams & Wilkins, Baltimore

Turner A, Foster M, Johnson S F (eds) 1996 Occupational therapy and physical dysfunction: principles, skills and practice, 4th edn. Churchill Livingstone, Edinburgh

Turner A, McCaul C 1996 The therapeutic use of activity In: Turner A, Foster M, Johnson S (eds) Occupational therapy and physical dysfunction. Churchill Livingstone, Edinburgh

Tyerman R, Tyerman A, Howard P, Hadfield C, 1986 The Chessington occupational therapy neurological assessment battery (COTNAB) Nottingham Rehabilitation, London

Tyldesley B, Grieve J I 1996 Muscles, nerves and movement, kinesiology in daily living, 2nd edn. Blackwell Scientific Publications, Oxford

UDSMR. Uniform data system for medical rehabilitation 1993 Guide for the uniform data set for medical rehabilitation (Adult FIM) Version 4.0, State University of New York at Buffalo. Buffalo, NY

Unsworth C 1993 The concept of function. British Journal of Occupational Therapy 56(8):287–292

Van Manen M 1995 On the epistemology of reflective practice. Teachers and Teaching: theory and practice 1(1): 33–50

Velozo C, Kielhofner G, Fisher G 1998 A user's guide to worker role interview (version 9). University of Illinois, Chicago

Wallston K A, Wallston B S, de Vellis R 1978 Development of the multidimensional health locus of control (MHLC) scales. Health Education Monographs 6:160–171

Ward G, McCaulay F, Jagger C, Harper W 1998 Standardized assessment: a comparison of the community dependency index and the Barthel Index with a elderly hip fracture population. British Journal of Occupational Therapy 61(3):121–127

Ware J E, Snow K K, Kosinski M, Gandek B 1993 SF 36 health survey manual and interpretation guide. The Health Institute New England Medical Centre, Boston, MA

Warmbolt J J 1996 Functional skills programme for the neurologically impaired client. The Psychological Corporation, London

Watson D E 1997 Task analysis: an occupational performance approach. American Association of Occupational Therapists, Bethesda.

Watts J H, Brollier C, Bauer D, Schmidt W, 1989, The assessment of occupational functioning: the second revision. Occupational Therapy in Mental Health 8(4):61–87

Weber M F 1998 The book of sorrows, book of dreams: a first person narrative. In: Neistadt M E, Crepeau E B (eds) Willard and Spackman's Occupational therapy, 9th edn. Slack, NJ

Whiting S, Lincoln N, Bahvani G, Cockburn J 1985 Rivermead perceptual assessment battery manual, NFER–Nelson, Windsor, Berkshire

Wilcock A A 1998 An occupational perspective of health. Slack, New Jersey

Wilcock A A 1998b Reflections on doing, being and becoming. Canadian Journal of Occupational Therapy 65(5):248–256

Williams J H, Drinka T J K, Greenberg J R, Farell-Holton J, Euhardy R, Schram M 1991 Development and testing of the Assessment of Livings Skills and Resources (ALSAR) in elderly community-dwelling veterans. The Gerontologist 31(1):84–91

Willier B, Rosenthal M, Kreutzer J, Gordon W, Rempel R 1993 Assessment of community integration following traumatic head injury. Journal of Head Trauma and Rehabilitation 2:75–84

Willson M (ed) 1996 Occupational therapy in short-term psychiatry, 3rd edn. Churchill Livingstone, Edinburgh

Wondrake R 1998 Interpersonal skills for nurses and healthcare professionals. Blackwell Science, Oxford

Yerxa E J, Burnett-Beaulieu S, Stocking S, Azen S P 1988 Development of the satisfaction with performance scaled questionnaire (SPSQ). American Journal of Occupational Therapy 42:215–222

Young M, Quinn E 1992 Theories and practice of occupational therapy. Churchill Livingstone, Edinburgh

Zemke R, Clark F (eds) 1996 Occupational science the evolving discipline. F A Davis, Philadelphia

Glossary and Appendix

Glossary

Acquisitional level

The middle area of the developmental level. At the acquisitional level, basic skill components are utilized in the performance of actions, interactions and reactions and simple performance components.

Action

An observable, intentional, goal-related piece of physical performance.

Activity

A series of linked episodes of task performance which takes place on a specific occasion during a finite period for a particular reason. An activity is composed of an integrated sequence of chained tasks. A completed activity results in a change in the previous state of objective reality or subjective experience.

Activity Analysis

An organized and structured process in which an activity is observed and described and broken down into its component parts in order to understand its structure, performance demand or therapeutic potential.

Adaptation

1. Any change in the occupational habits or organization of a person which is made in order to meet environmental demands and restore fit.

2. An alteration made by a therapist or client to an object or environment in order to provide therapy or to improve the client's ability to perform.

Affective reaction

One which is prompted by an emotional response to a situation, person or object.

Affordance

Anything which the environment can offer the individual which is pertinent to role challenge and can facilitate role competence. Aspects of the environment perceived by the person which combine with the person's effectencies to produce competence (Christiansen & Baum 1997).

Analysis

A logical, reductive process in the course of which something is minutely examined and broken down into simpler components.

Applied analysis

Describes and analyses an activity or task in order to use it as therapy.

Assessment

The process of collecting accurate and relevant information concerning an individual's personal situation and potential, abilities and needs, in order to improve specified areas of occupational performance or as a means of monitoring and measuring the outcomes of therapy or intervention.

Basic analysis

To describe an occupation, activity or task as a defined entity in order to understand its structure, purpose and organization and the basis for engagement.

Capacity

The immediate potential of the individual to perform tasks which support occupational performance (Christiansen & Baum 1997).

Clinical reasoning

The process of ongoing, interactive reasoning related to the therapist's clinical role and interaction with client(s) (Christiansen & Baum 1997).

The cognitive processes performed by the therapist when evaluating information concerning the client during the case management (OT) process.

Closed area

The area of the environment which is unknown to the individual and/or inaccessible to the individual. The outer closed area is located at the outer edge of the external environment and contains the unknown areas of the earth and the rest of the universe. The inner closed area is located in the internal environment and equates with the unconscious.

Cognitive reaction

A response to an external event or stimulus which has been produced by conscious processing within the brain.

Competence

Skilled and adequately successful completion of a piece of performance, task or activity.

Achievement of skill equal to the demands of the environment (Christiansen & Baum 1997).

Competency

A defined technique, procedure or related set of performances in which an occupational therapist should be able to demonstrate proficiency. A competency is usually performed in a specified situation to a required standard.

Constructive level

The upper area within the developmental level. At the constructive level, task stages are chained to form tasks and simple task chains are mastered.

Content analysis

Analysis of a task or activity which describes its structure and purpose.

COPE

Competent Occupational Performance in the Environment. An occupational performance model based on the concept of achieving a fit or balance between the abilities of the person and the demand of the environment and the task.

Core competency

In occupational therapy, a competency which is central to, and contributes to the definition of, professional practice.

Core process

In occupational therapy, one of the four processes which is central to professional practice, that is therapeutic use of self; assessment; analysis and adaptation of occupations; analysis and adaptation of the environment.

Core skill

A skill which is central to, and essential for, professional practice. Core skills are the building blocks of professional competencies and may be re-assembled in numerous configurations to meet the demands of practice.

DARE

Development; Adaptation; Rehabilitation and Education – see processes of change.

Demand analysis

Analysis of the ways in which, and the degree to which, a specific task or activity challenges the individual to respond with skilled performance knowledge or attitudes.

Developmental demand

The intrinsic nature of a task which requires that an individual must have reached a certain developmental level in order to perform competently.

Developmental level

The level of occupation at which the potential to perform is converted into skill, skills are acquired and the ability to perform a repertoire of simple productive tasks is mastered.

Dysfunction

A temporary or chronic inability to engage in the repertoire of roles, relationships and occupations expected of a person of a comparable age, gender and culture. An inability consistently to meet performance demands adaptively and competently.

Educational demand

The demand created by the intrinsic nature of a task for prerequisite learning, including skill acquisition, knowledge, attitudes and values.

Effectance

A subset of the individual's abilities pertinent to the task challenges posed by role demands (Christiansen & Baum 1997).

Effective level

The level of occupation at which productive, meaningful activities are performed in order to enable the individual to achieve an adaptive fit with the individual's environment, which enhances and maintains survival, health and well-being.

Environmental demand

The challenges presented by an environment which press the individual to respond by appropriate occupational performance.

Evaluation

The process of using clinical reasoning, problem analysis and decision-making to interpret the results of assessment in order to make judgements about the situation or needs of an individual or the success of occupational therapy intervention.

Exploratory area

The area of the environment which is accessible to the individual but which is outside the individual's usual resource area. In the external environment, the exploratory area contains new information, resources or experiences which may be used by an individual. In the internal environment, the exploratory area is the reservoir of creativity, invention and imagination.

Fit

Short for 'person–activity–environment fit': refers to the match among skills and abilities of the individual, the demands of the activity and the characteristics of the physical, social and cultural environment (American Association of Occupational Therapists' uniform terminology 1994, Neistadt & Crepeau 1998).

Fit is required if competent performance is to occur.

Function

Describes a behaviour related to the performance of a task (Christiansen & Baum 1997).

Functional

Having the ability to perform competently the roles, relationships and occupations required in the course of daily life.

Functional adaptation

An adaptation to a task or an environment which promotes and enhances function.

Functional performance

Performance which competently achieves the purpose and/or product of the task.

Grading

Measurable increasing or decreasing of activity by alteration of factors such as duration, size, degree of effort, amount of energy, attention, judgement or discrimination required. Used in physical rehabilitation to describe a specific, biomechanical or cognitive–perceptual form of therapeutic adaptation.

Human occupation

The total range of productive, purposeful and meaningful occupations in which people participate. The area of human life with which occupational therapists are concerned.

Immediate environment

That which is within arms' reach of the user.

Interaction

Intentional engagement of an individual with objects or people within the environment.

Intervention

Any action by the therapist on behalf of the client, other than that required in order to provide direct treatment (therapy).

Learning prerequisites

The knowledge, skills, attitudes or values which an individual must previously possess in order to be able to meet task demand.

Macroanalysis

Analysis at the organizational level, especially of roles and occupations.

Mesoanalysis

Analysis of patterns of performance across an extended timeframe (a week or longer).

Microanalysis

Analysis of performance components, actions, interactions and reactions or the content of the immediate environment.

Modality

A therapeutic activity or agent; the application of a therapeutic agent.

Near environment

The environment which at any moment surrounds the user and is easily accessible to the user.

Occupation

1. COPE – a form of human endeavour which provides longitudinal organization of time and effort in a person's life.

2. Occupational science – units of activity which are named in the lexicon of the culture (Zemke & Clarke 1996).

Occupation performance model

A model created by an occupational therapy theorist which describes and defines the parameters of human performance, usually in terms of work, leisure and self-care (or synonyms). Occupational performance is generated by the interaction of the individual's mental, physical, sociocultural and spiritual skill components within an environment.

Occupational form

The composition of objective physical and sociocultural circumstances external to a person that influence the individual's occupational performance (Nelson 1996).

Occupational storymaking

The process through which the therapist enables the client to understand an occupational life story and to script a new ending towards which it may be possible to work.

Occupational storytelling

The process through which the therapist facilitates the client's telling of personal occupational experiences throughout the client's lifetime in order to provide insights into and meanings of a current situation.

Occupational therapy

COPE – occupational therapy is concerned with the acquisition, maintenance or restoration of competent adaptive performance, in order to maintain health, to enhance well-being, and to enable the client to do the things the client wants or needs to do, in the environment the client uses.

Ontogenesis

The origin and development of an organism over time. In occupational therapy, the development of the individual's repertoire of occupational performance over time.

Organizational level

The highest occupational level at which roles and occupational performances are combined and organized.

Participation analysis

Analysis of the degree to which an individual actually engages in an activity, and the patterns which underlie such engagement.

PEOP model

Person–Environment–Occupational–Performance model: a generic term for a group of occupational therapy models having similar philosophy and content.

Performance area

One of the classifications of human occupation. In the American Association of Occupational Therapists' uniform terminology (1994), these are designated as: activities of daily living (ADL); work and productive activities; play or leisure activities. (For a full list of tasks under each heading refer to AAOT uniform terminology article.)

Performance component

(*syn* COPE: skill components) As designated by American Association of Occupational Therapists' uniform terminology (1994), the components of performance can be classified as: sensori-motor; cognitive integration and cognitive; psychosocial and psychological components. (For a full list of components refer to AAOT uniform terminology article.)

Performance context

Situations or factors that influence an individual's engagement in desired and/or required performance areas (AAOT uniform terminology 1994). These include temporal contexts (influence of time on the individual) and environmental contexts.

Performance demand

The intrinsic characteristics of a task combined with the performance situation and content of the environment which together require the performer to respond by producing relevant and specific occupational performance.

Performance episode

A finite period of time during which a piece of occupational performance takes place (normally, a period of between 1 minute and a number of hours).

Performance unit

(COPE taxonomy) The smallest component into which a task can be divided.

Person-centred (client-centred)

Collaborative partnership approaches which are based on humanistic values which emphasize the central role of the client in determining the goals of intervention, and the obligation of the therapist to enable and empower the client to achieve these goals.

POET

Acronym for Person–Environment–Occupation–Therapist, the core components of occupational therapy.

PRESS

The demand for performance created by the constituents of the environment.

Process

A description of the means whereby the purposes and products of an occupation may be carried out. A process links together routines, procedures and activities which have similar purposes or which combine to achieve a particular product.

Process driven

Use of occupational therapy theory which takes a problem-based approach. Using the structure of the occupational therapy process, the therapist works with the client to define a problem, set goals, and formulate solutions, subsequently selecting an appropriate frame of reference on the basis of this information (as distinct from theory driven in which a pre-selected theory directs the occupational therapy process).

Processes of change

Ways in which an individual may change over time in response to the environment. These include: Development; Adaptation; Rehabilitation and Education (DARE).

Proto-occupational level

The lowest level in the hierarchy which contains the potential for performance.

Rationale

A reasoned explanation and statement of the logical basis for practice.

Reaction

A response made by an individual to a perception of some object or occurrence in the environment.

Resource area

The area within the environment which contains material used by the individual during occupational performance. In the external environment, the resource area contains the places objects and organisms used by the person; in the internal environment, the resource area contains the knowledge, attitudes, values and skills (KAVS) available to the person.

Routine

An automated and habitual chain of tasks with a fixed sequence.

Self-efficacy

A belief in one's ability to perform a given task successfully. It predicts the likelihood that someone will attempt a given behaviour and continue working at it, despite possible difficulties, in new situations (Christiansen & Baum 1997).

Sensori-motor

A skill domain which includes the skills required to receive information from the environment and to move within it.

Sequence analysis

Analysis of the order in which task stages occur.

Situational element

A component of an activity which is subject to change in response to circumstances or the wishes and choices of the participant.

Skill component

COPE – a foundation skill which is required for occupational performance (see also performance component). Skills may be classified into three domains: sensori-motor; cognitive–perceptual; psychosocial.

Social reaction

A response which is directed or modified by the presence of others, and the social or cultural expectations and rules which apply to the situation.

Social role

The behaviour expected of a person occupying a particular status or social position.

Stable element

An intrinsic component of an activity which is unchanged each time the activity is performed.

Task

A self-contained stage in an activity, or a self-contained piece of performance with a completed purpose or product. Tasks chain to form activities.

Task analysis

The process of analysing task performance in order to understand its structure, sequence, purpose and demand.

Task demand

The intrinsic characteristics of a task which require the performer to produce a specified set of responses (knowledge, skill, attitude).

Task stage

A subsection of a task during which a small piece of performance is completed.

Taxonomy

A system of classification.

Technique

A method of doing something which implies skill and a systematic approach. In occupational therapy, a technique may be a creative or technical activity, or a special method of treating a client.

Therapeutic adaptation

An adaptation which is made to a task or an environment in order to enhance therapeutic benefits for the client.

Therapeutic alliance

The partnership between therapist and client in which both contribute actively, with mutual respect.

Therapeutic relationship

The relationship which develops between client and therapist during the process of therapy, through which the client is empowered and enabled to achieve specified goals.

Used environment

That part of the external environment in which a person habitually lives and moves around, and from which the resources for living, social and practical are obtained.

Variation potential

The scope for change and adaptation inherent in a task or activity.

Visibility

The degree to which the inherent purposes, products, and degree of knowledge and skill required for a task, activity or occupation are apparent to an observer.

Appendix
Assessment: sources of information

PSYCHOMETRIC TESTS, TESTS OF FUNCTION AND OTHER STANDARD TESTS (NOT SPECIFIC TO OCCUPATIONAL THERAPISTS)

Beech J R, Harding L 1990 Assessment of the elderly. Billing and Sons, Worcester

Bowling A 1995 Measuring disease. Open University Press, Milton Keynes

Bowling A 1997 Measuring health: a review of quality of life measurement scales, 2nd edn. Open University Press, Milton Keynes

Browder D M 1991 Assessment of individuals with severe disabilities. An applied behaviour approach to life skills assessment, 2nd edn. Brookes, Baltimore

McDowell I, Newell C 1996 Measuring health: a guide to rating scales and questionnaires, 2nd edn. Oxford University Press, Oxford

Milne D 1992 Assessment: a mental health portfolio. NFER-Nelson, Windsor

Wade D T 1992 Measurement in neurological rehabilitation. Oxford University Press, Oxford

Wilkin D, Hallam L, Doggett M A 1992 Measures of need and outcome for primary health care. Oxford University Press, Oxford

Wright S, Johnson M, Weinman J 1995 Measures in health psychology: A user's portfolio. NFER-Nelson, Windsor

MANAGEMENT PERSPECTIVE

Van Deusen J, Brunt D 1997 Assessment in occupational therapy and physiotherapy. W B Saunders, Philadelphia

Seed P, Kaye G 1994 Handbook for assessing and managing care in the community. Biddles, Guildford

SPECIFIC INFORMATION FOR OCCUPATIONAL THERAPISTS

Assessment list and samples. College of Occupational Therapists' Library (in production 1999)

CD-ROM on assessment. Canadian Association of Occupational Therapists (in production 1999)

Forer S 1996 Outcome management and program evaluation made easy: a toolkit for the OT practitioner. American Association of Occupational Therapists, Bethesda

Hemphill B J 1988 Mental health assessment in occupational therapy. An integrative approach to the evaluative process. Slack, New Jersey

SUPPLIERS OF PUBLISHED ASSESSMENTS

Readers should note that while every effort has been made to ensure that information is accurate at the time of writing, contact addresses may change.

Functional Independence Measure (FIM). Available from:
- Uniform Data System for Medical Rehabilitation (UDSMR), 232 Parker Hall, 3435 Main Street, Buffalo, New York 14214–3007
  e-mail: info@udsmr.org (general enquiries)
  Functional Assessment Information Service: farinfo@udsmr.org

SF-36 Health Survey Manual (Medical Outcomes Trust). Available from:
- The UK Clearing House, Nuffield Institute, 71–75 Clarenden Road, Leeds L52 9PL

Ann Arbor Publishers Ltd, PO Box 1, Belford, Northumberland NE70 7JX (Perceptual/visual/motor, speech and language) http://www.annarbor.co.uk

NFER-Nelson Publishing Co. Ltd, Darville House, 2 Oxford Road East, Windsor, Berks SL4 1DF

Thames Valley Test Co., 7–9 The Green, Flempton, Bury St Edmunds, Suffolk IP28 6EL
e-mail: tvtc@msn.com

The Psychological Corporation, 32 Jamestown Road, London NWI 7BY (OT and PT Catalogue and psychometric tests)
e-mail: tpc@harcourt.com

TESTS DEVELOPED BY OCCUPATIONAL THERAPISTS

MODEL OF HUMAN OCCUPATION

Assessment of Motor and Process Skills (AMPS) and other Model of Human Occupation (MOHO) tests and training videos:
- UK contact: 23 Regent's Place, Bradford-on-Avon, Wiltshire BA15 1ED
- The Model of Human Occupation Clearing House, University of Illinois at Chicago, Department of Occupational Therapy (M/C 811), College of Associated Health Professionals, 1919 West Taylor Street, Chicago,

Illinois 60612 (312) 996–6901
http://www.vic.edu/hsc/acad/cahp/OT/MOHO

Tests and information available include:

A user's guide to Worker Role Interview (version 9) (Velozo C, Kielhofner G, Fisher G 1998).

Work rehabilitation in mental health programs (Mallinson T 1998).

Work environment impact scale (WEIS) (version 2.0) (Moore-Corner R A, Kielhofner G, Olson L 1998)

A user's guide to the Assessment of Communication and Interaction Skills (ACIS) (version 4.00) (Forsyth K, Sulamy M, Simon S, Kielhofner G 1998)

A user's guide to the Volitional Questionnaire (VQ) (version 3) (de las Heras C G, Geist R, Kielhofner G 1998).

A user's manual for the Occupational Self-Assessment (version 1.00) (Baron K, Kielhofner G, Goldhammer V, Wolenski J 1998).

A user's manual for the Occupational Performance History Interview (version 2.00) (OPHI-II) (Kielhofner G, Mallinson T, Crawford C, Nowak B S, Rigby M, Henry A, Walens D 1998).

OTHER OT TESTS

Canadian Occupational Performance Measure (COPM) (manual and test). Available from
- College of Occupational Therapists (UK), London
- The Canadian Association of Occupational Therapists, 3rd Floor, 110 Eglinton Avenue West, Toronto, Ontario, Canada M4R 1A3.

Allen Cognitive Level tests. Available from:
- S and S Arts and Crafts, PO Box 513, Colchester, Connecticut 06415-1513
  phone: 1.800 243 9232
  e-mail: service@snswwide.com
  internet: http://www.snswwide.com
- Nottingham Rehabilitation Suppliers, Ludlow Hill Road, West Bridgeford, Nottingham NG2 6HD.

Westmead Home Safety Assessment (Clemson). Available from:
- Co-ordinates Publications, PO Box 59, West Brunswick, Victoria 3055, Australia
  Fax: 011 61 3 9387 4829

Various tests are also available from Nottingham Rehabilitation.

LIST OF OTHER ASSESSMENTS MENTIONED IN THE BOOK

Note. Tests marked * are to be found in the general publications previously listed. Where a specific source for the whole test is known, it is given. Otherwise, references refer to journal articles or books in which the test is mentioned, but not necessarily illustrated. Readers must be aware that published tests are covered by copyright and may not usually be copied for use without permission.

EXAMPLES OF TESTS AND MEASUREMENT OF SPECIFIC SKILL COMPONENTS AND TASK PERFORMANCE AT THE DEVELOPMENTAL LEVEL

See also tests listed in Christiansen & Baum (1997) (Ch. 9 Movement-related problems) and Neistad & Crepeau (1998) (Ch. 16 Evaluation of performance components).

Psychological tests, *see* Suppliers of published assessments

Mobility

Berg Balance Scale (Berg, Wood-DauPhinee and Williams 1995).
Scale reproduced in: Shumway-Cook A, Woollacott M 1995 Motor control. Williams & Wilkins, Baltimore.
Tinetti Balance and Gait Evaluation; reprinted in Journal of Gerontological Nursing 1995 June: 15–16.

Cognitive–perceptual tests (some movement components)

* Rivermead Perceptual Assessment Battery (PAB) (Bhavani et al 1985).
* Chessington Occupational Therapy Neurological Assessment Battery (COTNAB) (Tyerman et al 1986). Available from Nottingham Rehabilitation.

Tests of cognition/confusion

* Clifton Assessment Procedures for the Elderly (CAPE) (Pattie & Gilleard 1979).
* Middlesex Elderly Assessment of Mental State (MEAMS) (Golding 1989). Available from Thames Valley Test Co.
* Mini Mental State Evaluation (Folstein et al 1975).

Non-OT assessment of personal activities of daily living

*Barthel ADL Index (BI) (Mahoney & Barthel 1965)
*Functional Independence Measure (FIM) (UDSMR 1993).
Functional Skills programme for the Neurologically Impaired Client (Warmbolt 1996). Includes tracking system to evaluate progress in sub-skills. Manual available from The Psychological Corporation.

OT ASSESSMENTS OF PERSONAL ACTIVITIES OF DAILY LIVING AND SIMPLE IADL TASKS

Assessment of Motor and Process Skills (AMPS) (Fisher 1994). See MOHO list.
Structured Observational Test of Function (SOTOF) (Laver & Powell 1995). Available from NFER-Nelson.
Arndottir OT–ADL Neurobehavioural Evaluation (A-ONE) (Arndottir G 1990 The brain and behaviour: assessing cortical dysfunction through activities of daily living. Mosby, St Louis).
Allen Cognitive Level Test (ACL) (Allen 1985). Available from S and S Arts and Crafts and Nottingham Rehabilitation.
Bristol Activities of Daily Living Scale (Bucks R S, Ashworth D L, Wilcock G K, Siegfried K 1996 Age and Ageing 25: 113–120).
Kitchen Task Assessment (KTA) (Baum C, Edwards D E 1993 Cognitive performance in senile dementia of the Alzheimer's type: the kitchen task assessment. American Journal of Occupational Therapy 47: 431-436).
Functional Needs Assessment Treatment Guide (Dombrowski & Kane 1997). Includes evaluation of verbal communication, self-care, community skills and prevocational skills. Available from The Psychological Corporation.
Assessment of Communication and Interaction Skills (ACIS) (version 4.0). See MOHO list.

ASSESSMENT AT THE EFFECTIVE LEVEL

See also tests listed in Neistad & Crepeau (1998) (Ch. 15 Evaluation of occupational performance areas).

Functional/environmental assessments

Satisfaction with Performance Scaled Questionnaire (SPSQ) (Yerxa E J, Burnett-Beaulieu S, Stocking S, Azen S P 1988 American Journal of Occupational Therapy 42: 215–222).
*Community Integration Questionnaire (CIQ) (Wilier, Linn and Allen 1993).
Safety Assessment of Function and the Environment for Rehabilitation (SAFER Tool) Oliver R, Blathwat J, Brackley C Tamaki T 1993 Development of the safety assessment of function and the environment for rehabilitation (SAFER) tool. Canadian Journal of Occupational Therapy 60: 78–82; Letts L, Scott S, Burtney J, Marshall L, McKean M 1998 The reliability and validity of the safety assessment of function and the environment for rehabilitation (SAFER tool). British Journal of Occupational Therapy 61(3): 127–133).
Assessment of Living Skills and Resources (ALSAR) Williams J H, Brinka T J K, Greenberg J R, Farell-Holton J, Euhardy R, Schram M 1991 Development and testing of the Assessment of Living Skills and Resources (ALSAR) in elderly community-dwelling veterans. The Gerontologist 31(1): 84–91.

Community Dependency Index (CDI) Eakin P A,
Baird H E 1995 The Community Dependency Index: a
standardized measure of outcome for community
occupational therapy. British Journal of Occupational
Therapy 58(1): 17–22.

Canadian Occupational Performance Measure (COPM)
(Law M, Baptiste S, Carswell A, McColl M A, Polatajko H,
Pollock N 1994 CAOT, Canadian Association of
Occupational Therapists, Toronto). Available from College
of Occupational Therapists.

WORK ASSESSMENT

Northern Ireland Committee of College of Occupational
Therapists 1992 Employment assessment and preparation
in occupational therapy. Available from College of
Occupational Therapists. Contains various assessments,
for example: Vocational Guidance Form (Appendix VI);
Employment Evaluation Application Form; Job Suggestion
List (Appendix VII).

Guidelines for Work Interview (Cynkin S, Robinson A M 1990
Occupational therapy and activities health: towards health
through activities (Appendix H). Little Brown, Boston).

Worker Role Interview (Velozo, Kielhofner & Fisher 1998).
See MOHO list.

EXAMPLES OF ASSESSMENTS OF PERCEIVED SELF-EFFICACY, PERSONAL CAUSATION AND LOCUS OF CONTROL

Satisfaction with Performance Scaled Questionnaire (Yerxa
et al 1988).
*Self-Efficacy Gauge (Gage et al 1994).
*Role Adaptation Bereavement Inventory (Larson 1992).
*Life Experiences Checklist (Ager 1992).
Assessment of Occupational Functioning (Rev 2) (Watts et al
1989).
Occupational Case Analysis Interview and Rating Scale
(Kaplan & Kielhofner 1989). See MOHO list.

There are numerous tests of personality, stress,
locus of control and self-perception designed by
psychologists, including:

*General Health Questionnaire (Goldberg & Williams).
*Multidimensional Health Locus of Control Scale (Wallston
et al).
*Recovery Locus of Control Scale (Partridge & Johnson).
*Perceived Stress Scale (Cohen et al).
*Rosenberg Self-Esteem Scale (Rosenberg).

Therapists need to check whether any training
is required in order to use psychological tests.
  More general information is given in:

Treatment of Work and Productive Activities: Functional
Restoration, An Industrial Rehabilitation Approach
(Fenton & Gagnon 1998).
Foster M Life skills: working In: Turner A, Foster M,
Johnson S E (eds) 1996 Occupational therapy and physical
dysfunction, 4th edn. Churchill Livingstone, Edinburgh,
Ch 8, p 212–220

Engagement in Leisure

Baxter R, Friel K, McAtamney A, White B, Williamson S
1995 Leisure enhancement through occupational therapy.
College of Occupational Therapists, London. Contains
several leisure questionnaires, including:
Influences on Leisure Questionnaire (p 46)
Discovering Leisure Patterns (p 21)
Discovering Leisure Attitudes Questionnaire (p 16)
Getting Leisure in Balance Questionnaire (Baxter et al 1995:
48).
Understanding Leisure (p 37)
Your Needs - What are you looking for in your leisure
experience? (p 43)

ASSESSMENTS AT THE ORGANIZATIONAL LEVEL

Occupational and social roles

Role Checklist (Oakley et al 1986). See MOHO list for recent
version.
*Life Experiences Checklist (LEC) (Ager 1990).
*Role Adaptation, Bereavement Inventory (Larson 1992).
Life Pattern Grid (roles and relationships related to
occupations) (Fanning & Fanning in Baxter et al 1995).

Patterns of engagement in occupations

Idiosyncratic Activities Configuration Questionnaire
(Cynkin & Robinson 1990 (Appendix A)).
'Round the clock' participation diary (Baxter et al 1995: 44).

Other suitable assessments are given in the
MOHO list.

Index

Index